Pocket Guide to the American Board of Emergency Medicine In-Training Exam

Pocket Guide to the American Board of Emergency Medicine In-Training Exam

Edited by

Bob Cambridge, DO, MPH

Faculty of the Emergency Medicine Residency Program, and Assistant Director of Research, San Antonio Uniformed Services Health Education Consortium, San Antonio, TX. Former Chief Resident, Emergency Medicine Residency Program, and Clinical Assistant in Surgery/Emergency Medicine, University of Illinois College of Medicine at Peoria, Peoria, IL, USA.

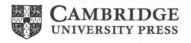

CAMBRIDGE
UNIVERSITY PRESS

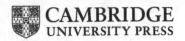

CAMBRIDGE
UNIVERSITY PRESS

Shaftesbury Road, Cambridge CB2 8EA, United Kingdom

One Liberty Plaza, 20th Floor, New York, NY 10006, USA

477 Williamstown Road, Port Melbourne, VIC 3207, Australia

314–321, 3rd Floor, Plot 3, Splendor Forum, Jasola District Centre, New Delhi – 110025, India

103 Penang Road, #05–06/07, Visioncrest Commercial, Singapore 238467

Cambridge University Press is part of Cambridge University Press & Assessment, a department of the University of Cambridge.

We share the University's mission to contribute to society through the pursuit of education, learning and research at the highest international levels of excellence.

www.cambridge.org
Information on this title: www.cambridge.org/9781107696266

© Cambridge University Press & Assessment 2013

First published 2013

A catalogue record for this publication is available from the British Library

Library of Congress Cataloging-in-Publication data
Pocket guide to the American Board of Emergency Medicine
in-training exam / edited by Bob Cambridge.
    p. ; cm.
Includes bibliographical references and index.
ISBN 978-1-107-69626-6 (pbk.)
I. Cambridge, Bob, 1980–
[DNLM: 1. Emergencies – Handbooks.   2. Emergency Medicine –
Handbooks.WB 39]
RC86.7
616.02´5 – dc23   2013007435

ISBN   978-1-107-69626-6   Paperback

Contents

List of contributors   vi
Preface   ix

1. **Cardiology emergencies**   1
   Marc D. Squillante and Ashley Anklam

2. **Respiratory emergencies**   33
   John Hafner

3. **Gastroenterologic emergencies**   54
   Gregory J. Tudor and Alex Koyfman

4. **Neurologic emergencies**   74
   Lisa Barker and Anthony J. Buecker

5. **Renal and urogenital emergencies**   86
   Guyon J. Hill and James F. Martin

6. **Endocrine, metabolic, and nutritional emergencies**   94
   Selina Jeanise

7. **Trauma emergencies**   104
   Rose Haisler and Theodor Schmidt

8. **Obstetrics and gynecology emergencies**   132
   Paul Matthews

9. **Pediatric emergencies**   141
   Teresa Riech

10. **Psychobehavioral emergencies**   153
    Paul Matthews

11. **Infectious emergencies**   159
    Mari B. Baker and Alex Koyfman

12. **Toxicologic emergencies**   174
    Robert Schwaner and Joshua Zavitz

13. **Environmental emergencies**   183
    Timothy Schaefer and Vivian Lau

14. **Procedures in emergency medicine**   194
    E. John Wipfler, III

15. **Rapid review**   210
    Richard Frederick and Andrew Vincent

Useful formulas   241
Index   242

Contributors

Ashley Anklam, MD
Clinical Assistant in Surgery/Emergency Medicine, University of Illinois College of Medicine, Peoria IL

Mari B. Baker, MD, FACEP
Clinical Assistant Professor of Emergency Medicine, University of Illinois College of Medicine, Peoria IL

Lisa Barker, MD, FACEP
Clinical Professor of Emergency Medicine University of Illinois College of Medicine Peoria IL

Anthony J. Buecker, MD
Clinical Assistant in Surgery/Emergency Medicine, University of Illinois College of Medicine, Peoria IL

Richard Frederick, MD, FACEP
Chairman, Department of Emergency Medicine, OSF St. Francis Medical Center Peoria IL

John Hafner, MD, FACEP
Clinical Assistant Professor of Emergency Medicine, University of Illinois College of Medicine, Peoria IL

Rose Haisler DO
Director, Lifeflight Aeromedical Transport University of Illinois College of Medicine Peoria IL

Guyon J. Hill, MD, FACEP, FAAEM
Faculty, Emergency Residency Program, San Antonio Uniformed Services Health Education Consortium, and Emergency Physician, Greater San Antonio Emergency Physicians, San Antonio TX

Selina Jeanise, DO
Emergency Medicine Physician, Emergency Medicine Residency Program, San Antonio Uniformed Services Health Education Consortium, San Antonio TX

Alex Koyfman, MD
Clinical Assistant in Surgery/Emergency Medicine, University of Illinois College of Medicine, Peoria IL

Vivian Lau, DO
Clinical Assistant in Surgery/Emergency Medicine, University of Illinois College of Medicine, Peoria IL

James F. Martin, MD, FACEP, FAAEM
Emergency Medicine Education Director, Monmouth Medical Center, Long Branch, NJ; Emergency Physician, Emergency Medicine Associates of NY and NJ

Paul Matthews, MD
Clinical Professor of Emergency Medicine University of Illinois College of Medicine Peoria IL

Teresa Riech, MD, FAAP
Director, Pediatric Emergency Department, OSF St. Francis Medical Center, Peoria IL; Clinical Assistant Professor of Emergency Medicine and Pediatrics, University of Illinois College of Medicine, Peoria IL

Timothy Schaefer, MD, FACEP
Assistant Residency Program Director, Emergency Medicine, OSF St. Francis Medical Center, Peoria IL

Theodor Schmidt, MD
Clinical Assistant in Surgery/Emergency Medicine, University of Illinois College of Medicine, Peoria IL

Robert Schwaner, MD, FACEP
Staff Emergency Medicine Physician and Toxicologist, Brookhaven Memorial Hospital Medical Center, Patchogue NY

Marc D. Squillante, DO, FACEP, FAAEM
Program Director, Emergency Medicine Residency, University of Illinois College of Medicine, Peoria IL; OSF St. Francis Medical Center, Peoria IL;
Clinical Associate Professor of Surgery/Emergency Medicine
University of Illinois College of Medicine
Peoria IL

Gregory J. Tudor, MD, FACEP
Assistant Clinical Professor of Surgery, Division of Emergency Medicine
University of Illinois College of Medicine
Peoria IL

Andrew Vincent, DO
Clinical Assistant in Surgery/Emergency Medicine, University of Illinois College of Medicine, Peoria IL

E. John Wipfler, III, MD, FACEP
Clinical Professor of Emergency Medicine
University of Illinois College of Medicine
Peoria IL

Joshua Zavitz, DO
Clinical Assistant in Surgery/Emergency Medicine, University of Illinois College of Medicine, Peoria IL

Preface

Emergency medicine is a broad discipline. There are many books covering all topics, providing on-line assistance and reference; there are preparatory books for the boards, both written and oral. There are even a few books intended as study tools for the inservice exam. However, almost exclusively, all these books are large and cumbersome. Emergency medicine doctors generally do not utilize big offices, and are often on the move. Unless something can be stuffed into a pocket, it gets tossed into a pile and forgotten. The goal of this book is to provide a concise study guide focused on the inservice exam, and which is small enough to be carried in a pocket.

The American Board of Emergency Medicine In-Training Examination (ABEMITE) is a two hundred and twenty-five question multiple-choice exam. The first twenty-five questions have visual cues (electrocardiogram tracings, radiograph reproductions, or photographs of physical exam findings) which are used to answer the question. The following two hundred questions are straightforward multiple choice. Emergency medicine residents have four and a half hours to complete the exam.

Not all questions that appear on an exam are scored. New questions have to go through a validation process and may appear in order to be field tested. If you get one right, great, but it will not improve your score. By the same token, if you get it wrong, that is ok, it will not hurt your score. However, there is no way to know which questions are scored and which questions are being tested. Assume that all questions are being scored.

The ABEMITE is administered to all ACGME and RCPSC accredited programs that elect to participate. The test takes place on the last Wednesday of February. Programs accredited by the AOA use a separate exam.

There is some correlation between the scores emergency medicine residents earn on the ABEMITE during their third year of residency and the passing rate on the first attempt of the written boards. The higher the score you get on the ABEMITE, the greater your chance of passing the written exam on the first attempt [1].

In emergency medicine, everything is important. But for the ABEMITE, some areas are more essential than others. If you are short on time and cannot review every section before the exam, focus on Cardiology, Pulmonology, Abdominal/GI, Trauma, and Pediatrics. The last chapter of the book is a rapid review which can be used throughout your study preparation, or as a last minute refresher right before the exam.

The breakdown of questions on the exam varies slightly year to year, but approximate topic percentages are as follows:

Signs and symptoms: ~10%
Cardiovascular: ~10%
Respiratory: ~10%
Trauma: ~10%
Abdominal and GI: ~8%
ENT: ~5%

Infectious diseases: ~5%

Nervous system: ~5%

Procedures: ~5%

Musculoskeletal: ~4%

OB/GYN: ~4%

Renal: ~4%

Toxicology: ~4%

Dermatology: ~3%

Endocrine: ~3%

Environmental: ~3%

Psychobehavioral: ~3%

Hematology: ~2%

Immunology: ~2%

The exam is constructed from topics outlined in the ABEM "Model of Clinical Practice of Emergency Medicine" [2]. This book has been constructed using the same topic list. The Model is reviewed every other year, with 2011 as the last review.

The Pocket Guide to the ABEMITE was developed to be a quick and thorough study guide for the ABEMITE; something small enough to easily carry, but thorough enough to cover nearly all of the topics found on the exam. The outline and table format makes it easy to quickly cover the essential information for each topic without having to slog through the unnecessary material found in most large textbooks. As opposed to question-and-answer reviews, this format also promotes rapid memorization.

This book was designed for emergency medicine residents taking the ABEMITE. In addition, the information contained in this book is also useful for other groups: emergency medicine residents preparing for their written ABEM certification exam, emergency medicine physicians preparing for the recertification examination, and residents from non-emergency medicine specialties who are preparing to rotate through the department and want an overview of emergency medicine.

References

1. American Board of Emergency Medicine. In-training Examination Overview [Internet]. East Lansing, MI: ABEM.org; [updated 4/10/2012; cited 9/18/2012]. Available from: http://www.abem.org/PUBLIC/portal/alias_Rainbow/lang_en-US/tabID_3427/DesktopDefault.aspx.

2. 2011 EM Model Review Task Force, Perina DG, Brunett CP, Caro DA, et al. The 2011 model of the clinical practice of emergency medicine. Academic Emergency Medicine. 2012; 19: e19–e40. doi:10.1111/j.1553–2712.2012.01385.x

Chapter 1

Cardiology emergencies

Marc D. Squillante and Ashley Anklam

1.1. Bradyarrhythmias

1.1.1. Sinus bradycardia

ECG: sinus rhythm, regular rate <60 beats per minute (bpm).

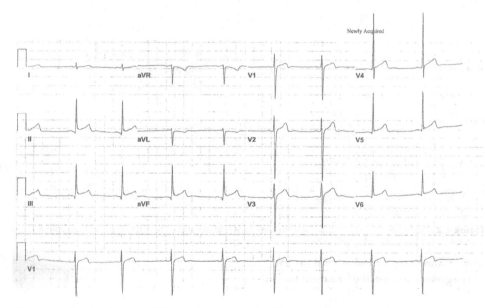

Figure 1.1. Sinus bradycardia at 53 bpm – 18-year-old male with syncope. Early repolarization also present.

Cause: hypothermia, medications, carotid sinus hypersensitivity, physically fit individuals.
Management: atropine for symptomatic or hemodynamically unstable. Pace if no response to atropine.

Pocket Guide to the American Board of Emergency Medicine In-Training Exam, ed. Bob Cambridge.
Published by Cambridge University Press. © Cambridge University Press 2013.

1.1.2. Junctional/ventricular escape rhythm

ECG: no P wave or inverted P wave; wide complex QRS if ventricular origin.
Cause: hyperkalemia, increased vagal tone, other causes as with sinus bradycardia.
Management: if symptomatic, treat underlying cause; pace as needed. Asymptomatic
bradycardia does not need treatment.

1.2. Conduction pathway blocks

1.2.1. AV blocks

1.2.1.1. First degree AV block

ECG: PR interval >200 msec with no variation in PR interval between beats, no beats are
dropped.

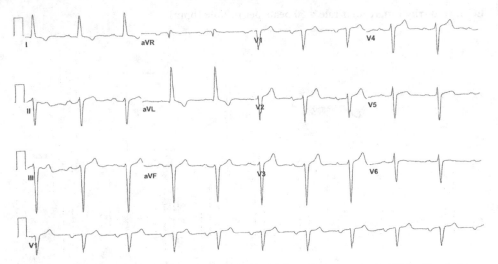

Figure 1.2. First degree AV block, left anterior fascicular block, left ventricular hypertrophy (LVH) – 66-year-old
man with history of hypertension (HTN), presents with syncope.

Cause: idiopathic, can be normal variant.
Management: no specific treatment needed.

1.2.1.2. Second degree AV block: Type I (Mobitz I or Wenckebach)

ECG: progressive PR lengthening until a P wave is not conducted, resulting in a dropped
   QRS. Pattern may repeat (often in P:QRS ratios of 3:2, 4:3).

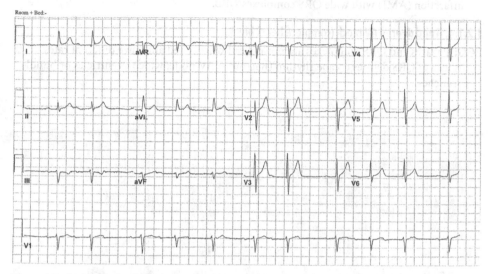

Figure 1.3. Second degree AV block – Type I (Mobitz I or Wenckebach). 58-year-old man with alerted level of
consciousness. Gradually increasing PR intervals seen before the dropped beats.

Cause: block at AV node level. Increased vagal tone, inferior MI, digitalis, rheumatic fever.
Management: will worsen with increased vagal tone or carotid massage and improves with
   atropine.

1.2.1.3. Second degree AV block: Type II (Mobitz II)

ECG: sinus P waves, PR interval constant, with intermittent non-conducted P waves and
   dropped QRS complexes (ratio of P:QRS 3:2, 4:3, can be 2:1). Usually have underlying
   chronic bundle branch block (BBB) (often left BBB [LBBB]).

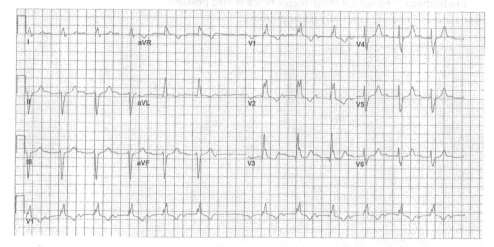

Figure 1.4. Second degree AV block – Type II. 104-year-old man with fever and altered mental status. First degree
AV block, RBBB, and left anterior fascicular block also present. PR constant before the dropped beats.

Cause: infranodal block. Seen in anteroseptal infarct, cardiomyopathy, degeneration of conduction system.

Management: pacing if symptomatic, prepare to pace in setting of acute myocardial infarction (AMI) with wide QRS complexes/BBB.

1.2.1.4. Third degree AV block (complete heart block)

ECG: P waves and QRS complexes are present but dissociated and have different rates. Width of QRS defines escape rhythm (narrow = AV node, wide = ventricles or bundle branches).

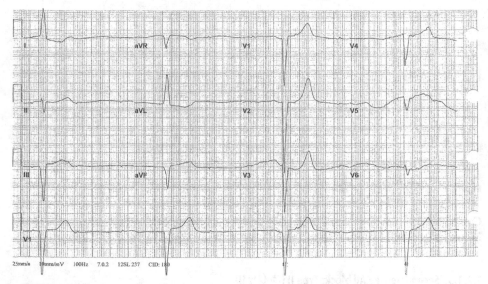

Figure 1.5. Third degree AV block (complete heart block) – 61-year-old man with weakness and near syncope. Sinus bradycardia with slow ventricular escape rhythm. LBBB also present.

Cause: acquired form is often secondary to ischemia/infarction, structural heart disease, or medications. Congenital third degree block is also possible.

Management: pacing, especially if symptomatic.

1.2.2. Bundle blocks

1.2.2.1. Right bundle branch block (RBBB)

ECG: wide QRS complex (>120 msec); M-shaped rSR' in V1 (or qR, RsR'); wide S wave in
I, V5–6.

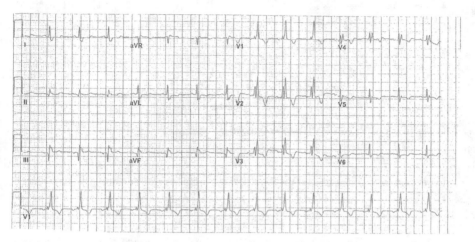

Figure 1.6. Right bundle branch block (RBBB) – 83-year-old man with weakness. Typical triphasic rSR' in V1–2, and wide S wave in I and V6. T wave inversion seen in the lateral V-leads, not due to the RBBB (consider lateral ischemia).

1.2.2.2. Left bundle branch block (LBBB)

ECG: wide QRS (>120 msec); broad, monophasic/notched R waves in I, aVL, V5–6; small
r waves with deep S waves in II, III, aVF, V1–3; ST-T changes opposite (discordant)
from terminal QRS.

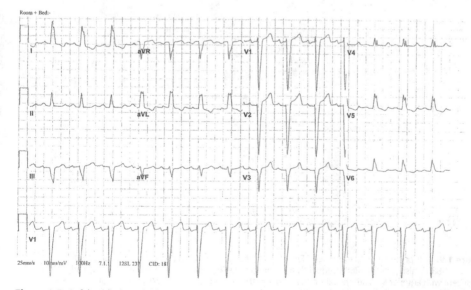

Figure 1.7. Left bundle branch block (LBBB) – seen in a 72-year-old female with near-syncope. Wide QRS, with broad monophasic notched R waves in I, aVL, V5–6. rS complexes in V1–2. Discordant ST-T changes seen in these leads (due to the LBBB).

1.2.2.3. Left anterior fascicular block

ECG: left axis deviation (−30 to −90 degrees); normal QRS interval; qR complex in aVL, rS in III.

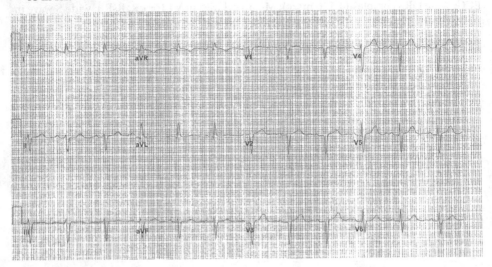

Figure 1.8. Left anterior fascicular block (LAFB) – seen in a 78-year-old patient with hypertension presenting with abdominal pain. Left axis deviation of −66 degrees, typical qR complexes in I, aVL, and rS complexes in II, III, and aVF.

Cause: HTN, valve disease, ischemia, cardiomyopathy, cardiac surgery, myocarditis.

1.2.2.4. Left posterior fascicular block

ECG: right axis deviation (+90 to +180 degrees); normal QRS interval (if no associated RBBB); rS in I, aVL; qR complex in III.

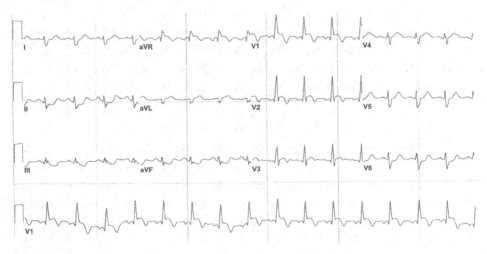

Figure 1.9. Left posterior fascicular block (LPFB) – from a 62- year-old man presenting with chest pain and dyspnea. RBBB is also present. (RBBB frequently accompanies LPFB.) Patient has ST elevation in the early V-leads, consistent with anterior MI. With the bifascicular block in the setting of an acute MI, patient is at high risk for worsening heart block. (Transcutaneous pacing should be ready.)

Cause: heart disease. Usually seen in association with RBBB. Implies more serious conduction system disease. In setting of AMI (usually anterior), may develop sudden complete heart block.

1.3. Tachyarrhythmias

1.3.1. Narrow complex tachycardias

Rate >100 bpm, QRS duration <120 msec.

1.3.1.1. Sinus tachycardia

ECG: consistent appearance of P waves, which are upright in most leads, rhythm regular, rate is >100 bpm.

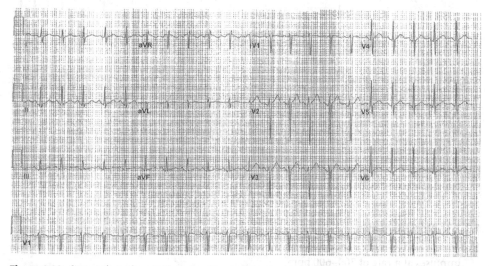

Figure 1.10. Sinus tachycardia – 130 bpm in a 52-year-old man with dyspnea.

Cause: anemia, congestive heart failure (CHF), sepsis, hypovolemia, panic, pain, pulmonary embolism.

Management: treat the underlying cause.

1.3.1.2. Supraventricular tachycardia

ECG: regular, narrow complex tachycardia, without depolarizing P waves preceding the QRS (P waves are buried within the QRS complex).

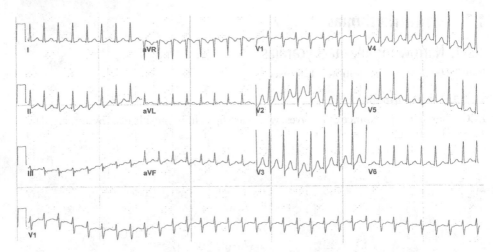

Figure 1.11. Supraventricular tachycardia at a rate ~190 bpm in a 58-year-old man with chest pain and palpitations. Small portions of retrograde P waves are seen at the end of the QRS complexes in leads II, III, and aVF (they are mostly buried in the QRS). ST depression is seen in the inferior and anterior leads. Successfully treated with adenosine.

Management: first attempt vagal maneuvers (carotid massage, Valsalva); if unsuccessful use 6 mg of adenosine. If still unsuccessful follow with up to 2 additional doses of 12 mg each. Synchronized cardioversion at 50–100 J is utilized for unstable patients.

1.3.1.3. Atrial fibrillation

ECG: no P waves, fibrillatory pattern followed by irregularly, irregular QRS response. Atrial impulses at a rate of 300–600 bpm.

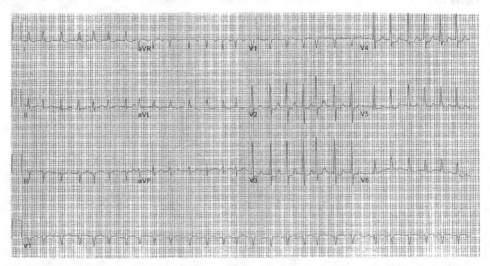

Figure 1.12. Atrial fibrillation – A-fib with rapid ventricular response (RVR) ~160 bpm in an 86-year-old man with dyspnea, and history of CHF and hypertension. Nonspecific ST-T changes also seen.

Cause: HTN, valvular heart disease, catecholamine excess, pericarditis, ischemic heart disease, acute alcohol intoxication ("holiday heart"), pulmonary embolism (PE), hyperthyroidism, lone atrial fibrillation (A-fib).

Types: rate controlled (the ventricular rate is <100 bpm); rapid ventricular rate (ventricular rate >100 bpm); new onset (<48–72 hours); paroxysmal (intermittent episodes that can last minutes to hours).

Management:

Chronic but rate controlled: due to risk of embolism from atrial thrombus, this type is managed by rate controlling as needed and treating triggers. Rate control is more crucial than rhythm control, especially in the elderly.

New onset (<48–72 hours): electrical cardioversion may be utilized. Pharmacologic cardioversion may be attempted with flecainide, procainamide, ibutilide, amiodarone, propafenone. Amiodarone, ibutilide or propafenone should be used with patients who have HTN, structural heart disease or ischemia.

New onset (> 48–72 hours) patient must be anticoagulated for >3 weeks prior to cardioversion. Pharmacologically rate control the patient.

Rate control medications: goal is HR 60–80 bpm and systolic blood pressure (SBP) over 90 mmHg. First line: IV β-blockers or calcium channel blockers (CCBs), such as diltiazem or verapamil. Second line is digitalis. Third line is magnesium sulfate. β-blockers and CCBs are most frequently employed in the outpatient setting.

Table 1.1 Rate controlling medications for atrial fibrillation

Agent	IV Loading dose	IV Maintenance dose
Diltiazem	0.25 mg/kg over 2 min (up to 25 mg) May repeat after 15 min 1 dose	5–15 mg/hr
Metoprolol	5 mg over 2 min, May repeat Q5 min x3 doses	None
Esmolol	500 mcg/kg over 1 min	50–200 mcg/kg/min
Amiodarone	150 mg over 10 min	0.5–1 mg/min
Digoxin	0.25 mg Q2 hours up to 1.5 mg total	0.125–0.375 mg IV/PO daily

Electrical cardioversion: indicated for unstable patients and patients with < 48–72 hours of A-fib. Synchronized conversion with 50–100 J is ideal, but synchronization is not always attainable. Must discuss risk of stroke related to cardioversion, recalling that the longer the A-fib has been present the greater the risk of stroke secondary to embolism from atria.

1.3.1.4. Atrial flutter

ECG: regular flutter waves at a rate of 250–350 per minute that have a "sawtooth" appearance seen best in II, III, aVF, V1–2, with a typical AV conduction ratio of 2:1 or 4:1.

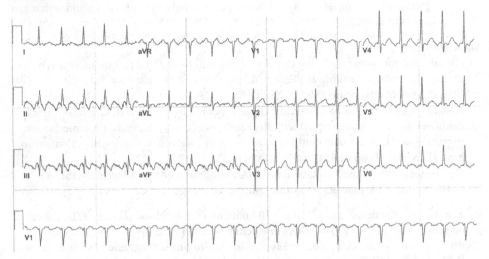

Figure 1.13. Atrial flutter – 67-year-old man with chest pain and dyspnea. The ventricular rate is ~125 bpm, and there is 2:1 AV conduction (common ratio). Sawtooth flutter waves are seen in leads II, III, and aVF (one at the end of the QRS, the other between the QRS complexes), at twice the ventricular rate.

Cause: thyroid disease, valve dysfunction, structural heart disease or heart failure.

Management:
Stable patient: control ventricular rate with CCB (preferably diltiazem) or β-blocker. Digitalis is second line or used for patients with chronic CHF.
Patient with ventricular rate >200 bpm: may indicate the presence of an accessory pathway. In this situation AV nodal blockers (CCB, adenosine, β-blockers, digitalis) must not be used – can lead to ventricular fibrillation (V-fib).

Electrical cardioversion: synchronized, 25–50 J for unstable patients or those with recurrent atrial flutter.

1.3.1.5. Multifocal atrial tachycardia (MAT)

ECG: at least 3 different P wave morphologies with HR >100 bpm, variable P'-P', P'-R and R-R interval.

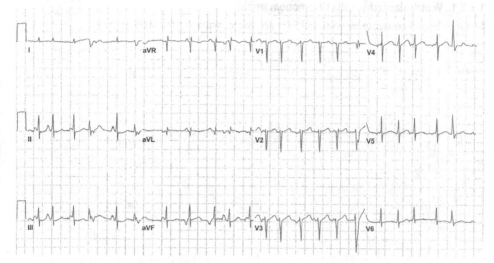

Figure 1.14. Multifocal atrial tachycardia (MAT) – 76-year-old man with dyspnea, cough, and wheezing from a chronic obstructive pulmonary disease (COPD) exacerbation. Note the multiple different P wave morphologies and irregular rhythm.

Cause: hypoxemia, pulmonary disease, electrolyte imbalance, drug toxicity, acid–base disturbance.

Management: correct underlying condition. If concern for MI, first line is CCB or β-blocker. Second line is magnesium.

1.3.2. Wide complex tachycardias

Rate >100 bpm, QRS duration >120 msec.

1.3.2.1. Ventricular tachycardia (VT; monomorphic)

ECG: at least 3 consecutive wide QRS (>120 msec) with a rate >100 bpm.

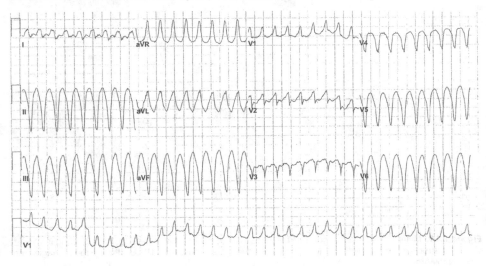

Figure 1.15. Ventricular tachycardia (monomorphic) – 64-year-old woman presents with dyspnea and near-syncope. History of MI and CHF. This is a regular, wide complex tachycardia, without P waves – in the setting of a patient with known structural heart disease, VT should be your primary consideration.

Cause: reentry mechanisms, premature ventricular contractions, most individuals will have underlying cardiac ischemia or heart disease, hypoxemia, hypercapnia, electrolyte imbalance.

Management: correct underlying cause then terminate dysrhythmia with amiodarone or lidocaine (first-line drug), procainamide or sotalol (second line), magnesium (third line). Electrical cardioversion is utilized for patients who do not respond to medications or are unstable. Start at 50–100 J then escalate up to 360 J.

1.3.2.2. Torsade de pointes (form of polymorphic VT)

ECG: often short episodes with rate >200 bpm and wide QRS with undulating axis.

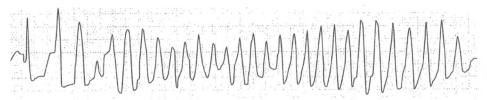

Figure 1.16. Torsades de pointes (form of polymorphic VT) – short run of torsades de pointes in patient with prolonged QT interval. Note the "twisting of the points" around a central axis during the dysrhythmia.

Cause: prolonged QT interval (hypokalemia, hypomagnesemia, MI, medications).

Management: in stable patient, treat the underlying cause and overdrive pace or employ a β-adrenergic infusion or IV magnesium. In unstable patients proceed to electrical cardioversion.

1.3.3. Antiarrhythmic medications

Table 1.2 Antiarrhythmic medications

	Mechanism of action	Drugs
Class 1A	Sodium channel blockers (intermediate speed) Slows conduction through the atria, AV node, and His Purkinje system	Quinidine, procainamide
Class 1B	Sodium channel blockers (fast speed)	Lidocaine, phenytoin
Class 1C	Sodium channel blockers (slow speed)	Flecainide, propafenone
Class 2	β-blockers	Propranolol, esmolol, metoprolol, most drugs ending in –lol
Class 3	Antifibrillatory	Bretylium, amiodarone, sotalol
Class 4	Calcium channel blockers	Verapamil, diltiazem

1.4. Assorted conduction abnormalities

1.4.1. Brugada syndrome

ECG: V1–3 have saddle-shaped ST elevation that can be transient, occasionally RBBB or first degree AV block as well.

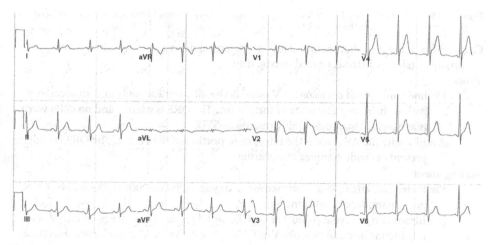

Figure 1.17. Brugada syndrome – typical pattern of coved ST elevation in V1–3. From a 44-year-old man with atypical chest pain and near-syncope.

Cause: sodium channel abnormality. Males and Asians most commonly affected.

Management: implantable defibrillator; can have syncope or sudden cardiac death with this syndrome.

1.4.2. Wolff–Parkinson–White (WPW) syndrome

ECG: may present in normal sinus rhythm or tachycardia (SVT, A-fib). Slurred upstroke of QRS (delta wave), with QRS interval >100 msec and PR interval <120 msec.

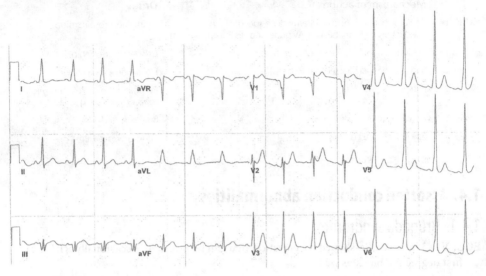

Figure 1.18. Wolff–Parkinson–White (WPW) syndrome – 26-year-old man treated with adenosine for SVT. This was the post conversion ECG. Note the short PR interval and delta waves seen in multiple leads.

Cause: often idiopathic, but can be related to structural disease such as mitral valve prolapse, tricuspid atresia or cardiomyopathy.

Types:
>   **Orthodromic (most common):** AV node is the anterograde route and an accessory path is the retrograde route of the circuit. The QRS is narrow and no delta wave is apparent. Most commonly presents as SVT.
>   **Antidromic:** the AV node is the retrograde portion of the circuit. The QRS is wide, presents as wide complex tachycardia.

Management:
>   **Orthodromic:** attempt vagal maneuver, if unsuccessful can utilize, β-blocker, CCB, procainamide, or adenosine.
>   **Antidromic:** must avoid β-blockers, CCB, and digoxin. These drugs block AV node conduction and can provoke V-fib. Use procainamide or amiodarone. Electrical cardioversion is indicated if medications fail or rate is >250 bpm.
>   **Unstable patient:** electrical cardioversion at 50–100 J, synchronized if possible.

1.4.3. Early repolarization

ECG: ST elevation usually seen in anterior leads, often diffuse, large amplitude T waves, J-point elevation or notching, usually <1/3 of total height of T wave. "Notch" at the end of QRS (J point) strongly suggests early repolarization (although not always present). ST segment is concave upward. Pattern stable on repeat ECGs (short term).

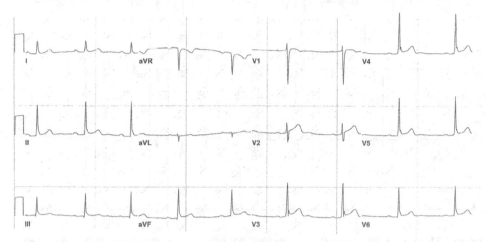

Figure 1.19. Early repolarization– diffuse ST elevation, and notching of the J-point in the inferior and anterior leads. From a 30-year-old man with atypical chest pain.

Management: none needed. Usually benign phenomenon but can be difficult to distinguish from AMI at times.

1.4.4. Pericarditis

ECG: Stage 1: diffuse ST elevation and PR depression. Stage 2: ST segments flatten, T waves flatten. Stage 3: symmetric T wave inversion. Stage 4: normalization.

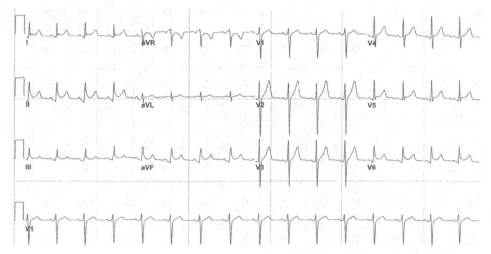

Figure 1.20. Pericarditis – diffuse concave ST elevation, with PR depression in multiple leads, and PR elevation in aVR. From a 43-year-old man with pleuritic, positional chest pain after a viral respiratory infection.

1.4.5. Electrical alternans

ECG: alternating amplitude and morphology of every other QRS complex; seen with cardiac tamponade.

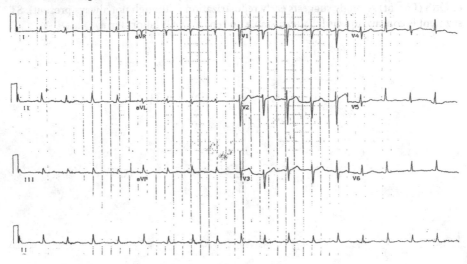

Figure 1.21. Electrical alternans – from a 67-year-old woman with breast cancer and a malignant pericardial effusion. Note the alternating heights and polarity of the QRS complexes.

1.4.6. Hypertrophic patterns

1.4.6.1. Left ventricular hypertrophy (LVH)

ECG: S wave in V1 + R wave in V5 or V6 that is >35 mm if age >40 years old; R wave in aVL >11 mm; ST-T changes with "ventricular strain" pattern.

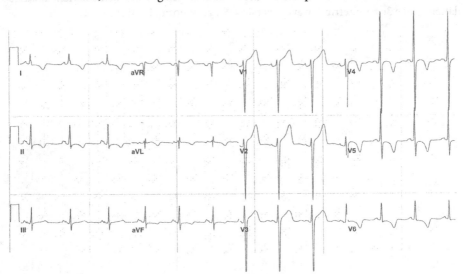

Figure 1.22. Left ventricular hypertrophy (LVH) – from a 44-year-old man with hypertension. Note the large precordial voltages (R in V1–2 + S in V5 > 35mm). Ventricular "strain" pattern (vs. ischemia) also noted particularly in the lateral limb and V-leads (ST-segment depression and T wave inversion).

1.4.6.2. Right ventricular hypertrophy (RVH)

ECG: tall R in V1 >6 mm; R: S ratio in V1 >1.

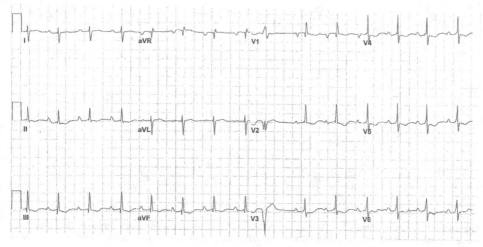

Figure 1.23. Right ventricular hypertrophy (RVH) – from a 70-year-old woman with pulmonary fibrosis, presenting with dyspnea and hypoxia. Note the large R wave in V1 and right axis deviation.

1.4.7. Electrical rhythms incompatible with life

For all of these rhythms, ACLS/PALS protocols should be followed for management.

1.4.7.1. Asystole

ECG: "flatline," no cardiac electrical activity.

1.4.7.2. Pulseless electrical activity (PEA)

ECG: organized cardiac activity, presentation may vary.
Clinical: electrical activity on ECG but no mechanical action of myocardium.
Causes: Hs and Ts (hypovolemia, hypothermia, hypoxia, hydrogen ion [acidosis], hyper/hypokalemia, hypoglycemia, trauma, thrombosis, tamponade, tension pneumothorax, toxins).
Treatment: ACLS/PALS, treat underlying cause.

1.4.7.3. Ventricular fibrillation

ECG: chaotic cardiac activity, with no clear P waves or QRS complexes.

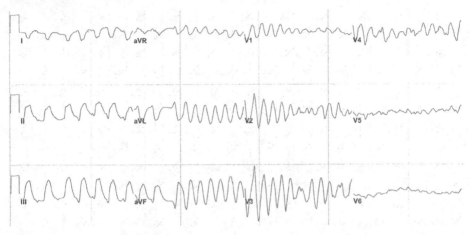

Figure 1.24. Ventricular fibrillation – V-fib develops (during the ECG) in a patient with an acute MI (ST elevation in II and III). Note the chaotic rhythm pattern consistent with V-fib, best seen in the V-leads. Patient was successfully defibrillated back to sinus rhythm.

1.5. Acute coronary syndromes

1.5.1. Acute MI overview

Table 1.3 Infarct patterns and localization

Location	Leads	Additional ECG considerations	Artery likely involved
Septal	V1–2		LAD
Anterior	V1–4	V1–4 (anteroseptal MI) V3–4 (anterior MI) V3–6 (anterolateral MI)	LAD
Lateral	I, aVL, V5–6		LCx, RCA, or LAD
Inferior	II, III, aVF	ST elevation in lead III greater than lead II (with ST depression in I, aVL) suggests RCA occlusion ST depressions in anterior leads V1–3 (posterior wall involvement), reciprocal depression in I and aVL	RCA (90%), LCx (10%)
Right ventricle	V1–2, V4R	ST elevation in right-sided V leads (V4R, V5R), in association with inferior MI. May see ST elevation in lead V1 also ST elevation greater in lead III than II suggests right ventricle MI Often have associated inferior and/or posterior MI	Proximal RCA, most often associated with inferior MI
Posterior	ST depression V1–2/3	ST segment depression in lead V1–3 T wave:S wave ratio >1 Posterior leads (V7–9) ST elevation	RCA or LCx
High grade	ST elevation in aVR	Diffuse ST depression in other leads	Left main trunk, triple vessel disease

LAD, left anterior descending; LCx, left circumflex; RCA, right coronary artery.

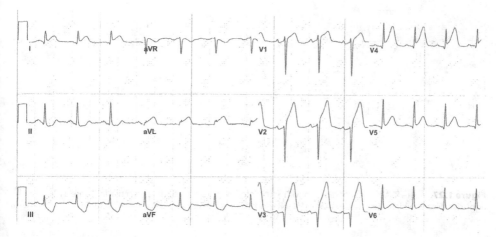

Figure 1.25. Acute anterior MI – from a 42-year-old male with severe chest pain. Anterior and lateral ST elevation (I, aVL, V1–5), with ST depression in the inferior leads. Hyperacute T waves (large, broad based) seen especially in leads V2–4. A proximal LAD occlusion was found and stented.

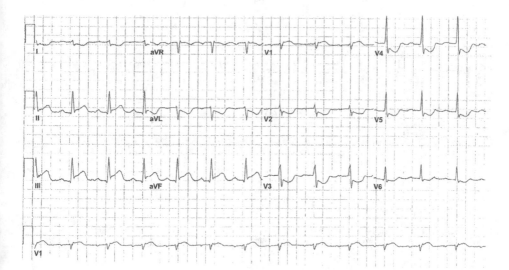

Figure 1.26. Acute inferior MI – from a 57-year-old man with chest pain. ST elevation in II, III, and aVF, reciprocal ST depression in I and aVL, with ST depression in V2–6 (posterior wall involvement). ST elevation in V1 may indicate RV involvement as well. Patient was found to have a proximal total RCA occlusion which was successfully stented.

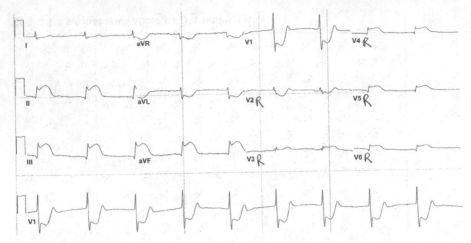

Figure 1.27. Acute RVMI – 71-year-old man with acute inferior–posterior MI. The precordial leads are all right-sided leads, which show ST elevation in V4–6R – indicative of RVMI and proximal RCA occlusion.

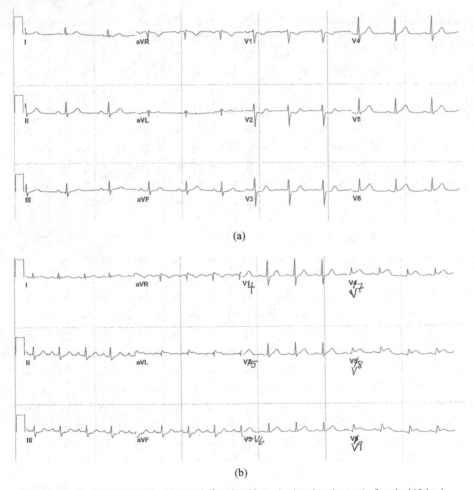

(a)

(b)

Figure 1.28. Acute posterior MI – 60-year-old female with waxing/waning chest pain. Standard 12-lead (a) showed ST depression in V1–3 without other changes. Posterior leads (b) showed ST elevation ~1 mm in V7,V8, and V9, consistent with posterior MI. Patient had successful percutaneous transluminal coronary angioplasty (PTCA) of culprit circumflex lesion.

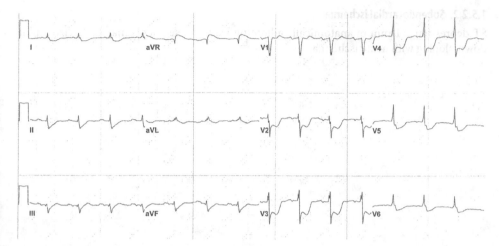

Figure 1.29. Left main coronary MI/occlusion – from a 68-year-old man who presented in cardiogenic shock with severe substernal chest pain. Note the diffuse ST segment depression, as well as ST elevation in aVR, findings suspicious for left main or triple vessel disease. Emergent angiography showed total occlusion of the left main coronary, as well as the right coronary artery. (Patient expired in cath lab.)

1.5.2. Additional infarct/ischemia ECG findings

1.5.2.1. Sgarbossa criteria for identifying AMI in presence of LBBB

ST elevation ≥1 mm concordant with QRS deflection (score 5).
ST depression ≥1 mm in leads V1, V2, V3 (score 3).
ST elevation ≥5 mm discordant with QARS deflection (score 2).
Score ≥3 gives specificity of AMI of 90%, sensitivity of 78%.

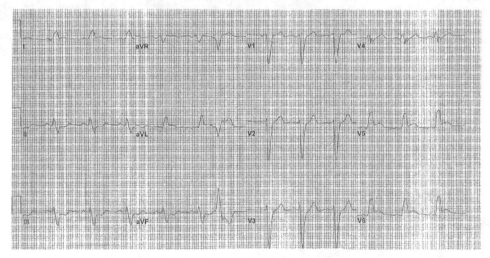

Figure 1.30. AMI with LBBB – 63-year-old man with chest pain. Concordant ST elevation is seen in leads I, aVL, and V5–6, as well as concordant ST depression in V3. Using the Sgarbossa criteria, this patient has an ECG diagnostic for STEMI. Patient was taken to the cath lab where an occluded LAD was successfully stented.

1.5.2.2. Subendocardial ischemia

ST depression ≥1 mm in anatomically adjoining leads. ST segments may be horizontal or down-sloping with acute ischemia.

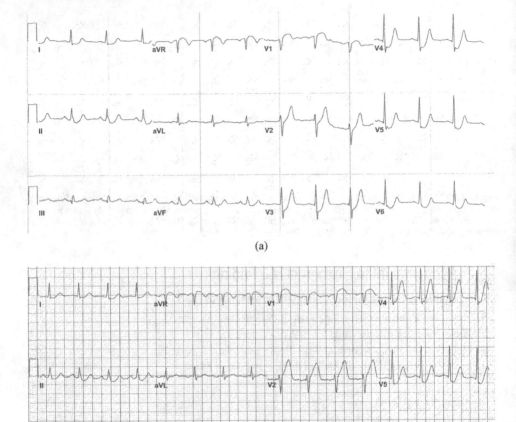

(a)

(b)

Figure 1.31. Subendocardial ischemia – 58-year-old man with severe chest pain. Diffuse ST depression (V2–6, I, II), with ST elevation in V1 (a). Repeat ECG (b) 12 minutes later on patient due to worsening chest pain. Patient has evolving anterior ST segment elevation MI. Note the hyperacute T waves in V2–4: tall, broad based, consistent with this evolving infarction. An occluded LAD was found at cath.

1.5.2.3. Hyperacute T waves

Tall, peaked, and slightly asymmetrical. Seen within minutes of myocardial injury/ischemia onset. May also see associated with hyperkalemia, LVH, early repolarization.

1.5.3. Acute coronary syndrome (ACS) and angina

Table 1.4 ACS types and characteristics

ACS type	Definition	High-risk characteristics
Acute myocardial infarction	Rise in serum cardiac markers (CK/Trop) with one of the following –ST or T wave changes –Abnormalities found on cardiac catheterization –Clinical picture consistent with ischemic pain	Pain similar to previous MI Angina worse than usual ECG changes
Unstable angina	–Angina at rest lasting >20 minutes –New onset of exertional angina within the past 2 months –Worsening of severity of angina within the past 2 months	Pressure or squeezing pain Feeling of "impending doom"
Stable angina	Chest pain with exercise, relieved by rest or nitroglycerin	

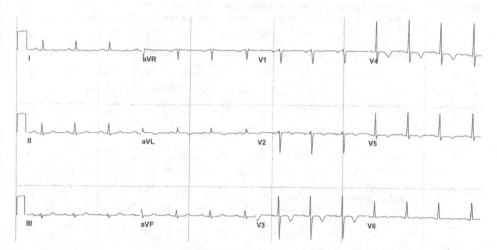

Figure 1.32. T wave inversion – 56-year-old man presented with classic history for unstable angina. Anterior T wave inversion in V2–5 (as well as in leads I and aVL) suspicious for ischemia were noted. His pain resolved with aggressive medical therapy in the ED, and a high-grade proximal LAD stenosis was found at cath, which was successfully stented. Wellens' pattern of T wave inversion in leads V2–3 (may also include V1 and V4), with deep symmetric inversions (most common), or biphasic T's (less common), can be seen in patients with proximal LAD occlusions. This is a special high-risk group of patients that may present pain-free, but require early angiography for successful treatment.

Risk factors for heart disease: smoking tobacco, diabetes, HTN, high cholesterol, family history.

Physical exam findings: new S3, worsening murmur, hypotension, rales from CHF, non-reproducible chest pain (however, if the pain is reproducible it does not rule out ACS).

Diagnosis:

Table 1.5 Cardiac biomarkers

Enzyme	Rise	Peak	Duration
Myoglobin	1–2 hours	4–7 hours	24 hours
CKMB	3–4 hours	12–24 hours	2–3 days
Troponin	3–6 hours	12–24 hours	7–10 days

Treatment: IV, oxygen, monitor; ABCs if patient is in extremis.

Table 1.6 Treatment strategies for ACS

Treatment strategy	Goal	Considerations	Absolute contraindications	Relative contraindications
Nitrates	Dilate the coronary arteries Reduce preload Minor afterload reduction	Can cause hypotension RV infarcts because they are volume dependent Treat hypotension with boluses of IVF	Hypotension (SBP <90 mmHg) Heart rate less than 50 bpm or greater than 100 bpm Medications for erectile dysfunction	
Morphine	Used for intractable pain and anxiety	Can cause hypotension	Opioid allergy	
Aspirin	Antiplatelet Chew 324 mg of non-enteric coated aspirin		Aspirin allergy Hemorrhage or potential aortic dissection	
Clopidogrel	Potent inhibitor of platelet aggregation	Can be given before going to cath lab as with aspirin Good if patient has aspirin allergy		
β-blockers	Antagonize catecholamine effect on the myocardium Decrease contractility and oxygen demand	Give in the first 24 hours In STEMI patients, if no risks for cardiogenic shock or other contraindications, can be considered	Signs of hypoperfusion SBP <100 mmHg HR <60 bpm	
ACE inhibitors	Helps to reduce afterload	Should be given within first 24 hours PO is as good as IV	Hypotension Volume depletion	
Heparin	Prevents clot formation	Use concurrently with tPA or after streptokinase to minimize systemic emboli		
Low molecular weight heparin	Prevents clot formation	No need for lab monitoring Lower rate of heparin induced thrombocytopenia		

Table 1.6 (cont.)

Treatment strategy	Goal	Considerations	Absolute contraindications	Relative contraindications
GIIb/IIIa inhibitors	Antiplatelet	Best in patients who will receive PCI		
Fibrinolytics	Indicated in individuals with >1 mm of ST elevation in two or more contiguous leads. Symptoms present for <6–12 hours		Active internal bleeding Suspected aortic dissection Known intracranial neoplasm History of hemorrhagic CVA History of non-hemorrhagic CVA in 3 months	Active peptic ulcer CPR >10 minutes Pregnancy Trauma, surgery, or internal bleeding within the past 2–4 weeks Uncontrolled BP (SBP >180/100) History of intracerebral pathology not in absolute contraindication list Noncompressible vascular puncture sites
Percutaneous coronary intervention (PCI)	Diagnosis and treatment of blockage	Results in better outcomes than fibrinolytics if delivered in a timely manner Should be treated with PCI within 90 minutes	Not indicated after fibrinolytics if symptoms resolve	

CVA, cerebrovascular accident; IVF, IV fluids; STEMI, ST elevation myocardial infarction.

1.5.4. Complications after MI

Table 1.7 Post-MI complications

Timeframe	Complication	Considerations	Treatment
Early	Accelerated idioventricular rhythm	Do not give lidocaine, can lead to asystole	None
	First degree AV block or Mobitz 1	Associated with inferior MI	None
	Mobitz 2 or third degree AV block	Associated with anterior MI	Pacemaker
Late	Dressler's syndrome	1 week to months post MI	NSAIDs
	Papillary muscle dysfunction/ ruptured chordae tendineae	Hypotension, CHF, new mitral murmur	Surgical
	Septal rupture	Sudden, dramatic clinical decline. New harsh, holosystolic murmur	Immediate cardiology consult. Vasopressors and inotropic medications. Balloon pump may be necessary

1.6. Heart failure

1.6.1. Types

1.6.1.1 Systolic heart failure

Pathophysiology: impaired contractility, ejection fraction (EF) <40%.
Causes: MI, anything that can cause myocyte dysfunction with contractility.

1.6.1.2. Diastolic heart failure

Pathophysiology: impaired relaxation, EF at least 60%.
Causes: HTN, hypertrophic or dilated cardiomyopathy, aortic stenosis.

1.6.1.3. Left-sided heart failure

Pathophysiology: fluid backup behind left ventricle (LV), leading to pulmonary congestion.
Symptoms: orthopnea, dyspnea.

1.6.1.4. Right-sided heart failure

Pathophysiology: fluid backup behind right ventricle (RV).
Symptoms: hepatomegaly, pedal edema.

1.6.2. Heart failure overview

Causes: HTN, pregnancy, infection, myocardial ischemia/infarction, anemia, pulmonary embolism, acute myocarditis or valve dysfunction, dysrhythmia.
Symptoms: include orthopnea, dyspnea, nocturia, paroxysmal nocturnal dyspnea.
Signs: clammy, crackles at the bases of lungs, wheezing, leg swelling.
Decompensated heart failure: jugular venous distension (JVD), rales, shortness of breath, orthopnea. This can be precipitated by CCB, β-blockers, NSAIDs, increased salt intake, medication noncompliance, arrhythmias, ACS, renal failure and uncontrolled HTN.
Diagnostics: B-type natriuretic peptide (BNP) level, chest X-ray (look for cardiomegaly, interstitial edema, pleural effusion, Kerley lines, enlarged pulmonary arteries which are suggestive of left-sided heart failure).
Treatment:
> **Diuretics:** indicated in decompensated heart failure and acute pulmonary edema. Loop diuretics (furosemide, bumetanide, ethacrynic acid) – provide symptomatic relief. Watch for hypokalemia, hypomagnesemia, hypovolemia. Potassium-sparing diuretics (spironolactone) decrease molarity. May cause hyperkalemia and gynecomastia.
> **Vasodilators:** indicated in decompensated heart failure and acute pulmonary edema. Nitroglycerin: reduces preload and afterload and decreases myocardial ischemia via vasodilation. Watch for hypotension.
> Nitroprusside: potent vasodilator, leading to decreased BP and improved cardiac output. Can lead to hypotension and thiocyanate toxicity (chronic use).
> **Angiotensin-converting enzyme (ACE) inhibitors:** decreases mortality and hospitalization in heart failure patients. Contraindicated in patients with bilateral renal artery stenosis, hypotension, hyperkalemia, angioedema, progressive azotemia or who are pregnant.
> **Angiotensin receptor blockers:** similar to ACE inhibitors but decrease incidence of cough and angioedema.

Beta blockers: help reduce sympathetic nervous system activity and reduce mortality. Contraindicated if hemodynamically unstable, class IV stable heart failure, bronchospasm, symptomatic bradycardia.

1.7. Cardiomyopathies

1.7.1. Dilated cardiomyopathy

Cause: idiopathic is the most common reason. Other causes include inherited, secondary to infection (viral and bacterial), post-myocarditis, pregnancy, or HTN. Also associated with tobacco or alcohol use, other toxins/drugs, collagen vascular disease.

Characteristics: dyspnea, chest pain, left heart failure.

Diagnostics: chest X-ray (look for cardiomegaly), ECG (nonspecific, poor R wave progression), echocardiogram (LV dilation, wall motion abnormality, EF <45%).

Management: remove offending agents (tobacco, alcohol, drugs). Treat with ACE inhibitors, nitrates, spironolactone, β-blockers, and implantable defibrillator.

1.7.2. Hypertrophic cardiomyopathy

Cause: autosomal dominant disease.

Characteristics: shortness of breath, chest pain, syncope, sudden death. Crescendo-decrescendo midsystolic murmur that becomes louder with squatting or Valsalva. Loud S4 gallop.

Diagnostics: chest X-ray (may be normal or can show LV or atrial enlargement), ECG (LVH, T wave inversions, ST abnormalities), echocardiogram (narrowing of left outflow tract, asymmetric LV with small ventricular chamber, limited septal wall motion).

Management: β-blockers improve symptoms by improving ventricular filling. Verapamil also increases filling.

1.7.3. Restrictive cardiomyopathy

Cause: infiltrative diseases (amyloidoisis, sarcoidosis), interstitial disease (post-radiation fibrosis), and some forms of endocarditis.

Characteristics: dyspnea, fatigue, palpitations, exercise intolerance, ascites.

Diagnostics: chest X-ray (cardiomegaly from atrial enlargement, pulmonary venous congestion, pleural effusions), ECG (nonspecific ST-T wave abnormalities, AV block, intraventricular conduction delay), echocardiogram (biatrial enlargement, thickened RV free wall, elevated RA pressure, normal to low diastolic chamber volume, normal or mildly reduced LV EF).

Management: diuretics, CCBs, cardiac transplantation.

1.8. Diseases of the pericardium and endocardium

1.8.1. Pericarditis

15–60 ml of fluid in the pericardial space normally.

Cause: viral, idiopathic, post-MI (Dressler's), neoplastic, infection, traumatic. Patients can also have myocarditis, leading to LV dysfunction.

History: pain is sharp, worse when supine, improved with sitting forward (tripod). Pleuritic pain is common.

ECG progression:

Stage 1: diffuse ST elevation and PR depression.
Stage 2: ST segments flatten, T waves flatten.
Stage 3: Symmetric T wave inversion.
Stage 4: Normalization.

Treatment: treat the underlying cause, NSAIDs for inflammation.

1.8.2. Pericardial tamponade

Pathophysiology: fluid accumulation in pericardial space prevents diastolic filling of right side of heart. Cardiac output drops, leading to syncope, hypotension, PEA, death.

Characteristics: hypotension and JVD.

Beck's triad: hypotension, JVD, muffled heart sounds.

Pulsus pardoxus: 10 mm decrease in SBP during inspiration.

Diagnostics: chest X-ray (enlarged cardiac silhouette), ECG (low voltage, electrical alternans), echocardiogram (ideal test; can visualize pericardial fluid and collapse of right atrium/ventricle during diastole).

Management: fluid resuscitation. Pericardiocentesis if unstable.

1.8.3. Infective endocarditis

Risk factors: calcified valve, rheumatic fever, congenital heart lesion, prosthetic valve, previous history of endocarditis, IV drug use.

Cause: mostly commonly bacterial, but can be viral or fungal.

Native valve: *Streptococcus, Staphylococcus, Enterococcus.*
IV drug use: *Staphylococcus aureus, Candida, Aspergillus.*
Immunocompromised: *Haemophilus aphrophilus, Actinobacillus, Aggregatibacter actinomycetemcoitans, Cardiobacterium hominis, Eikenella corrodens,* and *Kingella kingae* (HACEK group). Also *Candida* and *Aspergillus.*

Characteristics: malaise, fever, myalgias, cough, anorexia.

Diagnosis: three blood cultures taken from different puncture sites with at least a one hour gap between the first and last culture must be drawn. Labs may have elevation in sedimentary rate (ESR) or C-reactive protein. Chest X-ray may show heart failure. Look for conduction abnormalities on ECG. Transesophageal echo is very accurate test.

Duke criteria: list of major and minor criteria to help make a clinical diagnosis of infective endocarditis. Requires two major criteria, or one major and three minor criteria, or five minor criteria.

Major criteria: positive blood culture with typical organisms, evidence of endocardial involvement on echocardiogram.

Minor criteria: predisposing factors (see risks above), fever, evidence of embolism (such as Janeway lesions or splinter hemorrhages), immunologic problems (such as Osler's nodes), positive blood culture with a non-typical agent or serologic evidence of infection.

Management: initial antibiotic regimen.

Native valve: gentamicin and penicillin G plus either nafcillin or vancomycin.
Native valve plus IV drug use: vancomycin.
Prosthetic valve: vancomycin and gentamicin.

1.9. Valvular disease

Table 1.8 Valvular disease

	Causes	Presentation	Clinical findings	ECG	Considerations
Mitral regurgitation (chronic)	Rheumatic fever, dilated cardiomyopathy	May be tolerated for years, first symptom is usually exertional dyspnea	High-pitched holosystolic murmur with radiation to axilla	Left atrial and LV hypertrophy A-fib	Systemic emboli occur in 20% of patients without anticoagulation
Mitral regurgitation (acute)	Infective endocarditis, myocardial infarct (papillary muscle rupture), rupture of chordae tendineae	Dyspnea, tachycardia, pulmonary edema	Harsh, midsystolic murmur that radiates to the base	If acute, ECG changes are less likely. May have findings from underlying conditions	
Mitral stenosis	Most common is rheumatic fever	Exertional dyspnea, hemoptysis, orthopnea	Mid diastolic murmur with opening snap, loud S1, low to normal systemic BP, A-fib, pulmonary HTN	Left atrial enlargement (biphasic P wave in V1)	Straightening of the left heart border seen on CXR due to left atrial enlargement
Mitral valve prolapse	Congenital	Often asymptomatic, chest pain, palpitations, fatigue, non-exertional dyspnea	Midsystolic click		Give β-blockers for chest pain
Aortic regurgitation (chronic)	Rheumatic heart disease, congenital, syphilis, ankylosing spondylitis, rheumatoid arthritis	Palpitations (often while laying flat), chest pain, fatigue, dyspnea, may be asymptomatic for up to 20 years	Wide pulse pressure (>40 mmHg between systolic and diastolic) with a prominent ventricular impulse, head bobbing High-pitched, blowing diastolic murmur at left sternal border		
Aortic regurgitation (acute)	Majority of cases are caused by infective endocarditis, the remainder are caused by aortic dissection	Dyspnea, acute pulmonary edema	High-pitched, blowing diastolic murmur Soft, diastolic murmur		

(cont.)

Table 1.8 (*cont.*)

	Causes	Presentation	Clinical findings	ECG	Considerations
Aortic stenosis	Congenital is most common cause under 70 years old (bicuspid aortic valve is most common), rheumatic heart disease is second most common. Calcific degeneration most common cause over 70 years old	Classic triad is dyspnea, chest pain and syncope	Small amplitude pulse, narrowed pulse pressure. Crescendo-decrescendo systolic ejection murmur	LVH, LBBB, or RBBB in 10% of cases	Avoid nitrates, diuretics, vasodilators, strenuous activity

CXR, chest X-ray.

1.10. Hypertensive emergency

Definitions.

Hypertensive emergency: elevated BP with evidence of end-organ damage.

Hypertensive urgency: elevated BP with nonspecific symptoms and no acute end-organ damage.

Causes: stroke, pregnancy, pheochromocytoma, medication noncompliance, cocaine, amphetamines.

Characteristics: may complain of alterations to vision, chest pain, dyspnea or headache. Physical exam may reveal retinal hemorrhages and cotton wool spots. Patient can develop encephalopathy, hemorrhage or MI.

Diagnostics: chest X-ray (may reflect CHF, cardiomegaly), ECG (LVH), lab studies (hematuria on urinalysis; acute/chronic kidney injury).

Management: no treatment is needed for asymptomatic patients who have no evidence of end-organ damage. Treat symptomatic patients or those with damage. Goal is to lower mean arterial pressure by 25% within minutes to hours.

Labetalol and hydralazine are commonly employed. Alternatives include nitroglycerin, nicardipine, fenoldopam, nitroprusside.

Pheochromocytoma, cocaine overdose or monoamine oxidase inhibitor (MAOI) crisis should be treated with α-blocker (phentolamine) followed by β-blocker.

Pregnant patients can be treated with labetalol, hydralazine or nicardipine. Seizure prophylaxis with magnesium sulfate for eclampsia and severe preeclampsia.

1.11. Aortic pathology

1.11.1. Abdominal aortic aneurysm

Risk: family history of aneurysm, Marfan's syndrome, age >50, male, history of peripheral artery disease or other aneurysm, smoking, hyperlipidemia, and diabetes.

Presentation: abdominal or back pain which is often sudden and ripping/tearing in quality, syncope, nausea, or vomiting. Sudden death is possible with aortic rupture. Physical exam may reveal abdominal tenderness, Cullen sign (periumbilical ecchymosis) or Grey-Turner sign (flank ecchymosis) secondary to retroperitoneal hemorrhage.

Diagnosis: bedside ultrasound for unstable patient. CT with contrast ideal for stable patients. Forgo imaging if patient is likely to have ruptured aneurysm, go immediately to surgery.

Management: patient with ruptured aneurysm needs to be fluid resuscitated and emergently be surgically repaired. Aneurysms >5 mm have a higher risk of rupture.

1.11.2. Aortic dissection

Key point: diagnosis is imperative as the treatment for aortic dissection would make an MI or PE worse, and the treatment of MI/PE can be fatal if used in aortic dissection.

Risk factors: HTN, Marfan's, pregnancy, coarctation of aorta, bicuspid aortic valve, aortic stenosis, and syphilis.

Presentation: ripping, tearing, severe and abrupt chest or upper back pain. Some patients will have associated syncope. Physical exam reveals HTN or hypotension, unequal BP between bilateral or upper and lower extremities (>20 mmHg), blowing diastolic murmur suggestive of aortic regurgitation.

Diagnostics: chest X-ray may show mediastinal widening, irregular contour to the aorta, pleural effusion, left lung apical capping, depressed left mainstem bronchus, elevated right mainstem bronchus, deviated trachea. ECG is nonspecific, may see Q wave or nonspecific ST abnormalities. CT scan with IV contrast is quick with good sensitivity (93%) but renal issues may prevent its use. MRI has excellent sensitivity and specificity but the scan is not quick and the patient is not easily monitored during the study. Angiography is regarded as gold standard but a false lumen can lead to false negatives.

Management: goal is to decrease shear force on the aorta. Maintain SBP between 100 and 120 mmHg and HR between 50 and 60 bpm. β-blockers should be used before other antihypertensives to avoid reflex tachycardia. Esmolol is preferred because of its short duration of action and easy titration. Labetalol has the advantage of having α- and β-blocking effects so affects HR and BP. Once β-blockade is in place, nitroprusside or nicardipine can be used to lower BP.

1.11.2.1. Dissection classifications

1.11.2.1.1. DeBakey classification

Type I: originates in ascending aorta, propagates at least to the aortic arch and often beyond it distally.

Type II: originates in and is confined to the ascending aorta.

Type III: originates in descending aorta, rarely extends proximally but will extend distally.

1.11.2.1.2. Stanford classifications

Type A: involving ascending aorta. Can also include the arch and descending aorta. Treatment is surgical.

Type B: involving the descending aorta only. Treatment is medical.

1.12. Vascular occlusion

1.12.1. Deep venous thrombosis

Risk factors: post-operative state, previous history of deep vein thrombosis (DVT)/PE in patient or patient's family, cancer, immobilization, paralysis, age <40, estrogen use, pregnancy.

Diagnostics: D-dimer is a blood test that measures circulating cross-linked fibrin. Very sensitive, but not specific. Doppler ultrasound is very sensitive and specific.

Management: anticoagulation with heparin or low molecular weight heparin (LMWH) employed until warfarin reaches therapeutic level. Inferior vena cava (IVC) filter may be used if anticoagulation is contraindicated.

1.12.2. Pulmonary embolism – see Chapter 2

1.12.3. Arterial thromboembolism

Definition: detached thrombus that travels distal from the origin.

Cause: thrombus forming from MI, mitral stenosis rheumatic heart disease, and A-fib; or *in situ* thrombosis.

Characteristics: 5 Ps of arterial occlusion: pain, pallor, pulselessness, paresthesias and paralysis. Physical exam may reveal pulselessness and a cool, white or cyanotic limb distal to embolus/occlusion.

Diagnostics: duplex ultrasound is often test of choice; noninvasive method of measuring arterial blood flow. Angiography is the definitive test but carries the risk of contrast- and catheter-related adverse events. Magnetic resonance angiography (MRA) is able to pick up minimal changes in tissues before major structural changes occur.

Management: heparin should be started in the emergency department. Limb-threatening ischemia may need direct thrombectomy with bypass grafting. Surgical consult is warranted.

Bibliography

Marx JA, Hockberger RS, Walls RM, *et al.* *Rosen's Emergency Medicine: Concepts and Clinical Practice*, 7th edn. Philadelphia: Mosby Elsevier, 2010.

Neumar RW, Otto CW, Link MS, *et al.* Part 8: Adult advanced cardiovascular life support. 2010 American Heart Association Guidelines for Cardiopulmonary Resuscitation and Emergency Cardiovascular Care. *Circulation* 2010; **122**: S729–67.

Nishimura RA, Carabello BA, Faxon DP, *et al.* ACC/AHA 2008 Guideline update on valvular heart disease: Focused update on infective endocarditis; a report of the American College of Cardiology/American Heart Association Task Force on practice guidelines endorsed by the Society of Cardiovascular Anesthesiologists, Society for Cardiovascular Angiography and Interventions, and Society of Thoracic Surgeons. *J Am Coll Cardiol.* 2008; **52**(8):676–85.

Sgarbossa EB, Pinski SL, Barbagelata AB, *et al.* Electrocardiographic diagnosis of evolving acute myocardial infarction in the presence of the left bundle-branch block. *NEJM.* 1996; **334**(8): 483–5.

Tintinalli JE, Stapczynski JS, Cline DM, *et al.* *Tintinalli's Emergency Medicine: A Comprehensive Study Guide*, 7th edn. New York: The McGraw-Hill Companies, Inc., 2011.

Chapter 2

Respiratory emergencies

John Hafner

2.1. Arterial blood gas (ABG) interpretation

ABG interpretation is critical to evaluation of potential acid–base disorders. The following analysis plan is based upon "a practical approach," by R. J. Haber [1].

Rule 1: look at the pH. Whichever side of 7.40 the pH is on, that is the primary abnormality.

> **pH $<$ 7.40:** acidosis.
> > If $\uparrow PCO_2$ = respiratory acidosis.
> > If $\downarrow HCO_3^-$ = metabolic acidosis.
> **pH $>$ 7.40:** alkalosis.
> > If $\downarrow PCO_2$ = respiratory alkalosis.
> > If $\uparrow HCO_3^-$ = metabolic alkalosis.

Rule 2: is there appropriate compensation for the primary disorder?

> **Metabolic acidosis:** $PCO_2 = [1.5 \times (\text{serum } HCO_3^-)] + 8 \ (\pm 2)$.
> **Metabolic alkalosis:** $\uparrow PCO_2 = 0.6 \times \uparrow HCO_3^- \ (\pm 2)$.
> **Respiratory acidosis:** for each $\uparrow PCO_2$ of 10, $\uparrow HCO_3^-$ by 1 (acute) or 4 (chronic).
> **Respiratory alkalosis:** for each $\downarrow PCO_2$ of 10, $\downarrow HCO_3^-$ by 2 (acute) or 5 (chronic).

Rule 3: calculate the anion gap ($AG = Na^+ - (HCO_3^- + Cl^-)$). If the AG is ≥ 12 mmol/L, there is a primary metabolic acidosis regardless of pH or serum bicarbonate concentration. The body does not generate an anion gap to compensate for a primary disorder.

Rule 4: if there is a metabolic acidosis, calculate the excess anion gap (ΔAG = The total AG – normal AG [12 mmol/L] + HCO_3^-).

> If ΔAG is >30 mmol/L there is an underlying metabolic alkalosis.
> If ΔAG is <23 mmol/L there is an underlying non-anion gap metabolic acidosis.

Pocket Guide to the American Board of Emergency Medicine In-Training Exam, ed. Bob Cambridge.
Published by Cambridge University Press. © Cambridge University Press 2013.

Table 2.1 Etiologies of ABG abnormalities

Acute respiratory acidosis	CNS depression, neuromuscular disorder, acute airway obstruction, impaired lung motion (hemothorax, pneumothorax), severe pneumonia or pulmonary edema, thoracic injury/flail chest
Chronic respiratory acidosis with metabolic compensation	Chronic lung disease (obstructive or restrictive), chronic neuromuscular disorders, central hypoventilation
Acute respiratory alkalosis	Anxiety, hypoxia, lung disease, CNS disease, drug usage (salicylates, catecholamines, progesterone), pregnancy, sepsis, hepatic encephalopathy, mechanical ventilation
Metabolic alkalosis with respiratory compensation (urine chloride level low)	Vomiting, nasogastric suction, post-hypercapnia, diuretic usage
Metabolic alkalosis with respiratory compensation (urine chloride level normal or high)	Excess mineralocorticoid activity (Cushing's syndrome, Conn's syndrome, exogenous corticosteroids, licorice ingestion, ingested resin states, Bartter's syndrome), current or recent diuretic usage, excess alkali administration, refeeding alkalosis
Metabolic acidosis with respiratory compensation (normal anion gap)	GI bicarbonate loss (diarrhea, ureteral diversions), renal bicarbonate loss (renal tubular acidosis, early renal failure carbonic anhydrase inhibitors, aldosterone inhibitors) hydrochloric acid administration, post-hypocapnia
Metabolic acidosis with respiratory compensation (elevated anion gap)	Ketoacidosis (diabetic, alcoholic), renal failure, lactic acidosis, rhabdomyolysis, toxins (methanol, ethylene glycol, paraldehyde, salicylates, isoniazide, iron ingestion)

CNS, central nervous system; GI, gastrointestinal. [1]

2.2. Hypoxia

Defined as insufficient delivery of oxygen to tissue. Hypoxemia is a state of low oxygen in the blood (arterial oxygen). Hypoxemia is determined by measuring the partial pressure of oxygen in the arterial blood (P_aO_2).

2.2.1. A-a gradient

Pathophysiology: the A-a gradient is a measure of the difference between the alveolar concentration of inspired alveolar oxygen (P_AO_2) and the ABG measured arterial concentration of oxygen (P_aO_2); A-a gradient = $P_AO_2 - P_aO_2$.

$P_AO_2 = (P_{atm} - P_{water}) F_iO_2 - P_aCO_2/0.8$.

P_{atm} = atmospheric pressure (760 mmHg at sea level).

P_{water} = water pressure (76 mmHg).

F_iO_2 = the fraction of oxygen in the inspired gas (21% on room air).

P_aCO_2 = partial pressure of arterial carbon dioxide (measured from ABG).

If at sea level and inspiring room air, this equation can be simplified to: P_AO_2 = 145 mmHg – P_aCO_2.

A normal A-a gradient is < (patient's age divided by 4) + 4.

2.2.2. Hemoglobin oxygen saturation curve [2]

The hemoglobin oxygen saturation is determined by the oxygen–hemoglobin dissociation curve.

Rightward shift of the curve: increases the partial pressure of oxygen at the tissue level and unloads oxygen to the tissue. Increases the partial pressure of oxygen in the tissues during conditions of increased need, such as during exercise, or hemorrhagic shock.

Leftward shift of the curve: decreases the partial pressure of oxygen at the tissue level and binds it more in the lung.

Table 2.2 Causes of left and right shifts in oxygen–hemoglobin dissociation curve

	Left shift (high affinity for oxygen)	Right shift (low affinity for oxygen)
Temperature	Decrease	Increase
2,3-DPG	Decrease	Increase
PCO_2	Decrease	Increase
PCO	Increase	Decrease
pH (Bohr effect)	Increase (alkalosis)	Decrease (acidosis)
Type of hemoglobin	Fetal hemoglobin	Adult hemoglobin

2.2.3. Clinical hypoxemia

Hypoxemia results from one or a combination of mechanisms.

Table 2.3 Causes of hypoxemia

Cause of hypoxia	Pathophysiology	Clinical example
Hypoventilation	Associated with an increased P_aCO_2 and a normal A-a gradient	Narcotic overdose, head injury, spinal cord injury
Right-to-left shunt	Blood enters the systemic circulation without being oxygenated in the lungs. This results in an increased A-a gradient. Arterial oxygen levels will not increase with supplemental oxygen	Pulmonary atelectasis, vascular malformations, congenital heart disease
Ventilation/perfusion mismatch	Regional alteration of ventilation and/or perfusion affecting gas exchange and resulting in hypoxemia. Associated with an increased A-a gradient and improved with supplemental oxygen	Pulmonary embolism, pneumonia, COPD
Diffusion impairment	A condition that disrupts diffusion across the alveolar–blood barrier resulting in hypoxemia	Pulmonary fibrosis
Low inspired oxygen	Decreased ambient oxygen pressure results in hypoxemia. The A-a oxygen gradient is normal and improves with supplemental oxygen. P_aCO_2 may be low due to hyperventilation	High altitudes

COPD, chronic obstructive pulmonary disease.

Presentation: mild hypoxia: headache, fatigue, shortness of breath. Severe hypoxia: tachypnea, respiratory distress, cyanosis, poor coordination, altered mental status, loss of consciousness, seizures, coma.

2.3. Disorders of pleural/mediastinal space

2.3.1. Pneumothorax [3]

Definition: free air in the thoracic cavity

Pathophysiology: caused either by a defect allowing communication between the intrapleural space and the airway, or by a defect allowing communication between the atmosphere and intrapleural space. Pneumothorax causes a collapse of the affected lung with a decrease in lung capacity. Shunting with ventilation/perfusion (V-Q) mismatch can lead to hypoxemia. Progressive intrapleural air accumulation leads to increasing intrathoracic pressure, further collapsing the lung and shifting the mediastinum toward the contralateral side. Increasing intrathoracic pressure impairs cardiac venous return, leading to cardiovascular collapse and death.

Table 2.4 Types of pneumothoraces

Primary spontaneous pneumothorax	Pneumothorax not caused by trauma or any obvious precipitating factor, occurring in persons without clinically apparent lung disease
Secondary spontaneous pneumothorax	Pneumothorax not caused by trauma or any obvious precipitating factor, occurring in persons as a complication of preexisting lung disease
Iatrogenic pneumothorax	Pneumothorax resulting from a complication of a diagnostic or therapeutic intervention
Traumatic pneumothorax	Pneumothorax caused by penetrating or blunt trauma to the chest, with air entering the pleural space directly through the chest wall; visceral pleural penetration; or alveolar rupture due to sudden compression of the chest
Open pneumothorax	Pneumothorax caused by penetrating or blunt trauma to the chest, with air entering the pleural space directly through the chest wall (sucking chest wound)
Tension pneumothorax	Life-threatening condition occurring when a pneumothorax progresses, and the increasing intrathoracic pressure shifts the mediastinum toward the contralateral side, impairing cardiac venous return, and leading to cardiovascular collapse and death
Hemo-pneumothorax	The combination of a hemothorax and a pneumothorax

Presentation: sudden onset of pleuritic chest pain, tachycardia and tachypnea, hyperresonant chest sounds, or asymmetric chest excursion. Tension pneumothorax presents with respiratory distress, jugular venous distension (JVD), tachycardia, hypoxia, hypotension, and tracheal deviation.

Diagnosis: tension pneumothorax is a clinical diagnosis and treatment should not be delayed for X-ray confirmation.

Chest X-ray: shows a thin white pleural line separating normal-appearing lung with lung markings from a dark radiolucent peripheral area. A lateral width of 1 cm corresponds to about a 10% pneumothorax. Lateral decubitus and expiratory views may improve visibility of small pneumothoraces.

CT: more sensitive than chest X-ray, and may be helpful in difficult cases, such as blebs or severe COPD patients.

Bedside ultrasound: can evaluate for the absence of a normal lung and pleural interface. Signs of normal lung and pleura signs are lung sliding and comet tails, and their absence makes the ultrasound diagnosis of pneumothorax.

Treatment:

Table 2.5 Treatment of pneumothorax

Small (<20%)	Moderate	Moderate/large	Tension
In small pneumothoraces, reabsorption occurs at 1–2% per day and increases to 4% with 100% oxygen. If patient is reliable and clinically stable, observe for 6 hours, reimage to ensure the pneumothorax is not increasing then discharge with follow-up in 24 hours	In young healthy patients with a first episode who are clinically stable, simple catheter aspiration can be tried. Small pig tail catheters can also be inserted with aspiration and observation. Re-evaluate (clinically and with chest X-ray) prior to discharge. Chest tube thoracostomy if reaccumulation of the pneumothorax	Tube thoracostomy. 7–14 French tube for a primary spontaneous pneumothorax. 20–28 French tube for a secondary spontaneous pneumothorax. >28 French tube for a concomitant effusion/hemothorax or plans of positive pressure ventilation. Connect to water seal. Suction does not improve the rate of resolution	Emergent needle decompression followed by tube thoracostomy

Patients should not fly or go scuba diving until resolution is complete. If pneumothoraces are recurrent, refer to surgeon for potential pleurodesis or resection of bullae.

2.3.2. Pneumomediastinum

Pneumomediastinum is defined as free air or gas contained within the mediastinum.

Cause: can occur spontaneously from asthma, exertion, Valsalva, seizure, inhaled drugs, intubation, endoscopy. When it occurs spontaneously it is often benign and is self-limiting. Can also be acquired from an esophageal rupture, trauma, or pulmonary barotrauma.

Presentation: Hamman's sign (a series of precordial crackles synchronous with the heartbeat), chest pain, dyspnea, neck pain, subcutaneous emphysema, dysphagia.

Complications: infection, pneumothorax.

Diagnosis: on X-ray, vertical radiolucent lines at the heart border can be seen. Subcutaneous emphysema can be seen as radiolucent streaks in the soft tissues. Associated trauma or other causative etiologies may be seen. When the chest X-ray is non-diagnostic, additional studies such as a barium swallow, CT scan, or endoscopy may be needed.

Treatment: supportive, treat the underlying or associated condition.

2.3.3. Mediastinitis

Mediastinitis is a life-threatening infection of the mediastinal space.

Cause: most often related to esophageal perforation, but can spread from any head or neck infection. Infection moves through potential spaces: carotid sheath, prevertebral space from the skull to T3, or anterior to the prevertebral fascia, which extends down into the posterior mediastinum.

Presentation: recent history of an upper respiratory infection. Patient may have fever, chills, pleuritic chest pain, sore throat, or neck swelling. Consider the diagnosis if a patient develops sepsis or cardiovascular symptoms after endotracheal intubation or nasogastric (NG) tube placement (esophageal perforation).

Diagnosis: neck X-ray may show a widening of the prevertebral or retropharyngeal soft tissues (normal is 6 mm at C2 and 22 mm at C6). Chest X-ray may show mediastinal widening, pneumomediastinum, mediastinal air–fluid levels, or a pneumothorax.

Treatment: broad spectrum antibiotics with anaerobic coverage. Consult thoracic surgery.

2.3.4. Pleurisy

Inflammation of the pleura from any of several causes (trauma, infectious disease, cancer, rheumatic disease).

Presentation: chest pain described as sharp, worse with inhalation or coughing.

Diagnosis: clinical. Chest X-ray will be normal unless there are signs of the concomitant cause.

Treatment: anti-inflammatories and incentive spirometry to encourage good pulmonary function.

2.3.5. Pleural effusion

An accumulation of fluid between the visceral and parietal pleural surfaces. A parapneumonic effusion is pleural fluid that results from pneumonia or lung abscess, and can be either uncomplicated (resolves with antibiotics) or complicated (requires drainage for resolution). An empyema is defined as purulence in the pleural space.

Presentation: pleural effusions can be asymptomatic or produce respiratory distress if large or there is underlying lung disease. Decreased breath sounds, dullness to percussion, and a pleural rub can occur.

Diagnosis: chest X-ray shows fluid in the fissures or causing a blunting of the costophrenic angles when patient is upright (150–250 mL of fluid required). Apical capping may be seen when the patient is supine. Lateral decubitus film may reveal accumulations as small as 5–15 mL of fluid. Ultrasound and CT scans of the chest are helpful when the chest X-ray is equivocal.

Table 2.6 Diagnosis based on thoracentesis fluid analysis

	Transudate	Exudate
Pathophysiology	Increase in hydrostatic pressure or decrease in oncotic pressure in the pulmonary vasculature	Defective lymphatic drainage or increased capillary permeability
Causes	>90% are due to CHF Also caused by pulmonary embolus (most common cause of pulmonary effusion in patients under 40 years old), superior vena cava syndrome, cirrhosis, and nephrotic syndrome	Parapneumonic process is most commonly caused by pneumonia or lung abscess Other exudative pleural effusion causes include connective tissue disorders, abdominal infections, and uremia

Table 2.6 (cont.)

	Transudate	Exudate
Light's criteria	Fluid does not meet any of the three criteria for exudate	Pleural fluid to serum protein level ratio is >0.5 Pleural fluid to serum LDH ratio is >0.6 Pleural fluid LDH is >2/3 of the upper limit of a normal serum LDH.
Additional fluid tests	The fluid is body plasma and further testing is not helpful	Gram stain Culture for bacteria and fungi Fluid pH (<7.3 is more consistent with parapneumonic process, TB, malignancy, or rheumatoid etiologies; <7.0 is suggestive of empyema or esophageal rupture) Cell count (normal is <1000/µL WBC) Hematocrit (if the hematocrit is >50% of the peripheral blood hematocrit, the effusion is a hemothorax) Amylase (high in pancreatic disease, esophageal rupture) Cytology

CHF, congestive heart failure; TB, tuberculosis

Treatment: based on the etiology of the pleural effusion/pleurisy and the patient's condition. Chest tube placement for a pleural effusion is performed when necessary to diagnose a rapidly progressing pleural effusion or to stabilize a patient with cardiovascular or respiratory compromise.

Transient hypoxia can occur after pleural effusion drainage resulting from V-Q mismatch. Unless large volumes are removed, re-expansion pulmonary edema is rare.

If bacterial infection is suspected (empyema), start a broad spectrum antibiotic (clindamycin and a third-generation cephalosporin) and drainage with a large bore chest tube.

2.4. Pulmonary embolism (PE)

The estimated average annual incidence in the United States is 1 episode per 1000 registered patients, and as many as 300 000 persons die from PE annually [4]. Often underdiagnosed in the emergency department.

Pathophysiology: PE occurs when a venous thrombus originating in the deep veins of the extremities and pelvis embolizes to the lung. PE severity ranges from small asymptomatic emboli to massive embolism causing immediate death. 79% of PEs originate from a lower extremity thrombus [4].

Risk stratification: useful to determine the patient's pretest probability of having a pulmonary embolism. Can be determined using clinical gestalt, factoring in known PE risk factors, or by utilizing risk stratification criteria (Wells criteria for PE, Pulmonary Embolism Rule-Out Criteria (PERC) rule).

Table 2.7 Risk factors for PE

Risk category (Virchow's triad)	Specific risk [4]
Hypercoagulability	Factor V Leiden disorder Protein C or protein S deficiency Antithrombin deficiency Active cancer Antiphospholipid antibody syndrome Oral contraceptives/hormone replacement therapy (estrogens) Chemotherapy Polycythemia vera Pregnancy
Venous stasis	Immobilization/cast Spinal cord injury Pregnancy Reduced mobility/advanced age Major surgery
Venous injury	Trauma Central venous catheters Major surgery

Table 2.8 Wells' criteria for PE and PERC rule

Wells' criteria for PE [5] Clinical feature	Points
Clinical symptoms of DVT	3
Other diagnosis less likely than PE	3
Heart rate greater than 100 bpm	1.5
Immobilization or surgery within past 4 weeks	1.5
Previous DVT or PE	1.5
Hemoptysis	1
Malignancy	1

- >6 points: high risk
- 2–6 points: moderate risk
- <2 points: low risk

PERC rule: must be able to answer yes to all 8 questions [6]

Age <50 years	
HR <100 bpm	
Oxygen saturation on room air >94%	
No prior history of DVT/PE	
No recent trauma or surgery	
No hemoptysis	
No exogenous estrogen	
No clinical signs suggesting DVT	

- PERC applies to low-risk patients only
- If PERC rule is negative, <2% chance of PE

DVT, deep vein thrombosis

Symptoms/exam: highly variable presentation. Can be asymptomatic to full arrest. Dyspnea is the most common symptom. Pleuritic chest pain is the second most common symptom. Hypoxemia and tachypnea are common; tachycardia is seen in half of patients. Rales, wheezing, hemoptysis, fever, and JVD can also be seen. Large emboli can cause acute right heart failure.

Diagnosis: clinical testing depends on pretest probability. No testing for patients who are low risk by Wells' criteria and PERC rule negative [6]. D-dimer for patients who are PERC rule positive but low risk by Wells' criteria. If D-dimer negative, 0.5% risk of PE [5]. CT scan of chest or VQ scan for patients who are intermediate or high risk by Wells' criteria, or who are D-dimer positive.

> **ECG:** most common ECG in patient with PE is a normal ECG. Most common abnormality is sinus tachycardia. Classically, large PE causes symmetric anterior T wave inversion, S1Q3T3 pattern, or a new right bundle branch block.

> **Chest X-ray:** useful to identify alternative diagnoses. Rare classical findings include Hampton's hump (wedge-shaped opacity in the periphery of the lung with its base toward the pleural surface) or Westermark sign (lack of pulmonary vascular markings).

> **VQ scanning:** very sensitive but not very specific and the specificity is further reduced by airspace disease.

> **CT scan:** very sensitive and more specific, and can find other causes for symptoms, but cannot be used in patients with elevated creatinine levels (IV contrast).

Treatment: anticoagulation with heparin or low molecular weight heparin until warfarin is therapeutic. If patient is having or likely to have hemodynamic compromise or collapse, thrombolytics are beneficial.

Predictors of impending cardiovascular collapse: hypotension, tachycardia greater than systolic blood pressure, elevated B-type natriuretic peptide (BNP) or troponin, hypoxia on room air, right ventricular failure on ECG.

2.5. Asthma

Common disease affecting adults and children. One in 12 people (about 25 million, or 8% of the US population) had asthma in 2009 [7]. Asthma has the highest prevalence amongst children (aged 5–17 years old), females, and African Americans [8].

Pathophysiology: defined as a chronic inflammatory disease of the large airways resulting in episodic reversible airway obstruction. The bronchial airways are hyperresponsive to triggers. During an episode vascular congestion, bronchial wall edema, and thick secretions occur.

> **Early response:** occurs within one hour – caused by the release of preformed histamine from mast cell granules inducing bronchial smooth muscle constriction and airway edema.

> **Late response:** occurs 4–6 hours – cytokine generation causing prolonged bronchospasm and obstruction.

> **Airway remodeling:** repetitive and chronic airway inflammation causes airway wall thickening and fibrosis.

> **Status asthmaticus:** an acute exacerbation of asthma that does not respond to standard treatment of bronchodilators and corticosteroids.

Table 2.9 Risk stratification and increased risk for death

Asthma severity	Intermittent	Mild persistent	Moderate persistent	Severe persistent
Symptoms	2 or less days per week	More than 2 days per week	Daily	Throughout the day
Nighttime awakenings	2 times per month or less	3–4 times per month	More than once per week but not nightly	Nightly
Rescue inhaler use	2 or less days per week	More than 2 days per week, but not daily	Daily	Several times per day
Interference with normal activity	None	Minor limitation	Some limitation	Extremely limited
Lung function	FEV1 >80% predicted and normal between exacerbations	FEV1 >80% predicted	FEV1 60–80% predicted	FEV1 less than 60% predicted
Increased risk for death		1. History of sudden severe exacerbation 2. Prior intubation 3. Prior ICU admission for asthma 4. 1 admission for asthma in the past year 5. >2 visits to the ED for asthma in the past year 6. Admission or ED visit for asthma in the past month 7. Use of >2 MDI canisters per month 8. Current use of systemic corticosteroids or recent withdrawal 9. Comorbidities 10. Illicit drug use		

ED, emergency department; ICU, intensive care unit; MDI, metered dose inhaler. [9].

Symptoms/exam: cough, wheezing, dyspnea, chest tightness. As airflow worsens wheezing may become silent. Hyperresonance to percussion (from air trapping), prolonged expiratory phase of respiration may be seen. Lethargy, exhaustion, or confusion is worrisome for impending respiratory failure. Cyanosis is uncommon and late stage, as the respiratory alkalosis causes a left shift of the oxygen–hemoglobin dissociation curve and makes unloading of oxygen easier.

Diagnosis: forced expiratory volume in one second (FEV1) or peak flow can be measured and changes in the peak flow can be used to measure improvement with therapy. Chest radiographs are usually not helpful unless ruling out complicating conditions (i.e. associated pneumonia, pneumothorax). A pulsus parodoxus, or fall in inspiratory blood pressure >10 mmHg correlates with severe disease.

Treatment:

Table 2.10 Treatment medications for asthma

Class	Medication	Considerations
Inhaled β-agonist	Albuterol (2.5–5 mg)	Mainstay of emergency department treatment. Nebulizer and MDIs with a spacer are similarly effective.
Inhaled anticholinergics	Ipratropium bromide (0.5 mg)	Blocks secretions and bronchoconstriction. Maximum effect at 30–120 minutes
Subcutaneous adrenergic agents	Epinephrine (0.01 mg/kg of 1:1000 solution SQ)	For critical patients who are unable to inhale a sufficient dose of medication
IV adrenergic agents	Epinephrine (2–10 mL of 1:10 000 solution)	For critical patients who are unable to inhale a sufficient dose of medication. Use cautiously if >40 years old and any suspected cardiovascular disease.
Corticosteroids	Prednisone (2 mg/kg PO), Solumedrol (2 mg/kg IV, maximum of 125 mg)	Give to anyone with moderate to severe attacks, an incomplete response to initial treatment, and to those who have relapsed for a recent exacerbation. Oral course should be given for 3–10 days.
Smooth muscle relaxants	Magnesium sulfate (2–4 g IV over 20 minutes)	Possibly useful in severe attacks and may prevent intubation
Gas mixtures	Heliox	Increases laminar flow allowing nebulized medications to get farther into the bronchial tree

Intubation should be done in impending or actual respiratory failure. All efforts to avoid intubation should be sought. Continue nebulized medications.

Propofol and ketamine offer bronchodilator effects for rapid sequence intubation (RSI).

Permissive hypercapnia is acceptable: slower respiratory rate and prolonged expiratory times still allow for oxygenation and ventilation but prevent breath stacking, barotrauma and hypotension from trapped intrathoracic pressure. Use high F_iO_2, tidal volume of 6–8 mL/kg, low respiratory rate, and high inspiratory flow rate.

2.6. Chronic obstructive pulmonary disease (COPD)

Chronic obstructive pulmonary disease (COPD) is a heterogeneous group of slowly progressive diseases characterized by airflow obstruction that interferes with normal breathing [10]. The airflow limitation is not fully reversible, and patients typically have dyspnea with exertion and a chronic cough.

Two major clinical COPD patterns exist (often mixed).

Table 2.11 COPD clinical patterns

Type	Characteristics	Pathology
Bronchitic	Prominent cough, crackles from uncleared secretions, carbon dioxide retention, hypoxia, cyanosis, cor pulmonale, chronic JVD	Chronic bronchial mucus production and chronic cough. Often referred to as a "blue bloater." Chronic bronchitis is defined clinically as cough with sputum expectoration for at least 3 months a year during a period of 2 consecutive years.
Emphysematous	Pursed lip breathing, hyperinflated lungs, impaired diaphragmatic motion and flattening on chest X-ray, hyperresonance, quiet end expiratory rhonchi	Destruction of the terminal bronchioles with chronic air trapping. Often referred to as a "pink puffer"

Presentation: cough (with or without sputum production), dyspnea, chest tightness, and wheezing/rhonchi. In severe COPD exacerbation the carbon dioxide produced by the increased work of breathing becomes greater than the amount being cleared by respiration and the carbon dioxide sharply rises. Respiratory acidosis, hypercapnea, confusion, stupor, apnea and death follow.

Diagnosis:

> **Pulse oximetry:** useful for following trends and evaluating for hypoxia.
>
> **ABG:** can be useful if there is a baseline P_aCO_2 to compare to. Can also be used to look for response to treatment.
>
> **Capnography:** can monitor rise and fall of carbon dioxide levels.
>
> **Chest X-ray:** used to look for other potential causes of patient's symptoms (pneumonia, pneumothorax, CHF) which may also be treatable and help alleviate the exacerbation.
>
> **Sputum culture:** only if certain agents are suspected (*Legionella*, TB, pneumocystis pneumonia [PCP], fungus). Difficult to get an adequate sample unless intubated.
>
> **ECG:** evaluate for dysrhythmias and myocardial infarction.
>
> **Lab tests:** BNP may be helpful to rule out CHF. Conversely, elevated levels can be seen in both CHF exacerbation and right heart strain from cor pulmonale.

Treatment: oxygen use in COPD is often controversial because COPD patients are frequently hypercarbic and thus become dependent on the hypoxic drive. Providing additional oxygen supplementation may remove the hypoxic drive causing apnea. However, hypoxia should be corrected to 90%.

Table 2.12 COPD treatment strategies

Strategy	Indications	Considerations
β-Adrenergic bronchodilators	First-line therapy, although bronchospasm is not the cause of exacerbation	SaO_2 may initially drop as a V-Q mismatch transiently occurs
Antibiotics	Consider in COPD exacerbation, especially if evidence of infection is present	Macrolides, third-generation cephalosporins, TMP-SMX, respiratory fluoroquinolone (levofloxacin, moxifloxacin, gatifloxacin)

Table 2.12 (cont.)

Strategy	Indications	Considerations
Anticholinergics	Useful bronchodilator adjunctive agents when given with β-adrenergic bronchodilators	Effects peak in 1–2 hours
Systemic corticosteroids	Useful in decreasing airway inflammation	Short course (3–10 days) of prednisone 40–60 mg
Noninvasive positive pressure ventilation	Assists ventilation in patients with moderate to severe respiratory muscle fatigue with hypercarbia and some degree of hypoxemia	Contraindicated by abnormal mental status, hemodynamic instability, aspiration risk, imminent respiratory arrest
Invasive mechanical ventilation	Use in patients who do not respond to treatment and are not candidates for noninvasive methods	General indications include hypoxia, hypercarbia, acidosis, altered mental status and apnea

TMP-SMX, trimethoprim-sulfamethoxazole.

2.7. Airway infections

2.7.1. Acute bronchitis

Cough is the most common symptom for which patients present to their primary care physicians, and acute bronchitis is the most common diagnosis in these patients [11].

Cause: infection of the bronchial mucous membranes. Most common cause is viruses. Infection leads to inflammation, exudate and bronchospasm.

Symptoms/exam: cough (either productive or non-productive) of less than one week in duration is the most common symptom for acute bronchitis. The color of the sputum is non-diagnostic. Evidence of other infection patterns (pneumonia, sinusitis) should be absent. No lung sound abnormalities, associated hypoxia or respiratory distress.

Diagnosis: chest X-ray and laboratory testing is unnecessary unless suspicious of other infectious patterns (i.e. pneumonia).

Treatment: mainly supportive. Antibiotics do not significantly change the course, and may provide only minimal benefit compared with the risk of antibiotic use itself [11]. Patients with COPD, with structural lung disease or chronic bronchitis, or the elderly may benefit from antibiotics. Cough suppressants, expectorants, and inhaler medications are not recommended for routine use in patients with bronchitis (do not alter the disease course).

2.7.2. Bronchiolitis

Most common lower respiratory infection in children. Children less than 2 years old are most commonly symptomatic because of airway sizes. The infection leads to inflammation; mucus production and sloughed debris leads to airway obstruction.

Cause: most common infectious agent is the respiratory syncytial virus (RSV). The second most common is the infectious agent parainfluenza virus. Other infectious causes include adenovirus, rhinovirus, influenza, and mycoplasma.

Symptoms/exam: 3–5 days of nasal congestion and cough followed by fussiness and febrile episodes. Respiratory distress with retractions and nasal flaring as the process progresses. Wheezing is commonly heard.

Diagnosis: for bronchiolitis the diagnosis can be made clinically and with serial exams. Chest X-ray is helpful only if the patient is deteriorating or if the disease course is prolonged. RSV swabs can provide a diagnosis, but do not alter treatment course.

Treatment: for bronchiolitis nasopharyngeal suctioning should be performed to keep the upper airway clear of mucus. With a wheezing patient, a single trial of nebulized β-agonist can be done. If improvement is noted, the treatment can be continued. Corticosteroids, nebulized hypertonic saline, and nebulized epinephrine are controversial, and antibiotics are unnecessary. Hospital admission for children with bronchiolitis who are tachypnic or having respiratory distress, are unable to feed, those that are oxygen dependent or those under 3 months old.

2.7.3. Pneumonia

Risk factors for developing pneumonia: immunosuppression, impaired mucus clearing, bacteremia, or foreign body (i.e. endotracheal tube, NG tube, feeding tube).

Pathophysiology: oropharyngeal secretions are often aspirated into the lower respiratory tract. Pathogens can also be inhaled directly or hematogenous spread from other sites. Pathogens can be bacterial, viral or fungal.

Symptoms/exam: classic physical findings: chest pain, productive cough, purulent sputum, fever, and shortness of breath. Can also note rales, decreased breath sounds, rhonchi, and wheezing. Atypical pneumonia begins with flu-like illness and non-productive cough. Often has an accompanying headache and GI symptoms. Tachycardia, tachypnea, and hypoxia are associated with severe pneumonia.

Diagnosis: features seen on chest X-ray cannot specify exactly what infectious agent is involved. In addition, absence of findings on chest X-ray does not rule out pneumonia. Treat the clinical picture. Blood cultures are not often positive and rarely affect management. However, consider obtaining in patients with severe disease. Thoracentesis is helpful for patients with a parapneumonic effusion, and diagnostic studies should include cell count, differential, Gram stain, and culture.

Table 2.13 Chest X-ray appearance patterns in pneumonia

CXR finding	Empiric treatment should cover:
Segmental infiltration with air bronchograms	Pyogenic bacteria
Lobar infiltrate	*Streptococcus pneumoniae, Klebsiella*
Dense lobar infiltrate	*Klebsiella*
Patchy infiltrate	Viruses, *Mycoplasma, Chlamydia*
Interstitial pattern	*Mycoplasma*
Miliary pattern	TB and fungus
Dependent infiltrate	Aerobes and anaerobes assuming aspiration
Peripheral consolidations	*Staphylococcus aureus* as it may be hematogenous spread, septic emboli
Apical infiltrate	TB

CXR, chest X-ray

Treatment: antibiotics are chosen based on suspected infectious agent and patient population.

Table 2.14 Treatment for pneumonia

Category	Organisms	Treatment
Community acquired, outpatient	*S. pneumoniae, Mycoplasma pneumoniae, Chlamydophilia pneumoniae, Haemophilus influenzae, Legionella,* viruses	If healthy and no antibiotics for 3 months: macrolide alone (azithromycin, clarithromycin, or erythromycin) or fluoroquinolone alone (levofloxacin, sparfloxacin, grepafloxacin, trovafloxacin, or other fluoroquinolone with enhanced activity against *S. pneumoniae*) or doxycycline alone. If comorbidities (COPD, diabetes, chronic heart, liver, lung, or renal disease, malignancy, alcoholism, asplenia, immunosuppressive condition or drugs) or antibiotic use <3 months: fluoroquinolone alone (levofloxacin, sparfloxacin, grepafloxacin, trovafloxacin, or other fluoroquinolone with enhanced activity against *S. pneumoniae*); or amoxicillin/clavulanate or second-generation cephalosporin + macrolide (azithromycin, clarithromycin, or erythromycin)
Community acquired, inpatient	As above	β-lactam (cefotaxime, ceftriaxone, or a β-lactam/β-lactamase inhibitor)+ macrolide (azithromycin, clarithromycin, erythromycin); or fluoroquinolone alone (levofloxacin, sparfloxacin, grepafloxacin, trovafloxacin, or other fluoroquinolone with enhanced activity against *S. pneumoniae*)
Community acquired, ICU	As above plus *Pseudomonas*	If *Pseudomonas* unlikely: β-lactam (cefotaxime, ceftriaxone, or a β-lactam/β-lactamase inhibitor) + macrolide (azithromycin, clarithromycin, or erythromycin) or a flouroquinolone (levofloxacin, sparfloxacin, grepafloxacin, trovafloxacin, or other fluoroquinolone with enhanced activity against *S. pneumoniae*). If *Pseudomonas* likely: Antipseudomonal, antipneumococcal β-lactam, cephalosporin or carbepenem (cefepem, ceftazidime, imipenem, meropenem, piperacillin-tazobactam) + macrolide (azithromycin, clarithromycin, or erythromycin) or fluoroquinolone (levofloxacin, sparfloxacin, grepafloxacin, trovafloxacin, or other fluoroquinolone with enhanced activity against *S. pneumoniae*) + an aminoglycoside. If MRSA is suspected: add vancomycin or linezolid
Aspiration	Anaerobes, Gram-negative bacteria	Fluoroquinolone (levofloxacin, sparfloxacin, grepafloxacin, trovafloxacin, or other fluoroquinolone with enhanced activity against *S pneumoniae*) with either clindamycin or metronidazole, or penicillin/β-lactamase inhibitor (Ampicillin/sulbactam, ticarcillin/clavulanate, or piperacillin/tazobactam)

Table 2.14 (cont.)

Category	Organisms	Treatment
Healthcare associated (Hospitalization for 2 days or more in the preceding 90 days, residence in a nursing home or extended care facility, home infusion therapy [including antibiotics], chronic dialysis within 30 days, home wound care, family member with multidrug-resistant pathogen)	*S. pneumoniae, H. influenzae*, MSSA, Antibiotic-sensitive enteric Gram-negative bacilli (*E coli, Klebsiella pneumoniae, Enterobacter* species, *Proteus* species, *Serratia marcescens*), *Pseudomonas aeruginosa, Acinetobacter* species, *Legionella pneumophila*, MRSA	Antipseudomonal, antipneumococcal β-lactam, cephalosporin or carbepenem (cefepem, ceftazidime, imipenem, meropenem, piperacillin-tazobactam) + fluoroquinolone (levofloxacin, sparfloxacin, grepafloxacin, trovafloxacin, or other fluoroquinolone with enhanced activity against *S. pneumoniae*) or an aminoglycoside. If MRSA is suspected, add vancomycin or linezolid

MRSA, methicillin-resistant *Staphylococcus aureus*; MSSA, methicillin-sensitive *Staphylococcus aureus*.

2.7.3.1. Fungal pneumonia

Histoplasma: commonly in Ohio and Mississippi River valleys.
Coccidioides: commonly in southwest USA.
Blastomyces: commonly in Midwest.
Pneumocystis jiroveci: seen in immunocompromised patients.

2.7.3.2. Viral pneumonia

Frequently begins as upper respiratory infection. Cough is likely to be non-productive.
Signs: mild scattered rhonchi and chest X-ray consolidation is rare.
Common cause:
> **Infants, children:** RSV, parainfluenza, influenza.
> **Adults:** influenza.
> **Immunosuppressed:** cytomegalovirus (CMV).

2.7.4. Pulmonary tuberculosis

Pathophysiology: *M. tuberculosis* is an obligate intracellular, acid-fast, aerobic bacillus that grows slowly in the terminal airspaces of the lung [12]. Prefers upper lung infection, due to the presence of high oxygen; superior segments of lung most commonly involved, may progress to multiple lobe involvement. Activation can occur upon exposure or years later after bacteria have lain dormant.

Risk factors for infection: occupational exposure, living in endemic areas, homelessness, incarceration, immunosuppression, alcohol or drug abuse.

Clinical presentation: initially asymptomatic (in healthy patients), mild fever and malaise can occur during initial immune response. As disease progresses, constitutional symptoms occur, night sweats, headache, fatigue, weight loss. Variably productive cough is the most common symptom. Hemoptysis indicates severe lung damage (erosion into a blood vessel). Extrapulmonary TB symptoms can occur: pain in joints, GI symptoms, meningitis, bone pain.

Complications: pneumothorax, empyema, superinfection (e.g. *Aspergillus* forming a fungal ball in the cavitary lesion), hemoptysis, pericarditis.

Diagnosis: chest film has a high negative predictive value in immunocompetent patients. Serial exams are needed to distinguish active from latent infection. Sputum studies are diagnostic (if collected correctly): acid-fast bacilli are seen on direct microscopy of stained specimen. Culture confirms diagnosis but takes 1–2 weeks for results. Bronchoscopy or bronchioalveolar lavage may be needed for adequate sampling.

Chest X-ray patterns

> **Primary TB:** most often seen as an infiltrate in the middle or lower lung regions and can mimic community acquired pneumonia. Hilar and mediastinal lymphadenopathy may also be present.
>
> **Reactivation TB:** classically seen in the upper lung segments; cavitation may be present.
>
> **Miliary (disseminated) TB:** multiple small nodules.

Tuberculin skin testing: negative in up to 20% of patients with active disease.

Table 2.15 Interpreting the tuberculin skin test

Test is positive if induration	Patient groups
>5 mm	HIV patients, patients with close contact with confirmed case
>10 mm	Healthcare workers, other patients with risk factors, patients less than 4 years old
>15 mm	Everyone else

Treatment [13]:

> **First-line 6 month treatment regimen:** new patients with pulmonary tuberculosis should receive a regimen containing 6 months of treatment – 2 months of isoniazid + rifampicin + pyrazinamide + ethambutol; 4 months of isoniazid + rifampicin.
>
> **Alternative first-line continuation phase:** in populations with known or suspected high levels of isoniazid resistance – 2 months of isoniazid + rifampicin + pyrazinamide + ethambutol; 4 months of isoniazid + rifampicin + ethambutol.

Emergent presentation: massive hemoptysis. Intubate with large bore endotracheal tube. Place the patient with the affected lung dependent, or intubate the mainstem of the unaffected lung. Emergent pulmonary consult.

2.8. Irritants and asphyxiants

2.8.1. Occupational exposures

2.8.1.1. Pneumoconiosis

Progressive pulmonary fibrosis secondary to chronic dust inhalation. Many types depending on agent inhaled.

2.8.1.2. Silicosis

Seen in those working in sandblasting, mining, foundries, manufacture of abrasive soaps, metal grinding, and any industry with potential for aerosolized silica particles.

2.8.1.3. Asbestosis

Leads to lung cancer (specifically mesothelioma, which is frequently seen as pleural thickening on chest X-ray).

2.8.1.4. Farmer's lung

IgG-mediated vasculitis preceded by a transient IgE-mediated bronchoconstrictive wheezing.

2.8.2. Asphyxiants

Any gas can be an asphyxiant if it is present in enough quantity to displace oxygen.

F_iO_2 **of 15%:** tachycardia, tachypnea, dyspnea, ataxia, dizziness, confusion.

F_iO_2 **of 10%:** lethargy and cerebral edema.

F_iO_2 **<6%:** incompatible with life.

Treatment: majority are occupational exposures. Removing the patient from the exposure usually leads to improvement of symptoms unless sequelae of ischemia are present. Supplemental oxygen or hyperbarics if available.

2.8.3. Airway irritants

Irritants dissolve on contact with respiratory mucosa, leading to inflammation. The degree of water solubility determines the effects.

Table 2.16 Solubility of irritants

Solubility	Affects	Examples	Treatment
High	Eyes and upper airway	Ammonia, capsaicin (pepper spray). Ammonia forms ammonium hydroxide, which can cause bronchospasm and pulmonary edema	Decontaminate eyes with irrigation. Supportive treatment
Intermediate	Upper or lower airway	Chlorine, nitrogen oxide. Chlorine is a green-yellow gas and forms acids on contact, nitrogen oxide forms nitric acid in alveoli. Pulmonary edema can occur up to 72 hours later	Corticosteroids may prevent bronchiolitis obliterans. Observe for several hours prior to discharge
Low	Distal airways. Lack of odor usually leads to greater duration of exposure	Phosgene (smells like newly mown hay). Forms HCl in alveoli leading to diffuse capillary leak and pulmonary edema	Supportive care. Supplemental oxygen and inhaled bronchodilators. Consider admission as delayed sequelae are common

2.8.3.1. Smoke inhalation

The heat capacity of air increases with steam or soot. Thermal injuries are more likely.

Symptoms: cough, bronchospasm, stridor. Singed nasal hairs, soot in the sputum is highly suggestive of exposure.

Diagnosis: co-oximetry is more reliable than ABG and pulse oximetry to detect an associated carbon monoxide intoxication. A lactate concentration greater than 10 mmol/L with acidosis suggests cyanide toxicity.

Treatment: intubate early prior to respiratory decompensation. Corticosteroids are not indicated and may be harmful. Bronchodilators have no demonstrated benefit. Treat carbon monoxide and cyanide toxicity if present.

2.8.3.2. Organophosphates/nerve agents

Acetylcholinesterase inhibitor exposure leads to the cholinergic syndrome.

Symptoms: SLUDGE BAM syndrome (Salivation, Lacrimation, Urination, Diarrhea, GI upset, Emesis, Bronchorrhea/Bradycardia, Abdominal cramping, Miosis/Muscle fasiculations) (alternative mnemonic: "DUMBELS," Diarrhea, Urination, Miosis, Muscle weakness, Bradycardia, Bronchospasm, Emesis, Lacrimation, Salivation) as well as seizures, coma, respiratory depression, and apnea.

Treatment: decontaminate the patient first as these agents are absorbed by all routes and are high risk to providers, then oxygenate. Atropine will reverse the muscarinic effects and should be given until the secretions are dried (the quantity required can occasionally deplete a small pharmacy). Pralidoxime (2-PAM) will reverse weakness and other neuromuscular findings (nicotinic effects) and prevent "aging" (irreversible binding to occur between organophosphates and acetylcholinesterase).

2.9. Airway obstruction

Presentation varies based on location of obstruction.

Table 2.17 Airway obstruction

Location	Sound	Congenital causes	Acquired causes
Nasopharynx	Expiratory stridor, sonorous, gurgling, muffled "hot potato" voice	Micrognathia, Treacher-Collins, Pierre-Robin, choanal atresia	Retropharyngeal abscess, adenopathy, tonsillar hypertrophy, foreign body
Supraglottic	Inspiratory stridor, high-pitched, hoarse voice	Thyroglossal cyst, lingual thyroid	Croup, epiglottitis, foreign body
Glottic	Biphasic stridor	Laryngomalacia, laryngeal web	Vocal cord paralysis, papillomas, foreign body
Subglottic	Expiratory stridor, high-pitched	Subglottic stenosis, tracheomalacia, vascular ring	Bacterial tracheitis, croup, subglottic stenosis, foreign body

Foreign bodies can cause obstruction at any level. In adults airway obstruction occurs most commonly at the vocal cords. In children it occurs most commonly at the cricoid cartilage. Trauma or burns can also cause obstruction through direct injury or edema at any level.

Diagnosis: the fastest study is a PA and lateral chest X-ray. Also consider bedside fiberoptic nasopharyngoscopy, rigid or flexible bronchoscopy, CT, MRI, or esophagram for further evaluation.

Treatment: based on the location and type of obstruction.

2.10. Pulmonary tumors

Lung cancer is the leading cause of cancer-related mortality in the United States [14]. Lung cancer is divided into two categories: small cell lung cancer (SCLC) and non-small cell lung cancer (NSCLC). NSCLC accounts for 85% of the lung cancer cases in the United States. Radiographic abnormalities may appear prior to onset of symptoms. Often found incidentally. Symptoms indicate late disease.

Complications of tumors:

> **Local effects:** pericardial effusion with tamponade, spinal cord compression, pathologic fractures, airway obstruction, erosion into a blood vessel and hemoptysis.
>
> **Metabolic effects:** syndrome of inappropriate antidiuretic hormone secretion (SIADH), hypercalcemia.
>
> **Hematologic effects:** hypercoagulability leading to DVT/PE.
>
> **Treatment effects:** tumor lysis syndrome.
>
> **Local symptoms:** new cough, change in chronic cough, hemoptysis, postobstructive pneumonia, cavitation, lung abscess.
>
> **Invasive symptoms:** chest pain, pericardial tamponade, superior vena cava syndrome, Horner's syndrome, Pancoast syndrome (Horner's plus brachial plexus involvement).
>
> **Metastases:** brain, bone, liver are common sites. Supraclavicular and cervical lymphadenopathy often seen.
>
> **Paraneoplastic syndromes:** weight loss, fever, anorexia, anemia from marrow replacement, endocrine abnormalities (hypokalemia, hypercalcemia, hyponatremia).
>
> **Lambert–Eaton syndrome:** disease of neuromuscular junctions with proximal muscle weakness. 70% have malignancy, usually small cell cancer.

References

1. Haber RJ. A practical approach to acid-base disorders. *West J Med.* 1991; **155**: 146–51.
2. Morgan TJ. The oxyhaemoglobin dissociation curve in critical illness. *Crit Care Resusc.* 1999; **1**: 93–100.
3. Sahn SA, Heffner JE. Spontaneous pneumothorax. *NEJM.* 2000; **342**(12): 868–74.
4. Tapson VF. Acute pulmonary embolism. *NEJM.* 2008; **358**: 1037–52.
5. Wells PS, Anderson DR, Rodger M, *et al.* Excluding pulmonary embolism at the bedside without diagnostic imaging: management of patients with suspected pulmonary embolism presenting to the emergency department by using a simple clinical model and D-dimer. *Ann Intern Med.* 2001; **135**: 98–107.
6. Kline JA, Mitchell AM, Kabrhel C, *et al.* Clinical criteria to prevent unnecessary diagnostic testing in emergency department patients with suspected pulmonary embolism. *J Thromb Haemost.* 2004; **2**(8): 1247–55.
7. Center for Disease Control. Vital signs: asthma in the US, growing every year [Internet]. 2011 [Cited 2012 May 12]. Available from: http://www.cdc.gov/VitalSigns/Asthma/index.html.
8. American Lung Association Epidemiology and Statistics Unit Research and Program Services. Trends in asthma morbidity and mortality [Internet]. 2012 [Cited 2012 May 12]. Available from: http://www.lung.org/finding-cures/our-research/trend-reports/asthma-trend-report.pdf.

9. National Heart, Lung, and Blood Institute. Expert panel report 3 (EPR3): guidelines for the diagnosis and management of asthma [Internet]. 2007 [Updated Aug 2008; cited 2012 May 12]. Available from: http://asthma.about.com/gi/o.htm?zi=1/ XJ&zTi=1&sdn=asthma&cdn=health&tm= 575&gps=485_13_1790_888&f=00&su=p284. 13.342.ip_&tt=2&bt=0&bts=0&zu=http% 3A//www.nhlbi.nih.gov/guidelines/asthma/ asthgdln.htm.

10. CDC. Deaths from chronic obstructive pulmonary disease; United States, 2000 – 2005. *MMWR*. 2008; **57**(45): 1229–32.

11. Albert RH. Diagnosis and management of acute bronchitis. *Am Fam Physician*. 2010; **82**(11): 1345–50.

12. Lawn SD, Zumla AI. Tuberculosis. *Lancet*. 2011; **378**(9785): 57–72.

13. World Health Organization. Treatment of tuberculosis: guidelines (4th edn.) [Internet]. Geneva: 2010. [Cited 2012 June 5]. Available from: http://whqlibdoc.who.int/ publications/2010/9789241547833_eng.pdf.

14. Molina JR, Yang P, Cassivi SD, *et al.* Non-small cell lung cancer: epidemiology, risk factors, treatment, and survivorship. *Mayo Clin Proc*. 2008; **83**(5): 584–94.

Bibliography

American Thoracic Society. Guidelines for the management of adults with hospital-acquired, ventilator-associated, and healthcare-associated pneumonia. *Am J Respir Crit Care Med*. 2005; **171**: 388–416.

Aujesky D, Auble TE, Yealy DM, *et al.* Prospective comparison of three validated prediction rules for prognosis in community-acquired pneumonia. *Am J Med*. 2005; **118**: 384–92.

Center for Disease Control and Prevention: Division of Tuberculosis Elimination. Tuberculosis (TB) [Internet]. 2012 [Cited 2012 June 5]. Available from: http:// www.cdc.gov/tb/statistics/default.htm.

Fine MJ, Auble TE, Yealy DM, *et al.* A prediction rule to identify low-risk patients with community-acquired pneumonia. *NEJM*. 1997; **336**(4): 243–50.

Lim WS, van der Eerden MM, Laing R, *et al.* Defining community acquired pneumonia

severity on presentation to hospital: an international derivation and validation study. *Thorax*. 2003; **58**(5): 377–82.

Mandell LA, Wunderink RG, Anzueto A. Infectious Diseases Society of America/ American Thoracic Society consensus guidelines on the management of community-acquired pneumonia in adults. *CID*. 2007; **44**: S27–72.

National Center for Health Statistics. Deaths: Final Data for 2006. *Natl Vital Stat Rep*. 2009; **57**(14): 1–134.

Sethi S, Murphy TF. Infection in the pathogenesis and course of chronic obstructive pulmonary disease. *NEJM*. 2008; **359**(22): 2355–65.

Sokolove PE, Rossman L, Cohen SH. The emergency department presentation of patients with active pulmonary tuberculosis. *Acad Emerg Med*. 2000; **7**: 1056–60.

Chapter 3

Gastroenterologic emergencies

Gregory J. Tudor and Alex Koyfman

3.1. Abdominal wall pathology

3.1.1. Hernias

Definition: Protrusion of viscus from its usual cavity. As hernia progresses it can become incarcerated (irreducible with edema formation, but blood supply is still intact), or strangulated (incarcerated with compromise of blood supply and infarction).

Table 3.1 Comparison of hernia types and locations

Type	Location	Considerations
Direct inguinal	Through the floor of Hesselbach's triangle	Rarely incarcerates
Indirect inguinal	Through the internal inguinal ring	Most common type of hernia in men and women. Often incarcerates
Femoral	Into the femoral canal below the inguinal ligament	More common in women. Often incarcerates
Obturator	Through obturator foramen into medial thigh	Usually occurs in elderly women
Ventral	Through the abdominal wall, often at the site of a previous surgery	Rarely incarcerates
Umbilical	At umbilicus, where fetal vessels perforated abdominal wall	Seen commonly in infants, usually closes by 3 years of age. Rarely incarcerates
Spigelian	Lateral to rectus muscle	Very rare

Management: manual reduction and surgical referral; emergent surgical consultation if incarceration or strangulation is suspected.

3.2. Peritoneum

3.2.1. Spontaneous bacterial peritonitis

Table 3.2 Spontaneous bacterial peritonitis

Signs	Diagnosis	Treatment
Fever, ascites, abdominal pain, increased liver function tests	Paracentesis and culture. WBC count >500/μL with >250/μL neutrophils is suggestive. Culture is definitive	Treat with broad spectrum antibiotics. Cover the most common species (*Escherichia coli, Streptococcus*)

Pocket Guide to the American Board of Emergency Medicine In-Training Exam, ed. Bob Cambridge.
Published by Cambridge University Press. © Cambridge University Press 2013.

3.3. Esophageal disorders

3.3.1. *Candida* esophagitis

Seen in immunocompromised patients (diabetes mellitus [DM], corticosteroid use, HIV/AIDS); most common cause of esophagitis in HIV patients.

Presentation: impressive odynophagia/dysphagia.

Management: fluconazole x10 days. If no improvement refer to gastrointestinal (GI) for upper endoscopy to rule out herpes simplex virus (HSV) or cytomegalovirus (CMV).

3.3.2. Gastroesophageal reflux disorder (GERD)/esophagitis

Reflux of stomach juices through the gastroesophageal junction into the esophagus.

Presentation: chest pain; retrosternal burning (epigastric area to throat), worse with lying down, cough, wheezing, hoarseness.

Complications: bleeding; perforation; stricture; increases risk of developing Barrett's esophagitis.

Management: lifestyle adjustment. Antacid with H2 blocker or proton pump inhibitor. Refer to GI.

3.3.3. Caustic toxic effects

Results from ingestion. Alkali worse than acid. Effects depend on volume, concentration, and exposure time. Oral findings are not predictive of esophageal injury.

Alkali: liquefactive necrosis, damage can be ongoing.

Acid: coagulation necrosis by denaturing proteins, eschar stops further damage.

Complications: perforation; stricture; airway involvement.

Management: consult GI for upper endoscopy. ABCs as necessary. Avoid charcoal, lavage, or nasogastric (NG) tube placement.

3.3.4. Motor abnormalities

3.3.4.1. Achalasia

Most common cause of motor dysphagia (liquids and solids). Lower 2/3 esophagus without peristalsis, and hypertensive lower esophageal sphincter.

Presentation: chest pain, dysphagia.

Treatment: target is to improve lower esophageal pressure. Calcium channel blockers (CCBs) or nitrates can be used in the emergency department. Definitive treatment is dilation by GI.

3.3.4.2. Esophageal spasm

Presentation: chest pain mimicking angina. Triggered by (cold) food.
Treatment: nitrates/CCBs.

3.3.5. Induced esophageal trauma

3.3.5.1. Mallory–Weiss syndrome

Partial-thickness tear at the gastroesophageal junction, often from recurrent vomiting.

Presentation: mild to significant hematemesis.
Diagnosis: endoscopic visualization.
Treatment: supportive care (typically resolves spontaneously); vasopressin for refractory
bleeding.

3.3.5.2. Boerhaave's syndrome

Full-thickness perforation, typically left-sided, mid-thoracic. Has a high mortality rate.

Most common cause: iatrogenic from upper endoscopy procedure. Also can occur after
vigorous vomiting.
Presentation: chest or abdominal pain radiating to neck.
Diagnosis: chest X-ray (look for pneumomediastinum, pneumothorax, or left pleural
effusion); gastrografin swallow study; CT chest.
Management: IV fluids, broad spectrum antibiotics for infectious pneumonitis, emergent
surgery for drainage of chemical pneumonitis and repair of esophageal injury.

3.3.6. Esophageal diverticula

Definition: outpouching of esophageal lumen through wall of esophagus. If it goes through
all layers it is a true diverticulum; if only a single layer is involved then it is a
pseudodiverticulum. Zenker's diverticulum is occurrence at esophago-pharyngeal
junction.
Presentation: may present with chest pain, may complain of regurgitation of undigested
food, may lead to perforation. Halitosis and/or neck mass may be presenting features.
Treatment: refer to GI; emergent surgical consultation for perforation.

3.3.7. Esophageal foreign body

Most common areas of obstruction: at the level of the cricopharyngeal muscle (C6) commonly in children, at the level of the aortic arch (T4), at the gastroesophageal junction (T11)
commonly in adults. Once in the stomach, the object usually passes.

Table 3.3 Ingested foreign bodies

Impacted object	Considerations	Treatment
Meat	More common in elderly, usually in distal esophagus	Glucagon (1– 2 mg IV) may relax the lower esophageal sphincter. Refractory cases need endoscopy
Coins	Orient in the frontal plane on chest film	Coins lodged in upper esophagus should be endoscopically removed. Coins in lower esophagus can be watched for 12–24 hours, then removed if they do not pass into the stomach
Large objects	Objects larger than 2 x 5 cm are unlikely to pass through the stomach in children and should be removed	Endoscopic removal
Button battery	True emergency if impacted in esophagus. Burns occur within 4 hours, perforation can occur within 6 hours	Emergent endoscopic removal should be done if battery is impacted in esophagus. If it is in the stomach, it can be watched for 48 hours to see if it passes

3.3.8. Esophageal hernia

Two types, paraesophageal and sliding.

Presentation: symptoms similar to GERD; hemorrhage, incarceration, obstruction, and strangulation are complications.

Diagnosis: endoscopy or barium swallow.

3.3.9. Strictures and stenosis

Results from scarring from GERD or other chronic inflammation. Most commonly occur at the distal esophagus and may interfere with lower sphincter function. May actually decrease reflux symptoms (barrier) as dysphagia increases.

Presentation: food bolus impaction and/or progressive dysphagia.

Treatment: dilation.

3.3.10. Tracheoesophageal fistula (TEF)

Five types, esophageal atresia with distal TEF is most common (88%); highly associated with other malformations. May be missed during antenatal examination.

Presentation: intolerance of feedings, coughing with feeding. NG tube coils in esophagus.

Treatment: manage with head-up position, IV fluids, NG tube in pouch to lower suction, referral to pediatric surgery.

3.3.11. Varices

Dilated venous vessels found in patients with portal hypertension.

Presentation: hematemesis, may be large volume.

Treatment: initially is supportive (IV fluids, transfusions) and IV antibiotic prophylaxis decrease mortality. Consider octreotide (50 mcg IV bolus, then 50 mcg/hr for up to 5 days). Vasopressin can be used (second-line), but because it causes non-selective vasoconstriction, also give nitro to prevent coronary ischemia. Endoscopy is treatment of choice for active variceal bleeding. A Sengsten–Blakemore tube can temporarily contain variceal bleeding until endoscopy can be performed. In refractory cases an emergent transjugular intrahepatic portosystemic shunt (TIPS) can be considered.

3.3.12. Esophageal tumors

Esophageal cancer is 95% squamous cell, with Barrett's esophagus predisposing to adenocarcinoma.

Epidemiology: age greater than 40, men 3:1 over women, and poor survivability (high rate of metastasis).

Presentation: progressive dysphagia.

3.4. Stomach

3.4.1. GI bleeds

3.4.1.1. Upper GI bleed

Features: hematemesis or NG tube with coffee grounds/blood. BUN/creatinine ratio > 30 (sensitivity 70%, specificity 95%).

3.4.1.2. Lower GI bleed

Features: hematochezia or bright red blood per rectum (no guarantee of lower GI bleed as massive upper GI bleed can have hematochezia as well). Diverticulosis is most common cause of painless lower GI bleed in people over 60.

Treatment of GI bleeds: aimed at cause. Until cause determined, start omeprazole 80 mg IV bolus followed by drip at 8 mg/hr. IV fluids, type and cross for blood transfusion if patient is symptomatic or if hemoglobin (HGB) below 8 g/dL. Note that HGB/hematocrit may be normal during acute bleed and can take up to 6–12 hours to equilibrate.

3.4.2. Ulcers

Predisposing factors: NSAID use, aspirin, tobacco, caffeine, *Helicobacter pylori* infection.
Presentation: stomach ulcers cause epigastric burning shortly after eating. Duodenal ulcers cause epigastric burning a few hours after eating.
Complications: scarring from chronic ulceration can cause pyloric obstruction. Perforation is rare but possible. Hemorrhage also uncommon.
Treatment: antacids, H2 blockers and/or proton pump inhibitors, mucosal surface protectants. For patients with bleeding ulcers give IV proton pump inhibitors. If patient has *H. pylori* initiate antibiotic therapy (omeprazole/amoxicillin/clarithromycin or bismuth/metronidazole/tetracycline or lansoprazole/amoxicillin/clarithromycin).

3.4.2.1. *Helicobacter pylori*

H. pylori is a Gram-negative rod. 70% of peptic ulcer disease and gastric ulcers have associated infection.
Location: 80% in duodenum, 20% in stomach. Occurs from inability of the mucosa to resist the peptic acid in a focal area.

3.4.2.2. *Perforated peptic ulcer*

Surgical emergency. Epigastric pain becomes generalized, free air on UPRIGHT (or LATERAL) film, may give shoulder pain (referred from diaphragm irritation). Often sudden in onset.

3.4.3. Gastritis

Inflammation of stomach lining.
Causes: *H. pylori*, drugs including aspirin, NSAIDs, potassium and iron, corrosives, hypoperfusion states, viral infections.
Presentation: epigastric abdominal pain, nausea and vomiting.
Treatment: antiemetic medication, supportive care. Decreasing acid production (H2 blockers, proton pump inhibitor) and antibiotics are needed if *H. pylori* is suspected.

3.4.4. Congenital hypertrophic pyloric stenosis

Usually first noticed around the third to sixth week of life. Classically affected children are the firstborn male, white, with a family history of the condition.

Physiology: narrowing of pyloric canal secondary to pylorus muscle hypertrophy and hyperplasia.

Presentation: occasional vomiting after meals progressing to vomiting after every meal. Vomit is projectile and non-bilious; child is usually hungry after vomiting.

Diagnosis: "palpable olive" in right upper quadrant (RUQ) with peristaltic waves after feeding. Labs show hypochloremic, hypokalemic metabolic alkalosis progressing to acidosis (if dehydrated). Ultrasound is test of choice, looking for thickened and elongated pyloric canal. Upper GI series shows "string sign" as contrast passes through pylorus.

Management: IV fluids, electrolyte correction. Surgery is needed (pyloromyotomy).

3.4.5. Gastric foreign body

Gastric foreign bodies are generally asymptomatic. Sharp points may lodge or perforate. Large objects that are too large to pass (2.5 cm round objects or objects longer than 5 cm) need to be endoscopically removed. Over 75% of gastric foreign bodies pass spontaneously.

Treatment: if object has the potential to pass naturally, serial X-ray to confirm passage out of the stomach can be done. If signs of obstruction occur or if the object does not show progress, consult GI.

3.5. Liver and gallbladder disorders

3.5.1. Cirrhosis

Irreversible scarring of the liver.

3.5.1.1. Alcoholic

10–20% of chronic alcoholics will develop; relate to amount, duration, nutrition, and hereditary factors.

3.5.1.2. Biliary obstructive.

Much rarer, resulting from chronic extrahepatic biliary obstruction.

3.5.1.3. Drug-induced

Usually from hepatitis; non-homogeneous with regions of fibrosis of liver and loss of hepatocyte function interspersed with normal hepatic tissue. Increase incidence with increasing age (except aspirin and valproic acid). Mechanism is usually either direct hepatocellular necrosis (from anesthetics [e.g. halothane], antimicrobial agents [e.g. ketoconazole]), or cholestatic agents (e.g. haloperidol, chlorpromazine, steroids, and erythromycin). Much overlap in mechanism, many drugs are dose dependent (acetaminophen).

Presentation: jaundice, spider angiomata, gynecomastia, ascites, edema, testicular atrophy, hepatic encephalopathy. Encephalopathy caused by accumulation of toxins in the blood. Acute worsening can be precipitated by infection, sedative medications, hypoxia, hypoglycemia. Acute accumulation of ascites has the same precipitants as encephalopathy.

Treatment: supportive. Oral lactulose and neomycin can help.

3.5.2. Hepatorenal failure

Usually a complication of cirrhosis, often begins with spontaneous bacterial peritonitis.

Defined as acute renal failure in patients with histologically normal kidneys in someone with acute or chronic hepatic failure. There are 2 types. Type 1 is more serious, progressive oliguria and doubling of creatinine over 2 weeks. Type 2 has gradual impairment in renal function that may or may not improve.

Type 1 survival median time is one month.

3.5.3. Hepatitis

Table 3.4 Types of viral hepatitis

	Cause	Spread	Incubation	Course	Diagnosis	Treatment
Hep A	RNA virus	Fecal–oral, person to person, ingestion of contaminated water	15–50 days	Mild course, fulminant hepatic failure is rare	If within 2 weeks of exposure, immune globulin prophylaxis is available	Primarily supportive. Hospitalize for signs of encephalopathy, INR >3, bilirubin >20
Hep B	DNA virus	Percutaneous or sexual exposure	> months	Mild or fulminant. 5–10% will develop chronic hepatitis	HBsAg = active/infective HBsAb = immunity HBcAb IgM = recent infection HBcAb IgG = remote infection HBeAg = ongoing viral replication, very high infectivity	Chronic may be treated with interferon. Acute is supportive
Hep C	RNA virus	Percutaneous or sexual exposure	15–160 days	Most common cause of viral hepatitis in the USA. Milder illness than HBV, chronic state develops in 50–85%	Serology for virus	Interferon and ribavirin for chronic. Supportive for acute
Hep D	RNA virus	Requires co-infection with HBV. Primarily percutaneous spread		Higher rate of chronic infection and cirrhosis than with HBV alone		Supportive
Hep E	RNA virus	Fecal–oral	15–60 days	Similar to HAV but with higher rate of fulminant liver failure, especially during pregnancy	No chronic or carrier state	Supportive

HAV, hepatitis A virus; HBV, hepatitis B virus; INR, international normalized ratio.

Table 3.5 Causes of chemical-induced hepatitis

Chemical	Considerations	Signs and symptoms	Lab findings	Treatment
Alcohol	Most common form of chemical hepatitis	Presentation can range from acute hepatic failure to cirrhosis. RUQ pain, fever, weakness, nausea, jaundice, dark urine, hepatomegaly	Pancytopenia, increased transaminases (AST > ALT), INR elevation, hypoglycemia	Supportive, alcohol abstinence, vitamin K for coagulopathy
Halothane	Causes damage through a toxic metabolite	Abrupt onset of fever, rash, pain, jaundice		No specific treatment. 50% fatality rate
Methyldopa	Causes damage through a toxic metabolite	Abdominal pain, rash, arthralgias, lymphadenopathy	Jaundice	Supportive. Chronic hepatitis and cirrhosis may develop
Cholestatic drugs	Anabolic steroids, OCP, erythromycin, phenobarbital	Malaise, anorexia, nausea, vomiting		
Acetaminophen	>150 mg/kg is toxic	Initially asymptomatic, abdominal pain, vomiting, liver failure	Plot drug level on Rumack–Matthew nomogram to determine probability of toxicity	N-acetylcysteine

OCP, oral contraceptive pills.

Cytomegalovirus: most common opportunistic viral infection after transplant. Treat with ganciclovir.

3.5.4. Liver abscess

Presentation: RUQ pain, fever. Jaundice usually present with multiple abscesses, rare with single abscess.

Diagnosis: ultrasound and CT are diagnostic.

Treatment: antibiotics empirically, with most commonly needing surgical drainage.
Mortality is 15% in the absence of other disease.

3.5.5. Lab findings in liver disease

Indirect bilirubin is elevated when there is overwhelming supply of unconjugated bilirubin to hepatocytes (hemolysis) or hepatocellular injury resulting in inability of hepatocytes to conjugate a normal supply of bilirubin (hepatitis).

Direct bilirubin increases when there is an obstruction preventing the secretion of the conjugated bilirubin (gallstone obstruction, biliary atresia).

Transaminases are intracellular. Liver injury usually increases all transaminases. Marked elevations seen with viral hepatitis. AST:ALT ratio of greater than 2 is common in alcoholic hepatitis (alcohol stimulates AST).

PT prolongation may be sign of hepatic failure, but may also be vitamin deficiency.

Low albumin is a sign of global dysfunction.

LDH is not liver specific and may be elevated for multiple other reasons (e.g. hemolysis).

Serum ammonia levels do not reliably correlate with acute hepatic function deterioration in the cirrhotic patient (may serve as a marker of general decline).

3.5.6. Cholangitis

Bacterial infection of the biliary tract.

Common pathogens: *E. coli* (most common), *Klebsiella, Enterococcus, Streptococcus.*
Presentation: Charcot's triad (fever/chills, jaundice, RUQ pain); Reynold's pentad
  (Charcot's triad + altered mental status and shock).
Treatment: antibiotics (Gram negatives, enterococcal) + surgical drainage.

3.5.7. Cholecystitis

Most common cause of abdominal pain and surgical disease in elderly. Obstruction caused by (cholesterol) stone in cystic duct or common bile duct (CBD) leads to distention and inflammation of gallbladder. Infection can set in (*E. coli*). Can also be acalculous, occurring in 5–10%. Acalculous causes include trauma, DM, burn, post-operative, sepsis, post-partum. Acalculous cholecystitis has a higher risk of gangrene, perforation, and mortality.

Presentation: RUQ pain following fatty meals, nausea, vomiting. Pain radiates to
  infrascapular region.
Complications: gangrene; perforation; abscess; cholangitis.
Diagnosis: ultrasound (gallbladder wall thickening; pericholecystic fluid; CBD dilation); if
  ultrasound is negative, consider HIDA scan; no labs sensitive or specific.
Management: IV fluids, antiemetic medicine, antibiotics, surgical evaluation.

3.5.8. Cholelithiasis/choledocholithiasis

Gallbladder or CBD stones. No inflammation.

Presentation: may be asymptomatic or may have biliary colic (constant RUQ pain +/−
  vomiting 30 minutes after eating fatty meal) secondary to transient obstruction of cystic
  or CBD.
Treatment: IV fluids and antiemetic medicine. Referral to surgery as an outpatient.

3.5.9. Gallbladder tumors

Gallbladder polyps present in 5% of people. Identification of cancerous (adenocarcinoma) or precancerous (adenomyomatosis) is surgical decision for elective removal. Gallbladder cancer usually presents with symptoms of cholecystitis. Mass on ultrasound should be referred for surgical evaluation.

3.6. Pancreas

3.6.1. Pancreatitis

Infection or inflammation of the pancreas.

Most common causes: alcohol use (men) and gallstones (women) and idiopathic.

Less common causes: trauma, hypertriglyceridemia, hypercalcemia, drugs, infection (i.e. mumps, viral, mycoplasma), scorpion sting. Potential drugs that cause pancreatitis include: furosemide, thiazides, valproic acid, tetracycline, amiodarone, estrogen, indomethacin.

Presentation: epigastric pain radiating to the back, nausea, vomiting, dehydration, tenderness with guarding. Patients may have retroperitoneal hemorrhage (two suggestive physical findings are: Cullen's sign – periumbilical bruising; Grey-Turner's sign – flank bruising). Jaundice may occur with biliary obstruction.

Diagnosis: lipase elevation is specific and parallels the clinical course. CT scan can be used to detect hemorrhage, abscess, pseudocyst. Pancreatic calcifications may be visible on abdominal X-ray in patients with chronic pancreatitis.

Prognosis: estimate with Ranson's criteria. Half of the score is calculated at arrival (age over 55, glucose over 200 mg/dL, WBC over 16 000/μL, AST over 250 U/L, LDH greater than 350 IU/L.

Table 3.6 Calculating Ranson's criteria

Criteria at diagnosis	Criteria at 48 hours
Age >55 years old	HCT drop >10%
Glucose >200 (mg/dL)	BUN rise >5 (mg/dL)
WBC >16 000 (cells/mm²)	Base deficit >4 (mEq/L)
AST >250 (U/L)	Calcium <8 (mg/dL)
LDH >350 (U/L)	PaO$_2$ <60 (mmHg)
	Est. fluid sequestration >6 L

One point for each criteria met.

Number of Ranson's criteria met	Estimated mortality
≤2	Less than 5%
3–4	15–20%
5–6	40%
≥7	Over 99 % (some sources 100 %)

HCT, hematocrit

Treatment: IV fluids, keep the patient NPO, pain control, antiemetics. Antibiotics are only indicated for sepsis or concurrent infections (cholangitis). NG tube only for patients with intractable vomiting.

3.6.2. Pancreatic tumors

Second most common GI malignancy and fourth leading cause of cancer-related death in the USA. Less than 4% of patients survive to 5 years after diagnosis. Due to lack of characteristic signs and symptoms, most patients present late (vague abdominal pain and signs of obstruction of pancreatic ducts).

3.7. Small bowel

3.7.1. Bowel infections

3.7.1.1. Inflammatory bacterial infections

Diarrhea caused by inflammation from invasion by bacteria. Colon and distal small bowel are the primarily affected areas. Symptom onset is gradual. Diarrhea is usually bloody.

Table 3.7 Inflammatory bacterial infections

Bacteria	Transmission	Presentation	Treatment	Complications
Salmonella	Ingestion of contaminated eggs and poultry. Can occur person to person, or animal to person (e.g. pet turtles)	Gastroenteritis with bloody stools. Typhoid fever may develop (persistent fever, bradycardia, rose spot skin lesions, cramping without diarrhea)	Self-limited. Severe disease or immuno-compromised patients should get antibiotics. Fluoroquinolone is drug of choice followed by bactrim. Typhoid fever should be treated with ceftriaxone	
Shigella	Fecal–oral transmission	High fevers, cramping, diarrhea (bloody mucoid stools). Tenesmus is classically seen. In children febrile seizures are classic	Self-limited. Bactrim, ampicillin, and quinolones can be used in severe cases	Reiter's syndrome, hemolytic uremic syndrome
Campylobacter	Ingestion of contaminated poultry. Most common cause of bacterial diarrhea in the USA	Nausea, cramps, diarrhea, localized abdominal pain	Self-limited but can be treated with erythromycin (drug of choice)	Reiter's syndrome, hemolytic uremic syndrome, Guillain-Barré syndrome
Yersinia	Ingestion of contaminated water. Can occur as direct transmission from farm or wild animals	Fevers, cramps, diarrhea. May cause mesenteric adenitis or terminal ileitis	Self-limited but can be treated with bactrim, quinolones, ceftriaxone	Polyarthritis, erythema nodosum
E. coli	Enterohemorrhagic E. coli produces a cytopathic toxin. Infection caused by ingestion of undercooked beef or unpasteurized milk	Watery diarrhea early progressing to bloody diarrhea, nausea, vomiting, cramps, fevers	Antibiotics not recommended as it increases the chances of developing HUS or TTP	Hemolytic uremic syndrome, thrombotic thrombocytopenic purpura
Vibrio para-haemolyticus	Ingestion of shellfish and other raw seafood	Nausea, vomiting, cramps, diarrhea	Self-limited but quinolones or tetracyclines can be used in severe cases	

HUS, hemolytic uremic syndrome; TTP, thrombotic thrombocytopenic purpura.

3.7.1.2. Non-inflammatory bacterial infections

Primarily affects small bowel. Toxins are released by bacteria, which causes diarrhea. Diarrhea tends to be large volume and watery without blood.

Table 3.8 Non-inflammatory bacterial infections

Bacteria	Transmission	Presentation	Treatment
Staphylococcus aureus	Most common cause of food poisoning. Ingestion of protein-rich food, contaminated with staphylococci and preformed toxin	Rapid onset (4–6 hours), vomiting, cramps, diarrhea	Resolves spontaneously in a day
Bacillus cereus	Ingestion of contaminated fried rice	Rapid onset of nausea, vomiting, cramps. Diarrhea less common	Resolves spontaneously in 12–24 hours
E. coli	Enterotoxigenic E. coli is the most common cause of traveler's diarrhea. Fecal–oral transmission	Explosive watery diarrhea with cramps	Self-limited. Ciprofloxacin for 3 days and antidiarrheals can shorten the duration of disease
Clostridium perfringens	Ingestion of contaminated meat and poultry	Fever, chills, headache	Self-limited
Vibrio cholera	Ingestion of shellfish and other raw seafood. Incubation in 1–2 days	Rice water stools, abdominal distension	Aggressive IV rehydration and treatment of severe dehydration, hypokalemia, hyperchloremic acidosis. Quinolones shorten the duration of disease. Tetracycline, doxycycline, and bactrim can be used
Scombroid	Ingestion of heat-stable toxins in the dark meat of fish	Bacteria produce histamine. Facial flushing, redness, abdominal cramps, vomiting, diarrhea, palpitations, bronchospasm	H1, H2 blockers. Nebulized β-agonists. Use epinephrine if anaphylactoid reaction occurs
Ciguatera	Ingestion of neurotoxin that accumulates in fish that eat dinoflagellates	Reversal of hot/cold sensations, dysesthesias, parasthesias, weakness, vomiting, diarrhea, myalgias	IV fluids, antiemetics, pain medication, IV mannitol occasionally helpful
Aeromonas hydrophilia	Contaminated well water. Immunocompromised and children affected more often	Watery diarrhea, vomiting, cramps lasting for weeks	Quinolones, bactrim, tetracycline

3.7.1.3. Parasitic

Table 3.9 Parasitic bowel infections

Parasite	Transmission	Presentation	Treatment
Entamoeba histolytica	Fecal–oral transmission	Anything from asymptomatic to profuse bloody diarrhea, fevers, and severe cramps. Abscesses can form in liver, lung and brain.	Flagyl plus paromomycin
Giardia	Most common intestinal parasite in the USA. Ingestion of contaminated water. Fecal–oral transmission	Watery foul-smelling diarrhea, cramps, bloating, nausea	Flagyl, tinidazole
Cryptosporidium	Fecal–oral transmission. Most common cause of diarrhea in AIDS patients	Watery diarrhea, cramps, nausea	Generally self-limited. IV fluids, paromomycin, nitazoxanide. Immunocompromised patients can have malabsorption
Isospora	Fecal–oral transmission. Symptoms primarily occur in immunocompromised	Watery diarrhea, cramps, nausea, vomiting	Long course bactrim
Enterobiasis (pinworms)	Ingestion of pinworm eggs. Eggs develop in the bowel. The adult migrates to the anus and deposits eggs at night	Anal itching primarily at night	Mebendazole, pyrantel, repeat after 2 weeks. Treat all close relatives
Necator (hookworm)	Larvae in soil penetrate skin	Diarrhea, abdominal pain, fever, cough, iron deficiency anemia	Mebendazole, albendazole, or pyrantel

3.7.1.4. Viral bowel infections

Table 3.10 Viral bowel infections

Virus	Transmission	Presentation	Treatment
Rotavirus	Primarily seen in children <2 years old	Nausea, vomiting, diarrhea, URI symptoms	Supportive
Norovirus	Ingestion of contaminated food	Nausea, vomiting, diarrhea, abdominal pain, fever	Supportive
Adenovirus	"stomach flu"	Nausea, vomiting, diarrhea, low fever, malaise	Supportive

URI, upper respiratory infection.

3.7.2. Inflammatory bowel disease

Two primary types of inflammatory bowel disease are Crohn's disease and ulcerative colitis. These disorders are similar in nature but differ in nature and location of inflammation.

Table 3.11 Inflammatory bowel diseases

	Crohn's	Ulcerative Colitis
Appearance	Full-thickness bowel wall lesions with a "cobblestone" appearance	Superficial ulcers, crypt abscesses
Location	Skip lesions, can appear anywhere along GI tract	Involvement is continuous, always involves rectum
Presentation	Abdominal pain, cramping, diarrhea, fever, rectal fistula or prolapse. Occult blood and fecal leukocytes are common	Lower abdominal pain, diarrhea, bloody stools, fever
Complications	Stricture and obstruction, GI bleed, GI malignancies, perforation, arthritis, uveitis	GI bleeding, toxic megacolon, perforation, fistula. Increase in risk of colorectal cancer, arthritis, uveitis, erythema nodosum, pyoderma gangrenosum
Treatment	IV fluids, steroids, sulfasalazine, azathioprine, antibiotics. GI consult and admission for dehydrated patients, those with significant electrolyte abnormalities, or those with complications	If no complications, outpatient management with corticosteroids or sulfasalazine. Antibiotics and IV fluids if complications occuring. Antimotility agents dispose the patient to toxic megacolon

3.7.3. Small bowel obstruction

Causes: adhesions (most common), hernia, cancer.
Presentation: diffuse abdominal pain, abdominal distention, nausea, vomiting, hyperactive bowel sounds.
Diagnosis: abdominal X-ray shows centrally distended air-filled loops of small bowel and lack of air in large bowel, air–fluid levels seen on upright or decubitus views. CT abdomen with PO contrast can show transition point.
Management: keep patient NPO, place NG tube for GI decompression. Although most resolve spontaneously, surgical consultation may be necessary.

3.7.4. Paralytic ileus

Etiology: most common cause of obstruction. Caused by electrolyte abnormality, medication, infection.
Presentation: similar to small bowel obstruction, except hypoactive bowel sounds.
Diagnosis: abdominal X-ray (distended air-filled loops of small and large bowel).
Management: keep patient NPO, place NG tube for GI decompression. Address underlying cause.

3.7.5. Aortoenteric fistula

Entertain diagnosis in patient with any amount of GI bleeding with history of abdominal aortic aneurysm repair as the condition is seen primarily in patients who have had abdominal aortic aneurysm repair with graft placement. A fistula develops between the bowel and the abdominal aorta.

Presentation: usually massive, painless lower GI bleeding.

Treatment: emergent surgical consult, type and cross for blood.

3.7.6. Congenital anomalies

Most common causes of congenital anomalies causing small bowel obstruction: webs, duplications, and malrotation. Most congenital anomalies are surgically corrected, others require life-long medical management. Goal in the emergency department is not to correct the problem, but to identify and stabilize.

3.7.6.1. Malrotation

Small bowel is found predominately on the right side of the abdomen. Cecum is near the epigastrum. Bowel is prone to volvulus and obstruction. Children may present with failure to thrive, abdominal distension, vomiting. Treatment is surgical.

3.7.6.2. Intestinal malabsorption

Disruption of digestion and nutrient absorption; common cause is celiac disease. Patients present with weight loss, chronic diarrhea, abdominal distention and pain, growth retardation. Often have abnormal serologic tests. Diagnosis is made with abnormal small bowel biopsy, clinical improvement often seen on gluten-free diet.

3.7.6.3. Meckel's diverticulum

Most common congenital abnormality of small intestine; heterotopic gastric mucosa retained in small outpouching.

Rule of 2: occurs in 2% of the population, most patients present when they are younger than 2 years old, diverticulum is usually 2 cm long and 2 cm wide and located 2 ft from ileocecal valve.

Presentation: abdominal pain, vomiting, painless GI bleeding, obstruction (leadpoint for intussusception).

Diagnosis: Meckel's (technetium) scan.

Management: IV fluids. Keep patient NPO, place NG tube for GI decompression. Refer to surgery.

3.7.7. Small bowel tumors

Only 10% of small bowel tumors are symptomatic, benign lesions are 10 times as common as malignant. Lymphoma is most common primary malignant tumor of small intestine with 75% of these being malignant. Bleeding and obstruction are most common symptoms.

3.7.8. Intussusception

Most common cause of obstruction in children aged 2 or under.

Presentation: vomiting, abdominal pain, and bloody stools (containing mucus/blood mixture "currant jelly stool"); pain is episodic, lasting 15–30 minutes, then resolves. May be able to palpate mass.

Diagnosis: ultrasound, air-contrast or hydrostatic barium enema is both diagnostic and therapeutic.

3.7.9. Vascular insufficiency

Ischemic colitis is most common cause of intestinal ischemia; mesenteric ischemia is a medical emergency and often leads to bowel necrosis. May result from thrombosis or embolus from the superior mesenteric artery, mesenteric venous thrombosis or nonocclusive mesenteric ischemia.

Risk factors: consider in any patient with low flow state (hypovolemia, dialysis patient), patients older than 60 years, or patients with comorbidities (atrial fibrillation, congestive heart failure [CHF], recent MI).

Presentation: abdominal pain out of proportion to exam. Post-prandial pain (intestinal angina).

Diagnosis: CT is most commonly employed diagnostic, but still with low sensitivity 64%, specificity 92%. Angiography is study of choice. Serum lactate elevation common.

Treatment: pain control, IV fluids, surgical referral.

3.8. Large bowel

3.8.1. Infectious disorders

3.8.1.1. Antibiotic-associated diarrhea

Usually moderate in severity without cramps, fever, or fecal leukocytes. Most symptoms are self-resolving after withdrawal of offending drug.

3.8.1.2. *Clostridium difficile*

Can cause mild to severe disease. 3 types of severe disease: neonatal pseudomembranous enterocolitis, post-operative pseudomembranous enterocolitis, and antibiotic-associated pseudomembranous enterocolitis. *C. difficile* is the most common cause of diarrhea in hospitalized patients.

Diagnosis: Consider the diagnosis in anyone presenting with diarrhea developing after hospital discharge or within 2 weeks of antibiotic therapy. Diagnosis is confirmed with ELISA for *C. difficile* toxin.

Treatment: oral metronidazole, 500 mg QID for 10 days. Severe illness may require ORAL vancomycin 250 mg QID. Failed treatment may require colectomy.

3.8.2. Parasitic diseases

3.8.2.1. Amebiasis

Caused by *Entamoeba histolytica* and spread by asymptomatic carriers whose excrement contains encysted organisms. Travelers at risk, 1–3 weeks for incubation time.

Presentation: constipation alternating with diarrhea, abdominal pain, fever weight loss. May have liver, pericardium, lung, and brain extension of infection.
Diagnosis: stool for ova and parasites.
Treatment: metronidazole 500 mg TID for 10 days.

3.8.2.2. Giardiasis

Caused by *Giardia lamblia* infecting small bowel most commonly. Occurs world wide, common to rural areas with poor water sanitation or in daycare setting.

Presentation: abdominal cramping, flatulence, foul-smelling watery diarrhea (weight loss with chronic infection).
Diagnosis: stool for ova and parasites.
Treatment: metronidazole 250 mg TID for 10 days.

3.8.2.3. Ascariasis

Roundworm infection with *Ascaris* may lead to large worm burden.

Presentation: may be asymptomatic. Can also present with bowel obstruction, hepatic abscess, acute pancreatitis, appendicitis, or pneumonitis. Primary symptom may be cough from young worms being expectorated and migrating to lungs from esophagus/gut.
Treatment: mebendazole.

3.8.3. Appendicitis

Most common abdominal surgical emergency.

Causes: obstruction of the appendiceal lumen, adhesions, lymphoid hyperplasia. Seen most frequently in 10–30 year olds.
Presentation: vague visceral pain, nausea, anorexia, fever. Pain begins to localize to right lower quadrant after 24 hours. Depending on how the appendix lays, other presentations may occur (dysuria, low back pain, RUQ pain).
Diagnosis: primarily clinical. WBC count is elevated 80% of the time. CT and ultrasound can help make the diagnosis when clinical suspicion is moderate.
Treatment: surgery, antibiotics.

3.8.4. Necrotizing enterocolitis (NEC)

Most common cause of neonatal intestinal perforation and most common GI emergency in infancy; most cases develop in neonatal intensive care unit (NICU), therefore often NOT considered as an emergency department diagnosis. Given increasing financial pressures to release hospitalized patients sooner, important entity to consider in premature infants presenting to the emergency department.

Presentation: infants present with feeding intolerance and vomiting; 3 stages: first is feeding intolerance, emesis and/or ileus; second is definite NEC with dilated bowel loops and pneumatosis intestinalis (air in bowel wall); stage 3 is perforation (shock, abdominal distention, disseminated intravascular coagulation [DIC] and metabolic acidosis).
Treatment: NPO, decompression with NG tube and pediatric surgical consultation. Strictures, fistulas and short-gut syndromes can develop in those that survive.

3.8.5. Radiation colitis

May present as late manifestation, after cessation of treatment. Usually associated with total radiation dose of 45 Gy (4500 rad).

Course: begins with direct mucosal injury, progresses to a direct proctitis, leading to ulceration, stricturing, or fistula (bladder or vagina) formation.
Diagnosis: CT usually diagnostic, with appropriate history.

3.8.6. Large bowel obstruction

65% are caused by tumor, 15% by volvulus, 15% by diverticulitis. Infrequent causes include constipation, radiation colitis, and inflammatory bowel diseases.

Presentation: poorly localizable abdominal pain, distension. Occult blood in stool if tumor or inflammatory bowel disease is the cause.
Diagnosis: abdominal X-ray shows dilated loops of large bowel (>8 cm) or cecum (>6 cm).
Treatment: Keep patient NPO, place NG tube, surgical consultation.

3.8.7. Volvulus

Table 3.12 Volvulus

	Cecal	Sigmoid
Frequency	1/3 of cases	2/3 of all volvulus cases
Affected group	Seen in healthy patients 20–40 years old. Results from embryologic defect where large bowel is not properly attached to the abdominal wall	Classically seen in patients with chronic constipation. Constipation leads to stretching and redundancy of sigmoid
Presentation	Sudden onset of abdominal pain, distension, vomiting, obstipation	Gradual or sudden onset of abdominal pain with distension, nausea, vomiting, and obstipation
Abdominal X-ray	Shows dilated loop of bowel arising from right lower quadrant, markedly dilated cecum	Shows dilated loop of bowel arising from left lower quadrant

3.8.8. Diverticulosis

Small herniations of colonic mucosa. Generally occur at the weakest points, which tend to be where the blood vessels enter the mucosa. Seen most often in the sigmoid colon and in patients who eat a low-fiber diet (constipation patients). Diverticulosis is the most common cause of lower GI bleeding in adults and the most common cause of massive rectal bleeding in the elderly. Bleeding should be painless.

Diagnosis: made definitively with sigmoidoscopy or colonoscopy. Can often be seen on CT.
Treatment: primarily supportive. Mesenteric angiography can be done to allow for embolization in uncontrollable large-volume bleeding. Surgery done for extreme cases.

3.8.9. Diverticulitis

Inflammation of a diverticulum, occurring after obstruction of the diverticular neck. GI bleeding is seen in over half of cases, but massive bleeding is uncommon.

Presentation: alternating constipation and diarrhea, focal abdominal pain (left lower most common), fever. Urinary symptoms are common if diverticula are near the bladder. If diverticulum ruptures, peritoneal symptoms can develop.

Diagnosis: abdominal X-ray can detect signs of complications such as ileus, free air, obstruction. CT scan can show those signs plus inflammation and localize the diverticulitis.

Treatment: high-fiber diet, antibiotics, pain control if disease is mild. If complicated or process is advanced, IV antibiotics, pain control, keep patient NPO, and surgical consult for admission. Up to 40% of patients will require surgery either urgently or eventually.

3.9. Rectum and anus

3.9.1. Perirectal abscess

Types: perianal, intersphincteric, supralevator, ischiorectal, deep postanal. Abscess develops from obstruction of glands at the base of the anal crypts. Associated with inflammatory bowel disease, sexually transmitted diseases, and radiation. Infections are polymicrobial.

Presentation: pain, fevers, malaise. Bowel movements are usually painful.

Treatment: incision and drainage. Perianal abscesses can be drained in the emergency department. Other perirectal abscesses should be drained in the operating room.

3.9.2. Pilonidal cyst and abscess

Occurs at superior edge of buttock in midline. Seen most commonly in men less than 40 years of age. Ingrown hair penetrates skin, causing a foreign body reaction, leading to development of a sinus tract. The tract gets clogged and an abscess forms.

Treatment: bedside incision and drainage in emergency department, start on antibiotics for skin flora and refer to surgery for excision of sinus tract.

3.9.3. Proctitis

Inflammation of the rectum; commonly occurs from anal intercourse or local extension of vaginal secretions to infect the rectum. Most infections are sexually transmitted disease organisms.

Presentation: rectal pain.

Diagnosis: clinical. Very tender during rectal exam.

Treatment: culture, broad spectrum treatment, and search for other underlying disease are important.

3.9.4. Hirschsprung's disease

Pathology: absence of intramural ganglion cells in rectum, can extend to sigmoid or entire colon.

Presentation: no passage of meconium stool in newborn within 24–48 hours, abdominal distention, vomiting. Can lead to toxic megacolon.

Diagnosis: abdominal X-ray (obstruction); barium enema (dilated segment of proximal colon); rectal biopsy (lack of ganglion cells).
Management: IV fluids, surgery.

3.9.5. Anal fissure

Most common cause of painful rectal bleeding in children and adults.
Cause: constipation with passage of hard stools.
Presentation: mucosal tear in posterior midline (if not midline, consider serious pathology or non-accidental trauma); pain with bowel movement; blood streaks on stool.
Management: sitz baths, stool softener, fiber diet, pain relief.

3.9.6. Anal fistula

Usually the result of infection or inflammation which leads to communication between perianal skin and an adjacent structure (colon, bladder, or other local structures). Intersphincteric is most common location. Usually presents with pain. Treatment is surgical referral for excision of fistula tract.

3.9.7. Rectal and anal tumors

Colorectal carcinoma is third most common type of cancer, and second most common cause of cancer death in the USA. As age increased, incidence increases. Right-sided tumors usually present with anemia (occult bleeding, fatigue, dizziness, microscopic anemia). Disproportionately poor prognosis in older patients versus younger patients.

3.9.8. Foreign body

May be iatrogenic (tip of enema, broken thermometer) or patient placed; rectal foreign body can cause perforation, abscess, or obstruction. Not all are radio-opaque and may require small amount of rectal contrast to visualize location and distance. If less than 10 cm from anal orifice, may be feasible to remove in emergency department. May need to employ procedural sedation for removal.

Bibliography

Marx, JA, Hockberger RS, Walls RM, Adams J, Rosen P, eds. *Rosen's Emergency Medicine: Concepts and Clinical Practice*. Philadelphia: Mosby Elsevier, 2010.
Tintinalli JE, Stapczynski JS, Cline DM, *et al. Tintinalli's Emergency Medicine: a Comprehensive Study Guide*, 7th edn.

New York: The McGraw-Hill Companies, Inc., 2011.
Wolfson AB, Hendey GW, Ling LJ, *et al. Harwood-Nuss' Clinical Practice of Emergency Medicine*, 5th edn. Philadelphia: Lippincott Williams & Wilkins, 2009.

Neurologic emergencies

Lisa Barker and Anthony J. Buecker

4.1. Cranial nerve (CN) disorders

4.1.1. Bell's palsy

Etiology: unilateral facial nerve (CN VII) palsy – associated with upper respiratory infection (URI) or herpes simplex virus.

Presentation: ipsilateral paralysis and numbness of CN VII including forehead involvement. Loss of corneal reflex and loss of taste. Rapid onset within a few days. Pain behind auricle before other symptoms. Preceding or concurrent URI or herpes simplex virus. Possible swelling.

Diagnosis and differentials: clinical diagnosis as above, if in doubt CT/MRI for stroke/lesion.

Ramsay–Hunt syndrome: ipsilateral zoster rash face/ear canal/tympanic membrane (TM) and extreme pain.

Lyme disease: can cause bilateral palsy.

Acoustic neuroma: associated with hearing loss with facial weakness.

Stroke: unlike Bell's, stroke with spare forehead; also comes with other neurologic deficits.

Malignant otitis externa: suspect in diabetes or immunocompromised.

Peripheral neuropathy: suspect in diabetes.

Treatment: prednisone and acyclovir/valacyclovir for 7–10 days. Greater efficacy if started within 72 hours of symptoms. Artificial tears, eye patch/tape at night to prevent corneal abrasions. Up to 71% will recover without treatment, 84% of those regain nearly full function. Recurrence is rare and should prompt consideration of another etiology.

4.1.2. Trigeminal neuralgia (tic douloureux)

Etiology: blood vessel or mass compresses the nerve, leading to demyelination/symptoms in distribution of the trigeminal nerve (CN V). V_1 – ophthalmic, V_2 – maxillary, V_3 – mandibular.

Presentation: brief unilateral sharp pains in distribution of any or all branches of CN V. Most cases occur after age 50. Triggered by light touch, chewing, brushing teeth, cold air, etc. May elicit pain by tapping affected region. Spasms with pain.

Diagnosis: clinic diagnosis as above, if in doubt CT/MRI for stroke/lesion.

Pocket Guide to the American Board of Emergency Medicine In-Training Exam, ed. Bob Cambridge.
Published by Cambridge University Press. © Cambridge University Press 2013.

Treatment: carbamazepine first-line and increase dose. Gabapentin, baclofen, phenytoin, or other antiepileptic drugs if carbamazepine fails. Surgery for decompression of nerve or neurectomy.

4.2. Demyelinating disorders

4.2.1. Multiple sclerosis

Etiology: autoimmune disease leading to multifocal areas of central nervous system (CNS) demyelination, leading to slowed conduction and plaques at sites of myelin loss.

Presentation: occurs in women > men and white > non-white. Presents with relapsing and remitting neurologic deficits. Common initial symptoms are optic neuritis, diplopia, internuclear ophthalmoplegia, sensory loss, weakness, paresthesias. Lhermitte phenomenon – electric shock sensation down spine when flex neck. Uhthoff's phenomenon – temporary worsening of symptoms with body temperature increases (hot shower, exercise, etc.).

Diagnosis: 2 or more episodes needed to make definitive diagnosis. MRI shows white matter lesions. Cerebrospinal fluid (CSF) shows IgG/oligoclonal bands, increased protein.

Treatment: investigate and treat fevers, which further slow conduction in demyelinated areas. High-dose IV methylprednisolone followed by taper to shorten/reduce complications of exacerbations. Oral prednisone not recommended for optic neuritis. Plasma exchange second-line therapy. Immunomodulators (interferon-β) for relapsing-remitting disease.

4.3. Headache

Features that suggest more serious etiology: Sudden or "thunderclap" onset, worsened by Valsalva or exertion, new headache after 50 years of age, change in level of consciousness or focal neurologic deficits, history of fever, cancer or immunosuppression.

Table 4.1 Primary and secondary headaches

Primary headache disorders			
Type	**General**	**Symptoms**	**Treatment**
Cluster	Men > women May be triggered by alcohol intake	Unilateral sharp "boring" pain behind or around the eye, associated with tearing, rhinorrhea, facial flushing. Occurs multiple times a day for several days then does not occur for months	Sumatriptan SQ if presents acutely (within 2 hours) Oxygen (7–10 L/min) if prolonged symptoms IV DHE Prednisone taper
Tension	Most common type of headache	Tight band-like pain, dull. Often worse later in the day. No photophobia, nausea or vomiting	Ibuprofen or acetaminophen
Migraine	More common in women, many patients have family history	15% of patients have an aura ("classic migraine"), the rest do not ("common migraine"). Distribution of headache is varied, nausea, vomiting, photophobia	NSAIDs Prochlorperazine or metoclopramide 10 mg IV IV fluid bolus IV DHE or sumatriptan SQ if not taken in the preceding 24 hours May repeat DHE IV x1 for status migranosus Opioids are not recommended for management of migraines

(cont.)

Table 4.1 (cont.)

Secondary headache disorders			
Type	**General**	**Symptoms**	**Treatment**
Brain tumor	Primary lesion seen mostly before 50 years of age, metastatic lesion if over 50	Pressure, worse in the morning, nausea/vomiting	Consult neurosurgery Dexamethasone for cerebral edema
Carotid/vertebral artery dissection	Minor trauma or sudden neck movement causes injury to the vessel wall, intramural hemorrhage occurs, and thrombus can form	Sudden onset of head or neck pain, often with focal neurologic deficits. Ipsilateral Horner's syndrome and contralateral hemispheric symptoms can occur with carotid dissection. Vertigo, ataxia, diplopia seen with vertebral artery dissection	Stroke prevention with anticoagulation and antiplatelet therapy. MRI or angiography is needed for definitive diagnosis
Cerebral venous sinus thrombosis	Associated with hypercoagulable states, inflammatory disorders, neurosurgical procedures	Nausea/vomiting seizures Decreased LOC or focal neurologic deficits Eye exam abnormal with cavernous sinus thrombosis CT may be abnormal, MRV study of choice	Anticoagulation Thrombolysis for worsening symptoms
Chronic subdural	More frequent in elderly and alcoholics due to cerebral atrophy	Diffuse headache, constant. Associated with confusion, weakness and seizures	Consult neurosurgery
Hypertensive	HTN rarely causes headache until DBP >130 mmHg	Diffuse headache, worse in morning. If vision changes, confusion or vomiting occur, hypertensive encephalopathy should be considered and treated	Good blood pressure control. IV labetalol for hypertensive encephalopathy – reduce MAP by 25% over 60 minutes
Post-lumbar puncture	Most common complication of LP To decrease occurrence: use a small-gauge atraumatic needle (Whitaker, Sprotte). Keep needle bevel parallel to dural fibers	Bilateral throbbing headache worse in upright position, nausea, vomiting, neck stiffness	Bedrest, hydration, analgesics. Caffeine may be of benefit If prolonged (> 24 hours), a blood patch may be needed
Pseudotumor cerebri (idiopathic intracranial HTN)	Uncertain etiology Young overweight females Possibly related to thyroid disorders, vitamin A, chronic steroid use, oral contraceptives, and/or tetracycline	Nonspecific chronic headache Peripheral vision loss CN VI palsy Loss of venous pulsations, papilledema on fundoscopic exam CT may show small ventricles LP OP >20 cm H_2O (25 if obese). CSF otherwise normal	Goal is to decrease ICP. LP offers temporary relief. Acetazolamide (carbonic anhydrase inhibitor) frequently used. VP shunt if refractory to medication

Table 4.1 (cont.)

Secondary headache disorders			
Type	**General**	**Symptoms**	**Treatment**
Temporal arteritis	Inflammation of branches of the external carotid. Usually seen in elderly and associated with polymyalgia rheumatica. Exceedingly rare <50 years of age.	Sudden onset of severe unilateral headache, jaw claudication, ESR > 50 mm/hr, temporal artery tenderness in less than half of cases	Prednisone (60–120 mg/day). Referral for temporal artery biopsy. Possibility of vision loss mandates aggressive treatment

DBP, diastolic blood pressure; DHE, dihydroergotamine; ESR, erythrocyte sedimentation rate; HTN, hypertension; LOC, level of consciousness; LP, lumbar puncture; LP OP, lumbar puncture opening pressure; MAP, mean arterial pressure; MRV, magnetic resonance venogram; VP, ventriculoperitoneal.

4.4. Hydrocephalus

4.4.1. Normal pressure hydrocephalus

Etiology: transient intracranial pressure (ICP) change leads to ventricular enlargement, which normalizes ICP.

Presentation: elderly patient with urinary incontinence, dementia, and broad-based, slow gait ("Wet, Wacky, Wobbly").

Diagnosis: neuroimaging shows ventricular enlargement out of proportion to atrophy. Mini mental state exam and walking test improve with large volume (50 mL) lumbar puncture.

Treatment: if clinically improves with large volume lumbar puncture, periodic lumbar punctures may be done or a ventriculoperitoneal shunt may be placed.

4.4.2. Ventriculoperitoneal shunt obstruction and infection

Etiology: neurosurgically placed CSF drain from ventricle into the peritoneum for hydrocephalus. May obstruct or become infected. Shunt infections are most common within 6 months post placement. Common agents are *Staphylococcus epidermidis* and *S. aureus*.

Presentation: signs of increased ICP – headache, nausea, vomiting, irritability, lethargy, and/or papilledema; meningismus. Shunt tubing may be warm or tender.

Evaluation: CT brain to assess for increased ICP, shunt series to assess that drain is intact. Neurosurgery should be consulted for obtaining CSF from the shunt for CSF cultures and analysis.

Treatment: ventriculoperitoneal shunt malfunction requires shunt revision. Admit shunt infections for antistaph, antipseudomonal IV therapy: IV vancomycin + cefepime, ceftazidime, or meropenem.

4.5. CNS infections and inflammatory disorders

4.5.1. Transverse myelitis

Etiology: post-viral, toxic, autoimmune, or idiopathic cause of spinal cord dysfunction. Involves 3–4 spinal cord levels, incomplete cross-sectional involvement.

Presentation: back pain, weakness, paresthesias, sensory loss, paraplegia, and sphincter dysfunction below level of lesion.
Diagnosis: MRI to exclude compressive lesion. CSF non-diagnostic. ESR elevated.
Treatment: corticosteroids, 50% partially recover or better.

4.5.2. Encephalitis

Etiology: infection of the brain parenchyma with neurologic and potentially meningeal symptoms. Caused by a variety of viral agents (Epstein–Barr virus (EBV), herpes, rabies, etc.) and *Mycoplasma*.
Presentation: behavior and personality changes, fever, seizures, headache, lethargy, altered mental status.
Associated signs depends on causative agent:

Vesicular rash – herpes simplex virus (HSV), varicella zoster virus, Enterovirus.
Erythema multiforme – *Mycoplasma*.
"Slapped cheek" – Parvovirus.
Conjunctivitis – Adenovirus, St. Louis encephalitis.

Evaluation: lumbar puncture to rule out bacterial meningitis and identify virus by PCR.
MRI or CT with contrast (focal edema, temporal lobe lesions – HSV), EEG.
Treatment: acyclovir for HSV and herpes zoster, ganciclovir for cytomegalovirus.

Table 4.2 Bacterial CNS infections

	Organisms/etiology	Presentation	Treatment
Bacterial meningitis	Age-associated, see Table 4.4	Headache (87%) Neck stiffness (83%) Fever (77%) Altered mental status (69%)	Antibiotics per age group IV dexamethasone before antibiotics improves outcomes for *Streptococcus pneumoniae* infection
Intracranial abscess	Most often contiguous infection History of head surgery/trauma DM, alcohol use, immunocompromise, streptococci, staphylococci, bacteroides, enterobacteriaceae, anaerobes	Often well-appearing Fever in < 50% Contrast CT to diagnose	Neurosurgical CT-guided aspiration 3rd gen cephalosporin + metronidazole +/− vancomycin
Spinal epidural abscess	Hematogenous spread History of IV drug use, DM, immunocompromise, spinal surgery. Causative agents: *S. aureus* (50–60%) Streptococci, enteric Gram-negative, coagulase-negative staphylococci	Back pain (occurs in up to 70% of patients, 1/3 thoracic) Fever (50–60%) Weakness or paralysis of the lower extremities. Tenderness of vertebrae to percussion is most sensitive exam finding. MRI with contrast, elevated ESR, WBC. LP has no value but has potential harm.	Emergent neurosurgical consult Third/fourth generation cephalosporin + vancomycin

DM, diabetes mellitus.

Table 4.3 Comparison of types of meningitis

Type	Bacterial	Viral	Fungal
Appearance	High mortality rate without treatment. Patients appear toxic	Mostly benign except herpes which can make patient appear toxic	More indolent time course Often afebrile since patient usually immunocompromised
CSF study findings	WBC >1000/µL, 80% neutrophils, glucose <40 mg/dL, protein >200 mg/dL, positive Gram stain	WBC <1000/µL, 1–50% neutrophils, glucose >40 mg/dL, protein <200 mg/dL, negative Gram stain	Mononuclear pleocytosis Elevated protein Decreased glucose
Treatment	Antibiotics empirically based on likely pathogens. Give corticosteroids before antibiotics to reduce cerebral edema	Supportive care, acyclovir if herpes suspected	Organism specific Amphotericin most common. Zygomycosis and aspergillosis may require surgical debridement

Table 4.4 Empiric bacterial meningitis treatment

Age group	Suspected organism	Empiric treatment
Neonate	Group B streptococcus Listeria Gram-negative bacilli	Ampicillin (50 mg/kg) with either cefotaxime (50 mg/kg) or gentamicin (2.5 mg/kg)
1–3 months	Group B streptococcus Listeria Haemophilus influenzae S. pneumoniae Neisseria meningitidis	Cefotaxime (50 mg/kg) or ceftriaxone (100 mg/kg). Ampicillin (50 mg/kg) up to 8 weeks of age. Vancomycin if potential for resistant strain of S. pneumoniae
3 months–18 years	H. influenzae S. pneumoniae N. meningitidis	Ceftriaxone (100 mg/kg). Vancomycin if potential for resistant strain of S. pneumoniae
18–50 years	S. pneumoniae N. meningitidis	Ceftriaxone (2 g). Vancomycin if potential for resistant strain of S. pneumoniae
50 years, immuno-compromised	S. pneumoniae N. meningitidis Listeria, Gram-negative	Ceftriaxone (2 g) plus ampicillin (2 g). Vancomycin if potential for resistant strain of S. pneumoniae

4.6. Movement disorders

4.6.1. Parkinson's disease

Etiology: neurodegenerative disease caused by loss of dopaminergic neurons in the substantia nigra. Usually occurs after age 60. Generally idiopathic.

Presentation: depends on advancement of disease course. Early on in the disease process the symptoms are nonspecific. Tremors typically begin in one extremity intermittently. As the disease progresses the common findings are resting tremor; rigidity; paucity of movement; pill rolling movements of thumb and index finger; and cogwheel rigidity. Muscle fatigue. Depression and dementia follow.

Diagnosis: clinical diagnosis. Look for tremor, rigidity, akinesia, and postural instability.
Treatment: dyskinesia from L-dopa can lead to rhabdomyolysis, dehydration, and alkalosis. Rule out infection, or aspiration pneumonia in patients presenting with acute akinesia, confusion, or psychosis.

4.6.2. Dystonic reaction

Etiology: extrapyramidal side effects of antipsychotics, antidepressants, or antiemetics leading to intermittent spasmodic contractions of muscles of face, neck, and trunk.
Presentation: torticollis, tongue protusion (buccolingual crisis), upward deviation of eyes (oculogyric crisis), back arching (opisthotonos), trismus, laryngospasms. Movements may be exacerbated by stress/anxiety.
Diagnosis: clinical presentation; normal mentation; antipsychotic, antidepressant, or antiemetic therapy.
Perform slit-lamp exam to rule out Wilson's disease as etiology (look for Kayser–Fleischer ring at periphery of iris).
Treatment: ABCs. Benadryl and/or Cogentin are first line. Benzodiazepines are second line.

4.7. Neuromuscular disorders

4.7.1. Guillain–Barré syndrome

Etiology: acute inflammatory demyelinating polyneuropathy. Often occurs after infection (viral URI or *Campylobacter jejuni* gastroenteritis most common) or medication/vaccine administration.
Presentation: begins with parasthesias in the extremities. Progressive ascending symmetric muscle weakness occurs, and eventually respiratory muscles and cranial nerves affected. Absent deep tendon reflexes. Often normal sensation. Onset is rapid (hours to days).
Diagnosis and differentials: CSF often shows elevated levels of protein. May be normal early in disease course. Also consider Tick paralysis, Lyme disease, myelitis.
Treatment: ABCs, respiratory support if needed. IVIG, plasma exchange.

4.7.2. Myasthenia gravis

Etiology: autoimmune disease with antibodies to the acetylcholine receptors at the neuromuscular junction. Associated with thymomas. Exacerbation may be precipitated by antibiotics (fluoroquinolones, macrolides, aminoglycosides), iodinated contrast, β-blockers, calcium channel blockers.
Presentation: muscle weakness that improves with rest. Extraocular muscles usually affected first leading to ptosis (may improve with application of cold pack) and diplopia, weak eyelid closure.
As disease progresses, proximal muscles affected more than distal muscles. Myasthenic crisis progresses to respiratory distress.
Diagnosis and differential: clinical presentation + edrophonium test (administration of 1–2 mg IV relieves weakness in seconds). Check negative inspiratory force (NIF); respiratory support needed if <20 cm H_2O. Also consider Lambert–Eaton syndrome or botulism.

Treatment: ABCs for myasthenic crisis. Edrophonium test may cause severe bradycardia, hypotension, and bronchospasms. Treat with atropine. Plasma exchange, IVIG, steroid therapy. Longer-acting cholinesterase inhibitors.

4.7.3. Additional neuromuscular disorders

Table 4.5 Additional neuromuscular disorders

Cholinergic crisis	Appears similar to a myasthenic crisis except for additional SLUDGE symptoms (Salivation, Lacrimation, Urination, Defecation, GI upset, Emesis) (alternative mnemonic: "DUMBELS," Diarrhea, Urination, Miosis, Muscle weakness, Bradycardia, Bronchospasm, Emesis, Lacrimation, Salivation)
Lambert–Eaton syndrome	Autoimmune destruction of presynaptic voltage-gated calcium channels. 60% associated with malignancies, often small cell lung cancer. No cranial nerve symptoms, and strength improves with exercise
Botulism	Weakness begins with bulbar and ocular muscles. Deep tendon reflexes are absent unlike myasthenia
Familial periodic paralysis	Associated with hypokalemia (occasionally hyperkalemia)
Tick paralysis	Ascending weakness and paralysis. Removing tick is curative

4.7.4. Peripheral neuropathies

Etiology: most common cause is diabetes due to microvascular injury of nerves.
Presentation: distal to proximal, symmetric, "stocking glove" distribution, paresthesias and pain, decreased or loss of deep tendon reflexes. Dysphagia, gastroparesis, diarrhea. Incontinence, impotence.
Diagnosis and differentials: clinical findings and rule out other causes. Consider toxic neuropathy, alcoholic neuropathy, B12 deficiency, HIV neuropathy.
Treatment: initiation of treatment for pain control: tricyclic antidepressants (TCAs), carbamazepine, gabapentin. Glycemic control to prevent progression.

4.7.5. Mononeuropathies

Table 4.6 Mononeuropathies

Nerve	Injury location	Clinical presentation
Radial	Mid-humerus/axilla (Saturday night palsy)	Wrist/finger drop. Numbness over first dorsal interosseus muscles
Ulnar	Elbow	Paresthesias to fourth and fifth digits. Unable to adduct fingers or grasp with thumb. Claw hand – paralysis
Median	Wrist (carpal-tunnel)	Positive Tinel's/Phalen's, thumb weakness, thenar atrophy, pain/paresthesias palmar aspect thumb, index, middle, and ring fingers
Sciatic	Buttock	Unable to flex knee or flex/extend ankle (foot drop)
Lateral femoral cutaneous	Inguinal ligament	Pain/numbness upper thigh
Common peroneal	Proximal fibula	Foot drop, numbness between first and second toes

4.8. Seizure disorders

4.8.1. Febrile seizures

Etiology: spontaneously resolving convulsion in child aged 6 months to 5 years with concurrent febrile illness. Family history, previous febrile seizures, neurodevelopmental delays may increase risk of febrile seizures.

Presentation: simple: generalized seizure lasting less than 15 minutes and not recurring within 24 hours.

Complex: focal seizure lasting over 15 minutes or recurring within 24 hours.

Diagnosis: clinical diagnosis. MRI, EEG unhelpful. Identify source of fever or rule out meningitis and encephalitis. Lumbar puncture not uniformly valuable.

Treatment: ABCs, antipyretics, benzodiazepines, and antiepileptic drugs as below if complex and ongoing.

4.8.2. Neonatal seizures

Etiology/presentation: neonatal seizures are a neurologic sign of serious underlying problem such as hypoxic-ischemic encephalopathy, infection, malformation of cortices, stroke, metabolic derangement, or trauma.

Diagnosis and differential: investigation of cause: hypoxic-ischemic, infection, malformation of cortices, stroke, metabolic (congenital or acquired), or trauma. Confirmation by EEG.

Treatment: D10 2.5–5 mL/kg bolus for hypoglycemia. Phenobarbital (loading dose of 20 mg/kg). Phenytoin and benzodiazepines (doses below).

4.8.3. Types of seizures

Table 4.7 Types of seizures

Type	Considerations	Presentation	Treatment
Simple focal	Consciousness unimpaired	Focal motor twitching or sensory changes	Self-limited. Benzodiazepine if troublesome to patient
Complex focal	Consciousness affected. May progress to generalized	As above with loss of consciousness	Self-limited. Benzodiazepine if prolonged
Tonic–clonic	"Grand mal"	Tonic phase progresses to clonus lasting 60–90 seconds, followed by a relaxation phase. Always followed by a post-ictal phase	Immediate medication is not needed as most are only 2–5 minutes long. Load with phenytoin in ED (not indicated in patients using alcohol)
Absence	Seen in school aged children (5–12 years old)	Sudden onset, consciousness is affected, postural tone is not lost. May have rhythmic movements, then consciousness returns without post-ictal state	Ethosuximide if prescribed by neurologist
Eclampsia	Complication of pregnancy, seen most commonly antepartum	Hypertensive, tachycardic, hyperreflexive, clonus, edematous with proteinuria	Load with 6 g IV of magnesium followed by 2 g IV/hr. Monitor for respiratory depression. Use hydralazine if DBP >105 mmHg after termination of seizures

ED, emergency department.

4.8.4. Status epilepticus

Presentation: continuous seizure activity or recurrent series of seizures without intervening return to baseline function that lasts more than 30 minutes. Likelihood of status epilepticus increases once seizure is past 5 minutes in duration.

Diagnosis: ECG, check glucose level, electrolytes, CBC, LFTs, ABGs, troponin, antiepileptic drug levels, and Toxicology screen for cause and to rule out mimics. Consider isoniazid overdose.

Treatment: ABCs. Antiepileptic drugs as below.

4.8.5. Antiepileptic drugs in the emergency department

First line: lorazepam (0.05–0.15 mg/kg IV, max of 4 mg per dose), phenytoin (20 mg/kg, no more than 50 mg/min), fosphenytoin (20 PE/kg, no more than 150 mg/min). If no IV: diazepam (0.15–0.3 mg/kg, max of 20 mg PR), midazolam 0.2 mg/kg IM.

Second line: valproate (40 mg/kg over 10 minutes, repeat 20 mg/kg over 5 minutes if still seizing), phenobarbital (20 mg/kg at 50 mg/min), propofol (1 mg/kg load, then 1–2 mg/kg IV every 3–5 minutes, and then 1–15 mg/kg/hr).

Third line: barbituate coma.

4.9. Spinal cord disorders

4.9.1. Spinal cord compression

Etiology/presentation:

Table 4.8 Causes and presentation of cord compression syndromes

Syndrome	Etiology	Presentation
Central cord syndrome	Hyperextension (most common incomplete injury)	Upper extremity weakness is much greater than lower extremity weakness
Anterior cord syndrome	Hyperflexion or injury to anterior spinal artery	Dense paralysis, loss of pain and temperature. Sense of touch, position, and vibration are preserved
Posterior cord syndrome	Hyperextension injury with vertebral arch fractures	Impairment of light touch, proprioception, vibratory sensation
Brown-Séquard syndrome	Hemisection of the cord from penetrating injury	Ipsilateral paralysis below the injury along with loss of position, vibration, and touch. Contralateral loss of temperature and pain
Conus medullaris syndrome	Disc rupture, prolapse, tumor at L3–S1	Loss of bladder control, impotence, saddle anesthesia, spasticity of lower extremities
Cauda equina	Lumbar disc prolapse at lower lumbar, tumors	Low back pain, radicular leg pain, saddle anesthesia, lower extremity weakness, urinary retention and fecal incontinence

Diagnosis: MRI study of choice.

Treatment: methylprednisolone (30 mg/kg bolus followed by 5.4 mg/kg/hr) for patients over 13 with acute injury and neurologic deficit (no proven benefit and may put at risk of infection and avascuar necrosis). Neurosurgical consult.

4.10. Cerebrovascular events

4.10.1. Stroke

Table 4.9 Types of strokes

Type	Cause	Presentation	Treatment
Ischemic	Atherosclerosis leads to thrombotic strokes. A-fib, septic emboli and cardiomyopathy lead to embolic strokes	80% of all strokes are ischemic Focal neurologic deficits develop over minutes to hours	With thrombolytics: keep SBP <185 mmHg, DBP <110 mmHg. Use labetalol 10–20 mg IV or NTG paste 1 inch transdermal If no thrombolytics: nitroprusside to lower DBP 10–20% and keep MAP under 130 mmHg
Intracerebral hemorrhage	Atherosclerotic disease, hypertension	Patients are usually >50 years old Focal neurologic deficits	Nitroprusside to lower SBP under 180 mmHg and DBP under 105 mmHg. Seizure prophylaxis with phenytoin. Neurosurgical consult
Subarachnoid hemorrhage	Aneurysm rupture or AVM	Patients are often <50 years old Sudden onset of symptoms, rapid progression Worst headache of life, nuchal rigidity. No lateralizing symptoms Nearly half of patients have a sentinel event	Neurosurgical consultation, pain control, nimodipine to reduce vasospasm and risk of concurrent ischemic stroke

A-fib, atrial fibrillation; AVM, arteriovenous malformation; NTG, nitroglycerin; SBP, systolic blood pressure.

Table 4.10 Inclusion and exclusion criteria for IV tPA in ischemic stroke

Inclusion criteria	Age >18 and <80 Diagnosis of ischemic stroke with measurable deficits No CT evidence of intracranial hemorrhage Onset of symptoms < 3 hours
Exclusion criteria	*Absolute contraindications* Evidence of intracranial hemorrhage High suspicion for SAH even with normal CT History of intracranial hemorrhage Uncontrolled HTN (SBP remains >185 mmHg or DBP >110 mmHg) Known AVM, neoplasm, aneurysm Witnessed seizure at onset of stroke Active internal bleeding or acute trauma such as fracture Acute bleeding tendency such as: Platelets <100 000/μL Heparin within 48 hours with elevated PTT Current anticoagulant use with INR > 1.7 or PT >15 seconds Within 3 months of cranial/spinal surgery, serious head trauma, prior stroke *Relative contraindications* – weigh risks/benefits Only minor (low NIHSS such as <5) or rapidly improving stroke symptoms Within 14 days of major trauma or surgery Within 21 days of GI or urinary hemorrhage Within 3 months of MI Post-MI pericarditis Abnormal glucose (<50 or >400 mg/dL)

GI, gastrointestinal; INR, international normalized ratio; NIHSS, National Institute of Health Stroke Scale; SAH, subarachnoid hemorrhage; tPA, tissue plasminogen activator.

4.10.2. Transient cerebral ischemia

Description: brief episode of neurologic dysfunction due to cerebral hypoperfusion. Focal deficits last less than 24 hours without residual deficits. Half of cases are thought to be due to atherosclerosis of the carotid arteries or posterior circulation. Deficits are related to affected area.

Diagnosis: clinical diagnosis with negative CT findings and resolution of symptoms.

Evaluation/treatment: ECG – evaluate for atrial fibrillation; anticoagulation may lower stroke risk. Give aspirin but rule out hemorrhagic stroke first. Cardiac echo, lipids, and carotid Dopplers as inpatient or outpatient depending on patient risk stratification and hospital capabilities.

4.11. Intracranial tumors

Etiology: 50% of intracranial neoplasms are primary and 50% are metastatic. In children neoplasms are mostly infratentorial and in adults neoplasms are mostly supratentorial. Effects of tumors due to compression, direct invasion, hydrocephalus, and increased ICP.

Presentation: varies related to location, and effect on adjacent structures. Headache and weakness often present with an indolent time course. Seizures. If patient has hearing loss and vertigo consider acoustic neuroma. If patient has bitemporal hemianopsia consider pituitary adenoma.

Diagnosis: CT and/or MRI. Not all are malignant.

Treatment: ABCs in setting of acute decompensation. Treat increased ICP and cerebral edema with mannitol, hypertonic saline, and/or steroids. Neurosurgery consult.

Bibliography

Adams HP, Jr, del Zopp G, Alberts MJ, *et al.* Guidelines for the early management of adults with ischemic stroke. *Circulation.* 2007; **116**(18): e478–e534.

Arif H, Hirsch LJ. Treatment of status epilepticus. *Semin Neurol.* 2008; **28**:342–354.

Daroff RB, *et al. Bradley's Neurology in Clinical Practice*, 6th edn. Philadelphia: Elsevier-Saunders, 2012.

Easton JD, Savers JL, Albers GW, *et al.* Definition and evaluation of transient ischemic attack. *Stroke.* 2009; **40**(6):2276–93.

Gilden DH. Clinical practice: Bell's palsy. *NEJM.* 2004; **351**(13): 1323–31.

Johnston SC, Rothwell PM, Nguyen-Huynh MN, *et al.* Validation and refinement of scores to predict very early stroke risk after transient ischaemic attack. *Lancet* 2007; **369**(9558):283–92.

Marx, JA, Hockberger RS, Walls RM, Adams J, Rosen P, eds. *Rosen's Emergency Medicine: Concepts and Clinical Practice*. Philadelphia: Mosby Elsevier, 2010.

Tintinalli JE, Stapczynski JS, Cline DM, *et al. Tintinalli's Emergency Medicine: A Comprehensive Study Guide*, 7th edn. New York: The McGraw-Hill Companies, Inc., 2011.

Chapter 5

Renal and urogenital emergencies

Guyon J. Hill and James F. Martin

5.1. Renal failure

5.1.1. Acute renal failure (ARF)

Definition: the deterioration of renal function over hours to days leading to the accumulation of toxins, metabolic derangements, and irregularities of volume status.

Clinical: diagnosis of ARF (also known as acute kidney injury or AKI) difficult in early stages because many patients are asymptomatic until the disease is severe. More common to recognize symptoms of the underlying cause. Important to identify the cause as prerenal (most common in the emergency department), intrinsic, or postrenal because many causes are easily reversible.

5.1.1.1. Prerenal

Decreased perfusion to the kidney from hypotension, volume loss, microvascular or renal artery disease.

Causes: burns, vomiting, diarrhea, hemorrhage, sepsis or other causes of excessive fluid loss or decreased fluid intake.

5.1.1.2. Intrinsic

A result of disease within the kidney itself. Can be precipitated by medications, infection, toxins, or ischemia.

Causes: nephropathy from IV contrast dye, drug-induced acute interstitial nephritis from drug reactions, papillary necrosis, glomerulonephritis, and ischemic acute kidney injury.

5.1.1.3. Postrenal

Due to a mechanical obstruction to the outflow of urine.

Causes: prostatic disease, urinary catheter obstruction, or nephrolithiasis.

Testing and diagnosis: serum chemistry, urinalysis, and urine electrolytes should be obtained. Consider an ECG when there is concern for hyperkalemia. Imaging can help rapidly identify reversible causes. Bedside renal ultrasound may be useful to detect hydronephrosis due to mechanical obstruction. Noncontrast abdominal/pelvic CT can also provide this while helping identify location and cause.

Pocket Guide to the American Board of Emergency Medicine In-Training Exam, ed. Bob Cambridge. Published by Cambridge University Press. © Cambridge University Press 2013.

Treatment: immediate treatment focuses on the underlying cause. Administration of IV fluids can treat or improve outcomes in many forms of ARF due to hypovolemia. Crystalloids are preferable to colloids. Be aware of the potential for postobstructive diuresis in the setting of prolonged obstruction.

Outcomes: most frequent causes of death associated with the diagnosis of ARF are sepsis and cardiopulmonary failure. Complete obstruction can cause a permanent loss of renal function in 10–14 days. Up to 90% of cases presenting to the emergency department have a potentially reversible cause.

5.1.2. Chronic renal failure

Gradually worsening kidney function over months to years. Usually present due to superimposed process. Hyperkalemia and volume overload are most common conditions. Condition is irreversible barring transplant. Renally dose medications when necessary, avoid IV contrast and other nephrotoxic substances when possible.

5.1.3. Complications of renal dialysis

Table 5.1 Complications of renal dialysis

Condition	Presentation	Cause	Treatment	Considerations
Hypotension	Nausea, vomiting, orthostatic hypotension, or syncope	Frequent cause is excessive ultrafiltration from underestimation of the patient's ideal blood volume (dry weight)	Halt dialysis and place the patient in Trendelenburg position. Normal saline can be given in small amounts if necessary	Most common complication of hemodialysis
Hemolysis	Shortness of breath, chest pain, or back pain	Most frequently caused by problems with dialysis solution	Stop dialysis; clamp the dialysis lines to prevent return of hyperkalemic blood. Treat hyperkalemia and possible hypotension as necessary and admit	
Arrhythmias		Rapid fluctuations in hemodynamics and electrolytes	Follows the same algorithm as in a nondialysis patient except for any renal function-based dosing	Ventricular and supraventricular arrhythmias are common in dialysis either during treatments or between
Dyspnea		Preceding dyspnea may be simply volume overload. Dyspnea during a treatment may be a result of ischemic heart disease, bacteremia, allergic reactions, or other causes	Dependent on cause	Shortness of breath that begins following the initiation of dialysis is more concerning than dyspnea beforehand

(cont.)

Table 5.1 (cont.)

Condition	Presentation	Cause	Treatment	Considerations
Chest pain		Hypotension, angina, hemolysis, dialysis disequilibrium syndrome, or air embolism	Dependent on cause	Be cautious that many of the agents used to treat angina will contribute to hypotension
Dialysis disequilibrium syndrome	Nausea, vomiting, and hypertension. Can progress to cause seizure, coma, or death and usually occurs immediately following dialysis	Theorized to be cerebral edema caused by osmolar imbalance between the blood and the brain	Stop dialysis and administer mannitol	
Air embolism	Symptoms vary based on the position of the patient. In seated patients, air enters cerebral circulation first, causing neurologic symptoms. In recumbent patients, air enters right ventricle and pulmonary circulation first, which can lead to shortness of breath, cough, or chest pain		Clamp venous line and place patient in a supine position. Administer 100% oxygen	

5.2. Glomerular disorders

5.2.1. Glomerulonephritis

Inflammatory disorders characterized by hematuria and proteinuria. Ranges from mild (asymptomatic proteinuria) to severe (nephrotic syndrome, hypertension, impaired renal function requiring renal transplant).

Causes: immune-mediated, inherited, or post-infection disorders. Due to deposition of immune complexes in the glomeruli, which cause inflammation and complement activation, leading to sclerosis and fibrosis. Most common infectious cause is β-hemolytic streptococci but also seen with staphylococcal species. Other causes include hereditary nephritis, Berger disease (immunoglobulin nephropathy), membranoproliferative diseases, Henoch–Schönlein purpura, lupus, polyarteritis, and hemolytic uremic syndrome.

Clinical features: macro- or microscopic hematuria, red cell casts, proteinuria, systemic hypertension.

5.2.2. Hemolytic uremic syndrome

Most common cause of preventable acute renal failure in childhood.

Features: microangiopathic hemolytic anemia, acute nephropathy, and thrombocytopenia.

Typical vs. atypical:
  Typical: children 1 week into case of infectious diarrhea, often bloody, without fever; attributed to Shiga toxin-producing *Escherichia coli*, O157:H7.
  Atypical: older children and adults, difficult to distinguish from thrombotic thrombocytopenic purpura (TTP) due to extrarenal involvement; attributed to *Streptococcus pneumoniae* or Epstein–Barr virus (EBV).
  Treatment: supportive. IV fluids, analgesia, RBC and platelet transfusions, hemodialysis for acute renal failure. Avoid antimotility agents and antibiotics.

5.2.3. Nephrotic syndrome

Disease of an unknown cause resulting in loss of protein in the urine. Often preceded by a viral upper respiratory infection (URI). Can be primary syndrome or caused by systemic diseases (e.g. lupus, Henoch–Schönlein purpura) or infections.

Presentation: generalized edema (most common patient complaint).
Diagnosis: hypoalbuminemia, proteinuria. Gold standard is 24-hour urine protein.
Treatment: patients in hypovolemic shock should receive isotonic fluids even in presence of severe edema. Primary treatment is oral corticosteroids although response will vary with underlying cause.
Complications: primary are infection and thromboembolic events. Corticosteroids used in therapy increase risk of infection and coagulation factors are lost as protein in urine.

5.2.4. Renal tubular acidosis

Accumulation of acid in the body due to failure of kidney to acidify the urine.

Four types: distal, proximal, combined, adrenal.

Table 5.2 Types of renal tubular acidosis

Type	Location of defect	Cause	Lab abnormalities	Clinical issues
Type 1	Distal tubule	Failure of hydrogen ion secretion by α-intercalated cells	Hypokalemia, normal anion gap metabolic acidosis	Kidney stone formation, rickets, osteomalacia
Type 2	Proximal tubule	Failure of bicarbonate reabsorption by proximal tubular cells	Hypokalemia, phosphaturia, mild urinary acidification	Seen most often as part of Fanconi's syndrome (osteomalacia from phosphate wasting, glucose wasting, uric acid loss)
Type 3	Combined 1 and 2	Combined 1 and 2		Very rare
Type 4	Adrenal	Aldosterone deficiency or resistance to aldosterone effects	Hyperkalemia	Seen with drug use: spironolactone, trimethoprim, and more

5.3. Infection of urinary tract

5.3.1. Cystitis

Inflammation of bladder most commonly caused by a bacterial infection (urinary tract infection [UTI]) but that can also have other etiologies.

Symptoms: urgency, dysuria, suprapubic pressure, increased frequency, and hematuria.
Treatment: based on cause.

5.3.2. Urinary tract infection (UTI)

Infection of the lower urinary tract.

Uncomplicated UTI: occurring in a healthy, non-pregnant female with normal anatomy.
Complicated UTI: occurring in male patients, immunocompromised, pregnant women, structural or functional irregularities, extremes of age.
Diagnosis: positive leukocyte esterase, positive nitrite, or WBCs on urinalysis. Send urine culture on all children or patients with potential for complicated UTIs. Catheterized specimens should be obtained in infants and young children.
Cause: *E. coli* is predominant organism in uncomplicated but complicated UTIs could be caused by all manner of bacteria or fungi.
Treatment: for uncomplicated UTI treatment options include nitrofurantoin (5-day course), fosfomycin (single dose), or fluoroquinolones (3-day course). For complicated UTI treat for 5–14 days with a fluoroquinolone.
Complications: recurrent UTI, bacteremia, sepsis, pyelonephritis, renal abscess. Long-term complications can include renal scarring, renal failure, and papillary necrosis. Neonates, infants, and young children may need to be screened for structural abnormalities.

5.3.3. Pyelonephritis

Infection of the upper urinary tract that usually progresses from a UTI as an ascending infection.

Presentation: urinary symptoms plus costovertebral angle (CVA) tenderness, fever, chills, nausea, and vomiting.
Diagnosis: urinalysis findings are similar to those in UTIs with the possible addition of WBC casts. Urine cultures should be sent on all patients with suspected pyelonephritis. Patients may need CT imaging to rule out renal abscess or emphysematous pyelonephritis or renal abscess.
Treatment: most patients are candidates for outpatient management. Fluoroquinolones are the only recommended outpatient antibiotic for empiric therapy. Duration of therapy is 7 days. Other antibiotics can be used after susceptibility data are available. If clinical concern for additional decompensation, admit patient for IV antibiotics and IV rehydration.

5.4. Structural disorders of urinary tract

5.4.1. Calculus of urinary tract

First occurrence usually at age 30; rare after age 60, 7% under 16 years old.

Cause: urine saturation with solutes, lack of inhibitory substances, urinary stasis. Medication causes include indinavir sulfate, carbonic anhydrase inhibitors, triamterene, laxatives.
Stone composition: 75–80% are calcium often combined with oxalate and/or phosphate. 10–15% are struvite (magnesium-ammonium-phosphate) and are due to infection by urea-splitting bacteria. 10% are uric acid (due to gout). Cystine stones are rare (1%).

Probability of passage: depends on size, shape, location, and ureteral caliber. 98% of stones smaller than 5 mm, 60% of stones 5–7 mm, and 39% of stones greater than 7 mm pass within 4 weeks without intervention.

Common areas of obstruction: ureterovesicular junction (most common), pelvic brim, ureteropelvic junction.

Presentation: colicky flank pain radiating to the groin, nausea, vomiting, CVA tenderness. 85% have hematuria.

Diagnosis: urinalysis to evaluate for infection, kidney dysfunction, pregnancy, and hematuria (however, 24% of flank pain + hematuria have no radiographic stone). CT is sensitive and specific and is the study of choice. IV urography (pyelogram) can delineate renal anatomy and function. Plain abdominal radiographs are neither sensitive nor specific enough to rule the diagnosis in or out. Ultrasound is useful for determining hydronephrosis.

Treatment: pain and nausea control, antibiotics for concomitant infection, peripherally acting α-blocker (tamsulosin), urology referral. Average passage for 5–6 mm stone without treatment is 7 to 20 days.

5.4.2. Obstructive uropathy

Pain from pressure of hydronephrosis due to obstruction of ureter. In acute ureteral obstruction, renal blood flow (RBF) and renal pelvic pressure (RPP) increase. Within 4 hours, RBF normalizes, but RPP remains high. If obstruction remains long term, RBF will decrease below baseline, and RPP will remain high. If unrelieved, irreversible renal damage in 3 weeks of complete obstruction.

During acute obstruction, there is no rise in creatinine. Unaffected kidney compensates up to 185% of baseline capacity.

5.5 Male genital tract

5.5.1. Inflammation/infection

5.5.1.1. Balanitis/balanoposthitis

Balanitis: inflammation of glans penis.

Balanoposthitis: inflammation of glans and foreskin.

Cause: inadequate hygiene or external irritation. *Candida*, *Gardnerella*, and anaerobes potential causes.

Presentation: glans and apposing prepuce are purulent, excoriated, erythematous, edematous, malodorous, tender.

Treatment: soap, dry the area, antifungal creams, oral azole, and occasionally circumcision. If bacterial infection suspected, broad spectrum first- or second-generation cephalosporin.

5.5.1.2. Epididymitis

Symptoms: gradual onset, lower abdominal, inguinal, scrotal, or testicular pain. May have reduced pain with scrotal elevation (Prehn sign).

Cause: commonly bacterial in origin; type due to age.

Young boys: sterile reflux, coliform bacteria, often congenital abnormalities of lower urinary tract.

Men <40: sexually transmitted diseases, or associated problems (urethral stricture).

Men >40: urinary pathogens such as *E. coli* and *Klebsiella*.

Diagnosis: tender, retro-testicular scrotal mass, initially located at globus minor, but can be larger due to inflammation. 50% have pyuria. Ultrasound with normal testicular blood flow, can also show a reactive hydrocele.

Treatment: outpatient (most cases). 14 days of age-appropriate antibiotics. Admission if fever and clinical toxicity, suggestive of possible abscess. Scrotal support.

5.5.1.3. Orchitis

Symptoms: isolated inflammation of testicle, tenderness and swelling of couple days duration.

Causes: Bacterial orchitis almost always associated with epididymitis. Also consider mumps as possible cause, although less common in immunized population.

Treatment: pathogen specific as above.

5.5.1.4. Gangrene of the scrotum (Fournier's gangrene)

Cause: polymicrobial necrotizing fasciitis of perineal, genital, or perianal area. Microthrombosis of subcutaneous vessels, leading to gangrene of overlying skin. Usually spares testicles. Overall mortality approximately 40%.

Predisposing conditions: immunocompromised from diabetes (20–70%), alcoholism (25–50%).

Signs and symptoms: localized severe pain and swelling, crepitus, ecchymosis.

Treatment: fluid resuscitation, broad spectrum antibiotic coverage, surgical debridement, hyperbaric oxygen.

5.5.1.5. Prostatitis

Bacterial inflammation of prostate.

Symptoms: low back pain; perineal, suprapubic, genital discomfort; urinary symptoms; pain with ejaculation; fever; chills. Perianal tenderness, rectal sphincter spasm, prostatic tenderness or bogginess.

Risk factors: anatomic or neurophysiologic lower urinary tract obstruction; acute epididymitis or urethritis, unprotected rectal intercourse, phimosis, intraprostatic ductal reflux, indwelling urethral catheter.

Causes: *E. coli* (majority), pseudomonas, *Klebsiella*, *Enterobacter*, *Serratia*, *Staphylococcus*.

Diagnosis: clinical diagnosis, as urinalysis and culture may be negative.

Treatment: antibiotics for 14–30 days. Needs antibiotic with good prostate penetration (ciprofloxacin, trimethoprim-sulfamethoxazole).

5.5.1.6. Urethritis

Symptoms: purulent urethral discharge.

Diagnosis: clinical diagnosis, but able to confirm with pyuria or bacteriuria on first-void urine specimen.

Cause: usually due to *Neisseria gonorrhoeae* or *Chlamydia*; also herpes simplex, *Ureaplasma*, and *Trichomonas*.

Treatment: appropriate antibiotics or antiviral medications.

5.5.2. Structural disorders

5.5.2.1. Phimosis

Inability to retract foreskin proximally, over the glans penis.

Causes: infection, poor hygiene, injury or scarring.

Treatment: topical steroid for 4–6 weeks. Definitive cure is circumcision.

5.5.2.2. Paraphimosis

Inability to reduce a retracted foreskin distally. True urologic emergency as inhibition of blood flow to glans leads to necrosis.

Treatment: analgesia (topical or ring block at base of penis), oral anxiolytics. Compression of glans for several minutes, using fingertips or elastic bandage, with resultant retraction of foreskin. Trephinate glans (22 G or 25 G needle) to allow expression of edema fluid. Dorsally incise constricting band.

5.5.2.3. Priapism

Persistent, painful, pathologic erection. Can cause urinary retention. 35% of cases result in impotence.

Causes: impotence medications (intracavernosal injections, oral erectile dysfunction), antihypertensive medications (hydralazine, calcium channel blockers), mental health medications (chlorpromazine, trazadone, thioridazine), hematologic disorders (sickle cell).

Treatment: analgesia, terbutaline (0.25–0.5 mg SC in deltoid, repeat in 20–30 minutes), corporal aspiration followed by irrigation, transfusion (for sickle cell).

5.5.2.4. Torsion of testis

Emergency consideration for scrotal pain, due to potential for infarction and infertility.

Epidemiology and pathophysiology: incidence = 1 in 400 males under age 25 (annually). Occurs from abnormal fixation of the testes in the tunica vaginalis. Allows testes to twist, especially with growth or minor trauma; however, only 4– 8% associated with trauma.

Symptoms: acute, severe, lower abdominal, inguinal, or testis pain. Not positional, as pain is due to infarction secondary to ischemia.

Diagnosis: early examination, testis is firm, tender, often horizontal lie (rather than vertical), and elevated compared to contralateral side. Most sensitive finding (99% sensitive) is absence of cremasteric reflex on affected side. Ultrasound shows diagnosis with lack of blood flow seen on Doppler. Radionuclide scintigraphy can also be done.

Treatment: salvage is related to duration of symptoms before surgical correction. Excellent prognosis if onset is less than 6 hours; prognosis for testicle salvage rapidly decreases thereafter. Emergent urologic consult is needed. Manual detorsion can be attempted in emergency department. Performed with a medial-to-lateral motion ("opening a book"). Initial attempt should be 1 and ½ rotations. If pain worsens, attempt opposite rotation.

6

Endocrine, metabolic, and nutritional emergencies

Selina Jeanise

6.1. Fluid and electrolyte disturbances [1]

6.1.1. Calcium metabolism

Adult body contains about 1200 g of calcium. 99% in bone; remaining 1% about 50% bound to serum proteins, 10% complexed to anions, and 40% is in free ionized state. 10% of calcium that is reabsorbed in the kidneys is under the control of PTH. Serum calcium decreases, PTH stimulates increase in bone turnover and calcium is released. A rise in calcium stimulates calcitonin release and decreases parathyroid hormone (PTH) levels to decrease serum calcium.

6.1.1.1. Hypocalcemia

Four broad causes: PTH insufficiency, vitamin D insufficiency, PTH resistance, calcium chelation.

Findings of severe hypocalcemia: decreased cardiac contractility, bradycardia, hypotension, and symptomatic congestive heart failure (CHF). ECG is a poor predictor.

Signs and symptoms: anxiety, depression, psychosis, dementia. Declining calcium levels are associated with progressive neuromuscular hyperexcitability.

Chvostek's or Trousseau's sign: tetany associated with hypocalcemia. Chvostek's is elicited by tapping over the facial nerve, causing twitching of ipsilateral facial muscles. Trousseau's is carpal spasm caused by inflating a blood pressure cuff to 20 mmHg above systolic blood pressure (SBP) for 3 minutes.

Management: verify ionized calcium levels. If severe symptoms, initiate treatment prior to obtaining confirmatory levels.

> **Calcium chloride 10%:** 10 mL ampules contain 360 mg of elemental calcium.
> **Calcium gluconate 10%:** 10 mL ampules contain 93 mg of elemental calcium.

6.1.1.2. Hypercalcemia

Usually mild (<12 mg/dL) and asymptomatic.

Hypercalcemic crisis: levels >14 mg/dL usually associated with significant signs and symptoms.

Most common cause of hypercalcemia: primary hyperparathyroidism, often due to parathyroid adenoma, parathyroid hyperplasia, or parathyroid carcinoma. Malignancy is the most common cause in hospitalized patients.

Pocket Guide to the American Board of Emergency Medicine In-Training Exam, ed. Bob Cambridge. Published by Cambridge University Press. © Cambridge University Press 2013.

Signs and symptoms: very nonspecific. Fatigue, weakness, confusion, ataxia, coma, hypertension, sinus bradycardia, polyuria, polydipsia, dehydration, prerenal azotemia, nephrolithiasis, nausea, vomiting, constipation, ileus.

ECG findings: short QT, bundle branch block, AV block.

Treatment: IV fluid hydration and restore intravascular volume. Diuresis to enhance renal excretion of calcium. Treatment of the primary disorder.

6.1.2. Hyperkalemia/hypokalemia [1]

The adult human has between 2500 and 3500 mmol of potassium, 98% is intracellular. The normal range of serum potassium is between 3.5 and 5.0 mEq/L.

6.1.2.1. Hypokalemia

Relatively common, but life-threatening hypokalemia is uncommon.

Cause: decreased potassium intake, increased excretion, or cellular shifts.

Clinical manifestations: neuromuscular, cardiovascular, gastrointestinal (GI), renal system, and affects acid–base balance. Symptoms occur when levels fall below 2.5 mEq/L.

Treatment: IV or PO replacement.

6.1.2.2. Hyperkalemia

Cause: may be the result of increased potassium intake, enhanced potassium absorption, impaired potassium excretion, or shifts out of cells. First consideration with hyperkalemia is to determine if it is a false elevation due to laboratory error (hemolysis).

Signs: cardiovascular and neurological dysfunction are the primary manifestations of hyperkalemia.

ECG changes:

> **Moderate to high levels:** peaked T waves, QTc shortening, QRS widening, PR prolongation, decreased P wave amplitude.
>
> **Extremely high levels:** loss of P waves, right bundle branch block (RBBB) or left bundle branch block (LBBB) pattern, rhythm appears as sinusoidal waves, ventricular tachycardia, ventricular fibrillation, asystole.

Treatment: cardiac monitoring. Mnemonic: "C A BIG K Drop." Calcium chloride or calcium gluconate for cardiac stabilization, albuterol nebulizer, bicarbonate (50 mEq of sodium bicarbonate), insulin (10 units of regular insulin IV), glucose (1 ampule of D50 IV), kayexalate, dialysis. Treat underlying cause.

6.1.3. Hypernatremia/hyponatremia [1]

6.1.3.1. Hyponatremia

Serum sodium of less than 135 mEq/L.

Symptoms: lethargy, apathy, confusion, disorientation, agitation, depression, and psychosis. Focal deficits include ataxia and seizures. Other nonspecific signs and symptoms include muscle cramps, anorexia, nausea, and weakness.

Severe symptomatic hyponatremia: may require 3% normal saline. The sodium level should not be corrected to above 120 mEq/L or increased by more than 10 mEq/L in a 24-hour period to avoid central pontine myelinolysis.

Three categories:

6.1.3.1.1. Hypovolemic

Loss of both water and sodium with a larger relative loss of sodium.

Cause: may be due to vomiting, diarrhea, GI suction or drains, fistulas, and third spacing of fluids in burns, intra-abdominal sepsis, bowel obstructions, and pancreatitis. Renal causes include diuretic use, mineralocorticoid deficiency, renal tubular acidosis, and salt-wasting nephropathy.

Treatment: correct with isotonic saline (normal saline 0.9%).

6.1.3.1.2. Euvolemic

Cause: include syndrome of inappropriate antidiuretic hormone secretion (SIADH) which may be due to central nervous system (CNS) disorders, pulmonary disease, drugs, stress, pain, and surgery. Most often seen in psychiatric disorders when patients drink large amounts of water.

Treatment: restrict free water intake.

6.1.3.1.3. Hypervolemic

Occurs when sodium is retained but more water is retained than sodium. Seen with CHF, hepatic cirrhosis, and renal failure.

Treatment: fluid restriction, with possible addition of diuretics.

6.1.3.2. Hypernatremia

Serum sodium above 145 mEq/L.

Three categories:

> **Hypovolemic:** caused by diarrhea, vomiting, fistulas, diuretics, postobstructive diuresis. In all cases water is lost faster than sodium.
> **Euvolemic:** hyperventilation, diabetes insipidus.
> **Hypervolemic:** iatrogenic administration of hypertonic saline or sodium bicarbonate, mineralocorticoid excess as in Cushing's syndrome. In these cases sodium gains are greater than water gains.

Symptoms: anorexia, nausea, vomiting, fatigue, and irritability. Physical findings include lethargy, confusion, stupor, coma, muscle twitching, hyper-reflexia, spasticity, tremor, ataxia, or focal findings such as hemiparesis or extensor-plantar reflexes.

Treatment: do not correct faster than 1 mEq/L per hour. Free water deficit can be made up with D5W, or excess fluid can be removed in time with fluid restriction.

6.1.4. Magnesium metabolism [1]

6.1.4.1. Hypomagnesemia

One of the most common electrolyte deficiencies, often associated with hypokalemia.

Symptoms: nonspecific and inconsistent. Life-threatening signs include dysrhythmias and seizures.

Treatment: replace with or without symptoms if levels are less than 1.2 mg/dL. 2–4 g magnesium sulfate IV can be given over 30–60 minutes.

6.1.4.2. Hypermagnesemia

Rare due to the ability of the kidneys to excrete large amounts of magnesium. Elevated magnesium is almost always associated with renal insufficiency.

Symptoms: directly correlate with the levels

3mg/dL: nausea, vomiting, weakness, and cutaneous flushing.

Above 4mg/dL: hyporeflexia and decreased deep tendon reflexes.

5–6 mg/dL: hypotension and ECG changes such as QRS widening, QT prolongation, and PR prolongation.

Above 9 mg/dL: coma, respiratory depression, and complete heart block.

Treatment: discontinue all exogenous magnesium. Mild elevation requires observation. Moderate elevation should be treated with IV fluids and IV lasix. Severely elevated magnesium levels should be treated with IV calcium. Start with 100–200 mg of either 10% calcium gluconate (1 ampule contains 93 mg) or 10% calcium chloride (1 ampule contains 360 mg).

6.1.5. Phosphorus metabolism [1]

Essential component for ATP synthesis.

6.1.5.1. Hypophosphatemia

Mild 2.5–2.8 mg/dL, moderate 1.0–2.5 mg/dL, or severe <1.0 mg/dL.

Causes: renal loss (most commonly from diuretic use); glucocorticoid use; diabetic ketoacidosis (DKA); hyperglycemic hyperosmolar nonketotic coma (HHNC); insufficient intestinal absorption because of increased intake/starvation, vitamin D deficiency, chronic diarrhea, and nasogastric (NG) suctioning; respiratory alkalosis; sepsis; salicylate poisoning; hepatic encephalopathy.

Clinical presentation: signs and symptoms are most often due to inadequate ATP production resulting in fatigue, myocardial depression, hypotension, impaired pressor response, and ventricular dysrhythmias.

Treatment: mild or moderate may be treated with oral supplements. Severe hypophosphatemia is treated with IV phosphate.

6.1.5.2. Hyperphosphatemia

>5 mg/dL, rare in patients with normal renal function. May be due to decreased clearance (most often due to renal failure), increased endogenous load, or increased exogenous load.

Pseudohyperphosphatemia: may be caused by analytic methods; when clinically feasible confirm with repeat labs.

Clinical presentation: most often reflect associated hypocalcemia. Paresthesias, hyper-reflexia, tetany, myocardial depression (hypotension, bradycardia, left ventricular [LV] dysfunction), as well as acute heart block and death.

Treatment: supportive care and treatment of symptomatic hypocalcemia. In patients with normal renal clearance infuse isotonic saline to increase phosphate clearance. Dextrose and insulin to help drive phosphate into cells may be used as a temporizing measure. Aluminum-containing antacids are the mainstay of therapy to prevent hyperphosphatemia in chronic renal failure. In life-threatening situations, consider hemodialysis.

6.2. Glucose metabolism [2]

6.2.1. Diabetes mellitus (DM)

Most common endocrine disease. Diagnosed with random blood glucose >200 mg/dL or fasting blood glucose >140 mg/dL.

DM classifications

Type 1: abrupt failure of production of insulin with tendency to ketosis.

Type 2: low, normal, or elevated levels of insulin with development of insulin resistance, rarely develops ketosis.

6.2.2. Diabetic ketoacidosis (DKA)

Syndrome in which insulin deficiency and glucagon excess combine to produce a hyperglycemic, dehydrated, acidotic patient with profound electrolyte imbalance and some level of serum ketosis and/or ketonuria.

Causes: most common precipitating factor is infection. However, noncompliance with treatment, stroke, MI, pregnancy, hyperthyroidism, pancreatitis, and pulmonary embolism (PE) are also common precipitants.

Clinical presentation: polydipsia, polyuria, polyphagia, altered mental status, weakness, coma, headache, nausea/vomiting, and abdominal pain. Patient may exhibit Kussmaul's respirations and have "fruity smelling breath."

Evaluation and diagnosis: glucose >350 mg/dL, ketonemia and ketonuria, pH < 7.3, bicarbonate <15 mEq/L.

Treatment: 1–2 liters normal saline over first hour (children 20 mL/kg over first hour).

    Insulin: consider bolus of 0.1 U/kg regular insulin, then start a drip at 0.05–0.1 U/kg/hr. When glucose is under 300 mg/kL change maintenance fluid to D5W ½ normal saline.

    Correct acidosis: if pH is under 7.1, add 44–88 mEq/L of bicarbonate to first liter of IV fluids.

    Potassium replacement: if potassium >5 mEq/L then no replacement. If potassium <5 mEq/L then add 10 mEq/hr to IV fluids. Goal is a potassium of 4–5 mEq/L.

Complications: cerebral edema. Higher risk in young, and new-onset diabetics that receive excessive fluids.

    Treatment of cerebral edema: mannitol, elevate head of bed 30 degrees, intubate, and mildly hyperventilate.

6.2.3. Hyperglycemic hyperosmolar nonketotic coma (HHNC) [2]

Etiology: poorly controlled DM II.

Clinical presentation: altered mental status, seizure, coma. Patients are severely volume depleted.

Lab findings: glucose >600 mg/dL, osmolarity >315 mOsm/L, minimal acidosis and low to no ketones.

Treatment: aggressive IV fluid replacement (normal saline initially, then switch to ½ normal saline when hemodynamically stable with good urine output). Add D5 when glucose is under 300 mg/dL. Replace half of fluid deficit in first 8 hours and the remainder over 24 hours. Treatment with insulin, potassium are the same as with DKA. Treatment of acidosis begins when pH is under 7.0 with a goal of 7.1.

6.2.4. Hypoglycemia [2]

Clinical features: symptoms occur at blood glucose level 40–50 mg/dL. Sweating, shakiness, anxiety, nausea, dizziness, confusion, slurred speech, blurred vision, headache, hemiplegia, seizure, decerebrate posturing, lethargy, and coma.

Diagnosis: glucose level and clinical presentation.

Treatment: correct serum glucose IV or PO. For IV administration give D50 for adults, 2 mL/kg of D25W for children, and 5 mL/kg of D10W for infants. If unable to obtain IV access give 1–2 mg glucagon IM or SC; may repeat in 20 minutes.

6.3. Thyroid and parathyroid disorders [2]

6.3.1. Thyroid disorders

6.3.1.1. Hyperthyroidism/thyroid storm

Thyroid storm is a rare life-threatening disease that is most commonly seen in Graves' disease and is usually precipitated by a stressful event.

Symptoms: increased sympathetic nervous system adrenergic effects, causing fever, tachycardia, altered mental status, diaphoresis.

Clinical presentation: history of hyperthyroidism, with complaints of diarrhea, weight loss, proximal muscle weakness.

Physical exam findings: exophthalmos, widened pulse pressure, atrial fibrillation (A-fib), CHF, premature ventricular contractions (PVCs). The elderly may be lethargic with decreased mentation and have an apathetic facies.

Diagnostic criteria: fever, tachycardia out of proportion of fever, CNS dysfunction, cardiac or GI symptoms, exaggerated peripheral manifestations of thyrotoxicosis.

Confirmation of diagnosis: increased T4 and decreased thyroid-stimulating hormone (TSH).

Treatment:

1. **Beta-adrenergic blockade:** Propanolol 5 mg IV then 5 mg/hr and titrate for effect. Alternatively use reserpine (if β-blocker contraindicated).
2. **Inhibit synthesis:** propylthiouracil (PTU) 1000 mg PO then 250 mg Q4 hours. Alternatively, give methimazole 100 mg PO loading dose then 20 mg Q4 hours.
3. **Inhibit thyroid hormone release:** saturated solution potassium iodide 8 drops PO Q6 hours OR Lugol's solution 8 gtt PO, NG, or PR Q6 hours OR sodium iodide 500 mg in solution Q12 hours, OR if allergic to iodine, lithium carbonate 300 mg PO or NG Q6 hours.
4. **Inhibit T3 to T4 conversion/treat adrenal insufficiency:** hydrocortisone 300 mg IV then 100 mg Q6 hours OR dexamethasone 2–4 mg IV Q6 hours.
5. **Supportive:** IV fluid, antipyretics, cooling blankets, fans, ice packs, ice lavage. Lorazepam or diazepam as anxiolytic and to decrease central sympathetic outflow.

6.3.1.2. Acute thyroiditis

Thyrotoxic phase of subacute thyroiditis or painless thyroiditis. Acute cause is often bacterial infection.

If painful: other causes include viral infection or granulomatous disease (de Quervain's thyroiditis; associated with fever and increased erythrocyte sedimentation rate [ESR]).

If silent: causes include post-partum state, autoimmune or subacute lymphocytic thyroiditis.

Treatment: NSAIDs, aspirin, steroids.

6.3.2. Hypothyroidism

6.3.2.1. Myxedema coma

Severe, life-threatening hypothyroidism.

Symptoms: fatigue, weakness, cold intolerance, constipation, weight gain, and deepening of voice. Dry, scaly skin, nonpitting waxy edema of face and extremities, and thinning eyebrows.

Signs: parasthesia, ataxia and increased deep tendon reflexes, hypothermia, hyponatremia, hypoglycemia, hypotension, altered mental status.

ECG findings: bradycardia and decreased voltage.

Treatment: ABCs, warming, hypertonic fluid and furosemide for severe cases. Hydrocortisone 100 mg IV Q8 hours. Levothyroxine 300–500 mcg IV or L-triiodothyronine 25 mcg.

6.3.3. Thyroid tumors

Can be benign or malignant. Adenomas are almost always benign but can secrete thyroid hormone that is not under control of TSH. May be asymptomatic or symptomatic. Symptoms are same as hyperthyroidism and require the same emergent treatment.

6.3.4. Parathyroid disease

PTH increases calcium levels and decreases phosphorus levels.

6.3.4.1. Hyperparathyroid disease

Most common cause of elevated serum calcium. Hyperparathyroidism increases the production of PTH, causing hypercalcemia.

Cause: due to parathyroid adenomas or hyperplasia, or can be secondary to malignancy.

Treatment: Surgery versus medical surveillance.

6.3.4.2. Hypoparathyroidism

PTH insufficiency is either primary or secondary. Secondary is most common and is most often iatrogenic from removal of or disruption of the blood supply of the parathyroid glands, resulting most often in hypocalcemia.

Treatment: calcium and vitamin D supplementation.

6.4. Pituitary disorders and adrenal disorders [2]

6.4.1. Pituitary dysfunction

6.4.1.1. Anterior pituitary

Master gland that along with hypothalamus regulates the activity of many other endocrine glands. The anterior pituitary gland produces prolactin (PRL), growth hormone (GH), adrenocorticotropic hormone (ACTH), luteinizing hormone (LH), follicle-stimulating hormone (FSH), TSH.

6.4.1.2. Posterior pituitary

Secretes oxytocin and vasopressin. When not functioning, patient presents with polyuria and polydipsia reflecting loss of vasopressin secretion.

6.4.1.3. Panhypopituitarism

Etiology: surgery, radiation, tumors, infection, infiltration, autoimmune, ischemia, carotid aneurysms, cavernous sinus thrombosis, and trauma.
Deficiency effects:

TSH deficiency can cause hypothyroidism.
Gonadotropin deficiency can cause menstrual disorders.
ACTH deficiency can cause relative hypocortisolism with relative preservation of mineralocorticoids.
PRL deficiency causes failure of lactation.
GH deficiency can cause growth retardation in children and abnormal body composition in adults.

6.4.2. Pituitary tumors

Most are benign and do not cause symptoms. Often symptoms are from mass effect and include the following: headache, visual changes, decreased sense of smell, nasal drainage, and lethargy.

6.4.3. Adrenal disease [1]

6.4.3.1. Adrenal insufficiency (Addison's disease)

Adrenal glands are not producing enough steroid hormones.

Causes: adrenal dysgenesis, impaired hormone production, adrenal damage (autoimmune or trauma), steroid medication withdrawal.
Presentation: weakness, dehydration, hypotension, anorexia, nausea, vomiting, weight loss, and abdominal pain. Severe cases are considered Addisonian crisis.
Diagnosis: cosyntropin stimulation test. Draw baseline cortisol, give cosyntropin 0.25 mg IM/IV then repeat cortisol level in 1 hour (then 4, 8, and 24 hours). If persistently low, the problem is primary adrenal insufficiency. If levels are delayed in rising, then the problem is secondary insufficiency.
Treatment: replacement of steroids. If in crisis, give hydrocortisone IV and fluid boluses.

6.4.3.2. Cushing's disease [2]

Elevated levels of cortisol.

Presentation: central obesity, extremity wasting, back fat, rounded facies, bruising, proximal myopathy, wide striae, hypokalemia.

Diagnosis: dexamethasone suppression test. Measure ACTH and cortisol levels after low-dose and high-dose dexamethasone administration.

Table 6.1 Interpretation of dexamethasone suppression test

ACTH level	Cortisol level	Interpretation
Undetectable or low	Level not suppressed by high or low doses	Primary adrenal Cushing's syndrome
Normal to elevated	Level not suppressed by high or low doses	Ectopic ACTH source
Suppressed	Level not suppressed by low doses, but suppressed by high doses	Cushing's disease

6.4.4. Adrenal tumors

6.4.4.1. Pheochromocytoma

Catecholamine-secreting tumor.

Clinical presentation: hypertension, arrhythmias, tachycardia.

5 Ps: pressure, pain, palpitations, perspiration, and pallor.

Lab findings: hyperglycemia, hypercalcemia, erythrocytosis; diagnostic lab test is plasma metanephrine levels.

Treatment: first α-blockade then β–blockade; definitive treatment is surgical resection.

6.5. Nutritional disorders [1]

6.5.1. Wernicke–Korsakoff syndrome (WKS)

Medical emergency with mortality rate 10–20% that is often unrecognized. Thiamine-dependent enzyme, transketolase, is deficient or less active in many patients.

6.5.1.1. Korsakoff psychosis

Amnesic state, also known as ethanol-induced persisting amnestic disorder. Disorder with recent memory impairment, inability to learn new things, apathy and confabulation. Increased risk in patients over 40 and in those with many years of heavy ethanol abuse.

Diagnostic criteria for WKS: dietary deficiency, oculomotor abnormalities, cerebellar dysfunction, altered mental status or mild memory impairment.

Treatment: alcoholics with altered mental status should be treated, regardless of the above criteria. Give thiamine 100 mg IV, obtain rapid blood glucose for glucose level or give empiric dextrose 25 g IV, correct all electrolyte abnormalities.

References

1. Marx, JA, Hockberger RS, Walls RM, Adams J, Rosen P, eds. *Rosen's Emergency Medicine: Concepts and Clinical Practice*. Philadelphia: Mosby Elsevier, 2010.

2. Fauci, Kasper D, Longo DL, *et al. Harrison's Principles of Internal Medicine*. 14th edn. New York: McGraw-Hill Health Professions Division, 1998.

Bibliography

Agile Partners. *The Merck Manual: The Professional Edition*. West Point: Merck, 2009.

O. John Ma, *et al. Emergency Medicine Manual*. 6th edn. New York: McGraw-Hill, 2004.

Chapter 7

Trauma emergencies

Rose Haisler and Theodor Schmidt

7.1. Trauma basics

7.1.1. Mortality and trauma

7.1.1.1. Trimodal death distribution [1 p. 5]

First peak: 50%. Seconds to minutes after injury. Only prevention of the injury is effective.
Second peak: 30%. Minutes to several hours after injury (the so-called "golden hour" of care). Advanced Trauma Life Support (ATLS) protocol vital in assessing and treating injuries. The emergency department physician plays a critical role in community hospitals. Tertiary facilities typically have trauma services on call.
Third peak: 15%. Several days to weeks after injury. Often due to multiple system organ failure or sepsis.

7.1.2. Trauma center designations

Level I: all essential specialties/services available, all available in-house, all available 24/7.
Level II: most specialties/services available, most available in-house, most available 24/7.
Level III: some specialist available, available 24/7, resources available for resuscitation, surgery and intensive care unit (ICU).
Level IV: capable of preliminary trauma treatment, all except the most "simple" traumas transferred.

7.1.3. Primary survey ("ABCDEs")

A: Assess Airway with C-spine precautions.
Secure airway if: Glasgow Coma Scale (GCS) <8, severe shock, significant airway burn, concern for progressive airway obstruction in the setting of penetrating injuries to the neck or face.
B: Breathing and ventilation.
Assess presence/adequacy of respirations. Provide supplemental oxygen.
C: Circulation with hemorrhage control.
Control killer bleeds – external hemorrhage is identified and controlled by direct pressure or other means.
D: Disability (neurologic status).

Evaluate mental status. Common tools include AVPU responsiveness scale and Glasgow Coma Scale.

AVPU responsiveness scale: Alert and responsive; Verbal stimuli response; Painful stimuli response; Unresponsive.

GCS: see Table 7.1.

E: Exposure/Environmental control.

Completely undress patient, but keep warm with blankets and ideally have a dedicated trauma bay room with elevated temperature.

Table 7.1 GCS calculation

Eye opening	4	Spontaneous
	3	To voice
	2	To pain
	1	No response
Verbal	5	Oriented and alert
	4	Disoriented
	3	Nonsensical speech
	2	Moaning, unintelligible
	1	No response
Motor	6	Follows commands
	5	Localizes to pain
	4	Withdraws to pain
	3	Decorticate posturing
	2	Decerebrate posturing
	1	No response

7.1.4. Secondary survey ("head-to-toe exam")

Perform detailed head-to-toe physical exam:

Obtain AMPLE history if possible (Allergies, Medications, Past medical history/Pregnancy status, Last meal/Last menstrual period and Events leading up to injury/illness/injury mechanism).

7.2. Shock

7.2.1. Hemorrhagic

Hypovolemia from blood loss is the most common cause in the trauma patient.

Table 7.2 Blood loss characteristics by amount

	Class I	Class II	Class III	Class IV
Blood loss (mL)	<750	750–1500	1500–2000	>2000
Blood loss (% blood volume)	<15%	15–30%	30–40%	>40%
HR (bpm)	<100	100–120	120–140	>140
Pulse pressure (mmHg)	Normal or elevated	Decreased	Decreased	Decreased
RR (breathes per minute)	14–20	20–30	30–40	>40
Urine output (mL/hr)	>30	20–30	5–15	Minimal
Mental status	Slightly anxious	Mildly anxious	Anxious, confused	Confused, lethargic
Fluid replacement	Crystalloid	Crystalloid	Crystalloid and blood	Crystalloid and blood

RR, respiratory rate.

Estimating fluid/blood loss: adult blood volume: 7% body weight or 7 mL/kg (i.e. 70 kg has ~5 L blood). Pediatric blood volume: 8–9% body weight or 80–90 mL/kg.

Treatment: when large volumes of fluids are needed, give 3 to 1 ratio of crystalloid to blood loss. Give type-specific and crossmatched blood if needed for class II. Give type-specific blood for class III. Give type O blood for class IV. Type O blood is universal donor. Rh negative should be given to premenopausal females and children. Rh positive can be used in men and postmenopausal women.

7.2.2. Non-hemorrhagic shock in trauma

7.2.2.1. Spinal shock

Loss of neurologic function and autonomic tone below the level of a spinal cord lesion. Usually occurs with spinal cord injuries C6 or higher. Can mask hemorrhagic shock.

In patient with spine fracture but no neurologic deficits shock is more likely to be hemorrhagic.

Presentation: flaccid paralysis with loss of sensation, urinary incontinence, loss of deep tendon reflexes, and bradycardia, hypotension, hypothermia.

7.2.2.2. Shock secondary to cardiac output obstruction

Cardiac tamponade, tension pneumothorax/massive hemothorax.

7.2.2.3. Pump malfunction

Myocardial contusion/dysrhythmia, structural cardiac damage (penetrating trauma, traumatic papillary muscle rupture).

7.2.3. Shock assessment

Follow the response to fluids through vital signs, capillary refill, pulses, and urine output. Normal urine output is 0.5 mL/kg/hr in adults, 1 mL/kg/hr in children, and 2 mL/kg/hr in infants.

7.2.4. Blood products/transfusions

7.2.4.1. Initial lab tests

7.2.4.1.1. Type and screen

Test performs ABO grouping, Rh typing, antibody screen for non-ABO/Rh antibodies.

7.2.4.1.2. Type and crossmatch

Mixing of recipient's serum with donor RBCs, final compatibility test.

7.2.4.2. Transfusion products

7.2.4.2.1. Packed red blood cells (PRBC)

Features: most plasma removed. Can be washed (all plasma removed) if prior allergic reaction, leukocyte poor (if prior febrile reaction, transplant patient), or irradiated (if neutropenic patient or if they have had recent chemotherapy; helps to reduce graft-versus-host disease).

Indications: acute hemorrhage, symptomatic chronic anemia with hemoglobin (HGB) <7 g/dL, heart disease with HGB <10 g/dL.

Dose: 1 unit of PRBC = 250–350 mL volume (hematocrit [HCT] 70%). 1 unit raises HGB 1 g/dL or HCT 3% (Pediatrics 3 mL/kg similar rise). Give amount dependent on degree of loss.

Cautions: large transfusions can lead to hypothermia, high potassium, low calcium, dilutional thrombocytopenia.

7.2.4.2.2. Fresh frozen plasma (FFP)

Contains all coagulation factors normally present in blood. Useful for treating deficiencies of factors II, V, VII, IX, X, XI.

Indications: bleeding/coagulopathy of unknown cause, reversal of warfarin toxicity, coagulation deficiency if concentrates unavailable, disseminated intravascular coagulation (DIC), thrombotic thrombocytopenic purpura (TTP), patient receiving massive transfusion, liver failure and bleeding.

Dose: 1 unit of FFP = 200–250 mL volume. Give 10–15 mL/kg for adult. Give 5–8 mL/kg to reverse warfarin. Pediatrics: give 10–25 ml/kg.

7.2.4.2.3. Platelet concentrate

1 unit raises platelets 5000 to 10 000/μL.

Indications: platelets <100 000/μL and active bleeding; platelets <50 000/μL and procedure (i.e. central venous line, surgery), trauma; platelets <10 000/μL, consider giving prophylactically; bleeding and qualitative platelet defects (i.e. uremia, aspirin therapy).

Dose: 4 to 6 units. Pediatrics: give 1 unit/10 kg.

7.2.4.2.4. Cryoprecipitate

Contains factor VIII, XIII, vWF, fibrinogen, fibronectin.

Indications: low fibrinogen < 100 mg/dL and bleeding.

Dose: 10 unit pool = 100–200 mL. Give 10–20 units per transfusion. Pediatrics: give 2–4 bags/10 kg.

7.2.4.2.5. Factor VIII (Hemophilia A) and factor IX (Hemophilia B)

Amount replaced depends on severity of injury.

Factor VIII: 1 unit/kg will increase activity 2%. Typically with trauma or if history is unclear, dose to 100% activity.

Factor IX: 1 unit/kg will increase activity 1%. Similar administration to factor VIII.

7.3. Head trauma [2–4]

Cause of half of all trauma deaths. Over 50 000 patients die each year from traumatic brain injury (TBI).

Motor vehicle accidents (MVAs) are the most common cause of TBI that results in hospitalization; violence is the major cause of TBI-related death.

General signs and symptoms of traumatic brain injury: severe headache, altered level of consciousness, vomiting, change in pupil size or reactivity, Cushing's reflex (hypertension, bradycardia), uncal herniation (unilateral pupil dilation and loss of reactivity, contralateral hemiparesis, rapidly deteriorating mental status).

Intracranial pressure (ICP): normal <10 mmHg; over 20 mmHg needs treatment; over 40 mmHg life-threatening.

Injuries can overwhelm the body's ability to autoregulate ICP.

Cerebral perfusion pressure (CPP) = Mean arterial pressure (MAP) – Intracranial pressure (ICP).

7.3.1. Direct intracranial injuries

7.3.1.1. Cerebral contusion

Bruise on surface of brain, most commonly base of the frontal lobes or anterior edge of temporal lobes.

Signs and symptoms: vary with location of injury.

7.3.1.2. Subarachnoid hemorrhage

Most common site of bleeding after head trauma (44%).

7.3.1.3. Subdural hematoma (SDH)

30% of severe TBI. Occurs from tearing of bridging veins. Occurs most commonly in parietal location and is more common in the elderly.

Radiographic appearance: convex hyperdensity that follows curve of the skull.

7.3.1.4. Epidural hematoma

Less common than SDH, only 1% of patients with TBI.

Mechanism: occurs from blow to the temple with fracture of the temporal bone and injury to the middle meningeal artery.

Clinical course: patient with a brief "lucid interval" prior to decompensating.

Radiographic appearance: hyperdense, biconvex, ovoid/lenticular.

Have better outcomes than SDH when recognized and treated appropriately because there is less parenchymal damage to the brain than the SDH, which is the result of stronger rotational forces that result in greater degree of axonal injury.

7.3.2. Diffuse intracranial injuries

7.3.2.1. Mild TBI

GCS 13 to 15.

Cause: acceleration/deceleration or rotational force. Often associated with sports. Does not require loss of consciousness for diagnosis.

Symptoms: amnesia for event, transient disorientation, headache, dizziness, vomiting, unsteady gait.

7.3.2.2. Moderate TBI

GCS 9 to 12. Can still usually follow commands. Can have significant intracranial pathology. Requires careful observation to prevent secondary insult.

7.3.2.3. Severe TBI

GCS <8. Unconscious. Associated with severe intracranial injuries and pathology.

7.3.2.4. Diffuse axonal injury (DAI)

Cause: shearing forces stretching and twisting the axons. This causes damage and swelling of the axons. Causes disruption of cortical physiology. No specific acute focal lesion is seen on CT despite coma. In some cases MRI may be more specific. Occurs in 50% of all comatose head-injured patients.

Severity of the injury is determined by the clinical course.

7.3.2.4.1. Mild DAI

Coma <24 hours.

7.3.2.4.2. Moderate DAI

Coma >24 hours.

7.3.2.4.3. Severe DAI

Prolonged coma and neurologic abnormalities.

7.3.3. Diagnosis and treatment of intracranial injury [2]

Stabilize airway and treat shock. Immediate CT head if patient condition and stability allows. Prompt neurosurgical consultation.

7.3.3.1. Emergency department interventions while awaiting neurosurgery

Goal is to maintain MAP of 80–90 mmHg. Avoid hypotension, hypertension and hypoxia. Elevate the head of bed to 30 to 45 degrees (this can reduce ICP by 50%). Mild brief hyperventilation can be a helpful temporizing measure in a patient with an acutely elevated ICP or herniation (goal of $PaCO_2$ 30 to 35). Steroids are NOT indicated.

7.3.3.2. Pharmacologic adjuncts

Mannitol (0.25–1 g/kg): Effect within minutes peaks at 60 minutes lasts up to 8 hours.
Hypertonic (3%) saline 0.1 to 1 mL/kg.
Barbiturate coma: reduces cerebral metabolic demands.

7.3.3.3. Surgical interventions

Evacuation of hematoma: done for all epidural hematomas, SDHs with mass effect and midline shift >5 mm, focal neurologic findings, posterior fossa location, or increased ICP. Some intraparenchymal hemorrhage is amenable to surgical evacuation.
Other interventions: ventriculostomy, decompressive craniectomy.

7.3.3.4. Indications for head CT in minor head trauma [2]

Loss of consciousness, altered mental status, signs of basilar skull fracture (Battle's sign – bruising behind the ears; raccoon eyes), repetitive questioning or amnesia, any focal neurologic findings, severe headache and persistent vomiting, highly focused blunt trauma (e.g. hammer strike), post-traumatic seizures, anticoagulation, elderly.

7.3.4. Scalp lacerations

Can be a significant source of hemorrhage.

Treatment: must irrigate, cleanse, and explore these wounds carefully for foreign bodies as infected scalp wounds have the potential to cause serious intracranial infections.
Control of bleeding can be obtained by: local injection with lidocaine with epinephrine, raney scalp clips applied to the wound edges. Update tetanus shot.
Closure of the wound: large lacerations of the galea must be closed. Skin, dermis, and galea can usually be repaired in a single layer with interrupted or vertical mattress sutures. Staples can be used for simple lacerations that do not involve the galea.

7.3.4.1. Scalp avulsions

Because the scalp is so very vascular even very large scalp avulsions tissue flaps can survive.

7.3.5. Facial fractures [2–4]

Up to 60% of patients with significant facial trauma have other injuries; 50% have associated brain injury. In urban areas up to 70% of facial fractures are from assault.

The most commonly fractured facial bone is the nose followed by the mandible.

7.3.5.1. LeFort fractures

7.3.5.1.1. LeFort Type I

Transverse fracture through the maxilla above the teeth and may be unilateral or bilateral. Nasal bridge remains stable, maxilla is mobile.

7.3.5.1.2. LeFort Type II

Pyramidal in shape; extends superiorly in the midface and involves the nasal bridge, maxilla, lacrimal bones, and orbital floor and rim. Nasal bridge and maxilla are mobile. Involves medial orbital wall.

Traumatic telecanthus can be seen with eyes moving apart because of ligamentous disruption. May have cerebrospinal fluid (CSF) rhinorrhea.

7.3.5.1.3. LeFort Type III

Craniofacial dysjunction: rare. Fractures start at the bridge of the nose and extend posteriorly along the medial wall of the orbit through the ethmoids along the maxillary floor of the orbit and through the lateral orbital wall and finally through the zygomatic arch. Nasal bridge, maxilla, and zygoma are mobile.

Markedly swollen eyes, "dish" face with flattening and elongated appearance. Frequently associated with CSF leak.

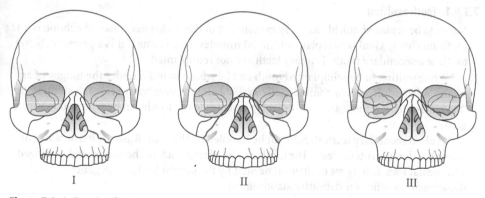

I   II   III

Figure 7.1. LeFort classifications.

LeFort management: pain control, prophylactic antibiotics, nasal packing for epistaxis, ice for swelling, consult maxillofacial surgery.

7.3.5.2. Zygomaticomaxillary complex (ZMC) fracture

Zygoma attaches in 4 places temporal, frontal, maxillary, and sphenoid.

Appearance: classic "tripod," diastasis of zygomaticotemporal and zygomaticofrontal sutures, fracture of the infraorbital foramen, causes facial flattening.

Signs and symptoms: anesthesia in the infraorbital nerve distribution, can have associated globe injuries, enophthalmos.

Treatment: maxillofacial evaluation to prevent late complications such as enophthalmos, diplopia, malunion, permanent nerve damage.

7.3.5.3. Mandible fractures

Second most common facial fracture. Mandible is a ring structure, which frequently fractures in two places. Most common sites are the condyle, body then angle.

Clinical presentation: patients complain of malocclusion of teeth and inability to bite down properly, trismus, and facial swelling.

Treatment: open fractures need antibiotic coverage against oral flora, clindamycin or penicillin, refer to oral maxillofacial surgeon.

7.3.6. Dental injuries [2, 4]

Table 7.3 Classification of tooth fractures

Ellis class	Injury	Consideration
1	Enamel only	No hot or cold sensitivity. No treatment needed
2	Enamel and dentin	Cover the dentin, and patient needs dental follow-up in 24 hours
3	Enamel, dentin, and pulp	Blood seen. Immediate dental referral needed

7.3.6.1. Tooth avulsion

Needs to be replaced quickly as every minute out of the socket decreases likelihood of the tooth surviving. Goal is to replant within 30 minutes. Determine if it is a primary (baby) tooth or a secondary tooth. Primary teeth are not reimplanted.

While waiting to be reimplanted tooth can be stored in milk, under the tongue of an awake, sober adult, or in a commercially available tooth preservative (Hank's solution or "Save-a-Tooth"); if these are not available or plausible the tooth can be wrapped in moist gauze.

Avulsed secondary teeth should not be handled by the root. Rinse in sterile water or saline but don't scrub to clean. The tooth can be placed back in the socket and stabilized with dental wax. Emergent evaluation needed by the dentist in the emergency department or office for definitive stabilization.

7.3.7. Orbital fractures [2, 4, 5]

Orbital floor is the most common site for fracture.

Mechanism: rapid increase in intraorbital pressure usually caused by a blunt trauma. Causes fracture in the inferior and medial wall, the weakest part of the orbit. Contents of the orbit, specifically infraorbital nerve and inferior rectus, can herniate through the fracture.

Symptoms: diplopia and pain on upward gaze, hypoesthesia of the ipsilateral cheek and upper lip, periorbital subcutaneous emphysema, epistaxis, extraocular muscle movement deficit.

Diagnosis: CT scan of facial bones.

Treatment: decongestants and antibiotics to cover sinus flora. Caution the patient against blowing their nose. Refer to ophthalmology or ENT for close follow-up. Emergent evaluation by ophthalmology if any evidence of muscle or nerve entrapment as this may require prompt surgical repair.

7.3.8. Eye injuries [2, 5]

7.3.8.1. Hyphema

Blood in the aqueous humor of the anterior chamber.

Cause: direct trauma with disruption of the vessels of the iris or ciliary body.

Symptoms: pain, photophobia, and decreased visual acuity.

Hyphema grades:

Grade 1: layering blood occupying less than ⅓ of the anterior chamber.
Grade 2: layering blood occupying ⅓ to ½ of the anterior chamber.
Grade 3: layering blood occupying ½ to less than the total anterior chamber.
Grade 4: total occlusion of the anterior chamber.

Treatment: emergent ophthalmology consultation. Bedrest and eye rest with elevation of the head of bed to 45 degrees. Medications may include topical β-blockers, topical α-agonist, topical carbonic anhydrase inhibitor, topical steroids.

Major complication: rebleeding 2 to 5 days out from initial injury.

7.3.8.2. Corneal abrasions

Causes: direct injury to eye, foreign bodies under the eyelid, accidental injury by rubbing or scratching, and contact lenses.

Symptoms: eye pain and irritation, photophobia, fluorescein dye uptake on slit lamp or blue light exam.

Treatment: topical ophthalmic antibiotics, cycloplegics for photophobia.

7.3.8.3. Corneal laceration

Cause: foreign bodies or high-velocity projectiles.

Symptoms: eye pain and irritation, photophobia, loss of vision.

Clinical findings: loss of anterior chamber depth, teardrop-shaped pupil, hyphema, positive Seidel's sign (leaking aqueous humor washes away fluorescein; waterfall appearance).

Treatment: emergent ophthalmology consultation for operative repair. May need imaging to exclude intraocular foreign body.

7.3.8.4. Corneal burns

Acids: chemicals with pH <2 more concerning. Causes coagulative necrosis and shallower burns.

Alkalis: worse than acidic burns. Chemicals with pH >12 more concerning. Causes liquefactive necrosis and deeper burns.

Clinical presentation: eye pain, redness and swelling of the eyelid, punctate keratitis on slit lamp exam, chemosis, corneal edema and opacification.

Treatment: copious irrigation with recheck of pH until pH is neutral and then recheck again 10 to 15 minutes after completion of irrigation to confirm. Analgesics and cycloplegics. Topical antibiotics ointment and, depending on the severity, close ophthalmology follow-up or emergent evaluation in the emergency department.

7.3.8.4.1. Ultraviolet light– "welder's burn"

Symptoms: similar to corneal abrasion.

Signs: ultraviolet keratitis (multiple punctate areas of uptake across the cornea). Can happen after exposure to welding torch without protective glasses.

Treatment: same as corneal abrasion.

7.3.8.5. Traumatic iritis

Occurs after a blunt injury to the globe causing contusion and inflammation of the iris and ciliary body resulting in spasm.

Signs and symptoms: deep aching eye pain and photophobia (direct and consensual), ciliary flush and flare and cell in the anterior chamber, small and poorly dilating pupil.

Treatment: long-acting cycloplegics and topical steroids. Usually resolves in a week.

7.3.8.6. Eyelid lacerations

Can be repaired in the emergency department if it does not involve the lid margins, the levator muscles, canthal tendons, or lacrimal ducts. Any concern for more than a simple superficial laceration warrants ophthalmology consultation.

7.3.9. Otologic trauma

7.3.9.1 Earlobe injury

Hematoma of the auricle can lead to necrosis of the cartilage. Hematomas should be evacuated and a pressure dressing applied. If the earlobe is lacerated into the cartilage, sutures should go through the skin and perichondrium, but not through the cartilage itself.

7.3.9.2. Tympanic membrane perforation

Seen in a majority of blast injury patients with other severe injuries. Also seen with foreign body insertion into the ear canal.

Treatment: most heal spontaneously, but patients should follow up with ENT. Give patients strict dry ear precaution instructions.

7.4. Neck trauma

7.4.1. Anatomy

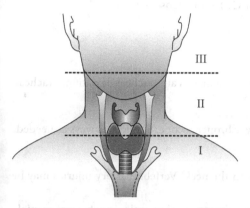

Figure 7.2. Zones of the neck.

Table 7.4 Zones of the neck

Zone	Anatomic location	Structures	Workup for injury
1	Sternal notch to cricoid cartilage	Proximal common carotid artery, vertebral artery, subclavian artery, mediastinal vessels, lung apices, esophagus, trachea, thyroid, thoracic duct, spinal cord	Angiography, endoscopy, bronchoscopy
2	Cricoid cartilage to angle of mandible	Carotid artery, vertebral artery, larynx, trachea, esophagus, pharynx, jugular vein, vagus nerve, recurrent laryngeal nerve, spinal cord	Surgical exploration
3	Angle of mandible to base of skull	Distal carotid artery, vertebral artery, distal jugular veins, salivary and parotid glands, cranial nerves IX–XII, spinal cord	Angiography, laryngoscopy

7.4.2. Penetrating neck trauma

Evaluate for platysmal penetration. If present, surgical evaluation is needed as deep structures can be injured.

Signs: hemoptysis, dyspnea, airway obstruction, subcutaneous air, focal neurologic deficits, expanding hematoma, hemorrhage.

Treatment: control bleeding by direct pressure. Blind clamping is not recommended as other structures can be injured in the attempt. Airway management if needed by intubation or surgical airway. Further workup based on the location of injury. (See Figure 7.2.)

7.4.3. Blunt neck trauma

Delayed airway occlusion can occur. Intubate early. Suspect C-spine injury in blunt neck trauma.

7.4.3.1. Pharyngoesophageal injuries

Uncommon. Cervical esophagus most affected. Most frequently missed neck injury.

Signs: hematemesis, odynophagia, subcutaneous emphysema, blood in saliva or nasogastric tube.
Diagnosis: contrasted swallow study (X-ray or CT), esophagoscopy.
Treatment: antibiotics, surgery.

7.4.3.2. Laryngotracheal injury

Mechanism: direct blow to anterior neck.
Signs: hoarseness, stridor, trouble breathing, subcutaneous air, tracheal deviation. Tracheal disruption is commonly seen at the cricoid.
Diagnosis: CT scan or X-ray in stable patients.
Treatment: if intubation indicated, attempt over bronchoscope. Surgical airways as needed.

7.4.3.3. Vascular neck injuries

Carotid is the most commonly injured artery in the neck. Vertebral artery injuries may be clinically occult.

Signs: expanding hematoma, pulse deficit, hemothorax, focal neurologic deficits of cranial nerves, Horner's syndrome.
Diagnosis: controversial. Angiography (gold standard) is slow. Computed tomography angiography (CTA) can miss certain lesions. Magnetic resonance angiography (MRA) expensive, not always available.
Treatment: if dissection is present, anticoagulate and initiate antiplatelet therapy. The goal of therapy is to prevent clot formation at the site of dissection. The dissection will usually heal spontaneously. Should be done with input from consulting service.

7.5. Chest trauma

Accounts for 20–25% of civilian deaths from trauma. Hypoxia is the most serious threat, as an intact chest wall is needed for ventilation.

7.5.1. Aortic dissection and disruption

Cause: high-speed deceleration. MVA, fall from great height. Occurs most often at the attachment of the ligamentum arteriosum just distal to the left subclavian (aortic isthmus). Most patients die at the scene.
Symptoms: substernal or interscapular pain, dyspnea, dysphagia.
Signs: harsh systolic murmur, pulse deficits, pseudocoarctation, paraplegia, hoarseness.
Diagnosis:
   Chest X-ray (CXR) findings: superior mediastinal widening, obliteration of aortic knob, rightward deviation of esophagus and trachea, downward deviation of left mainstem bronchus, left apical pleural cap, widened paraspinous stripes, widened paratracheal stripe.
   CT scan: fast, accurate.
   Aortography: old gold standard.

Management: β-blockers (i.e. esmolol) reduce pulse pressure, thereby shear force. Maintain systolic blood pressure (SBP) 100–120 mmHg. Sodium nitroprusside as second agent. Operative repair emergently.

7.5.2. Esophageal perforation

Occurs with iatrogenic trauma (endoscopy, stricture dilations), burns, foreign bodies, penetrating and blunt trauma, spontaneous/post-emetic.

Symptoms: pleuritic pain worsened by swallowing, neck flexion.

Signs: mediastinal air on X-ray or Hamman's crunch on auscultation, subcutaneous emphysema.

Diagnosis: incidental X-ray findings include mediastinal air, left-sided pleural effusion, pneumothorax, widened mediastinum. Definitive diagnosis with esophagography (standard) or helical CT with dilute oral contrast.

Treatment: Airway maintenance, antibiotics, emergent surgical consult.

7.5.3. Tracheobronchial injury

Mechanism: blunt chest trauma (intrathoracic, near carina most common), knife wound (neck), gunshot (anywhere).

Clinical features: massive air leak, hemoptysis, subcutaneous emphysema, Hamman's crunch.

Diagnosis: bronchoscopy, CT.

Treatment: intubate over a bronchoscope if possible, surgery.

7.5.4. Diaphragmatic injury

Occurs from high-velocity injury, MVA, fall from great height, or penetrating trauma. 70–80% occur in left hemidiaphragm, often missed initially. The liver prevents herniation of bowel contents on the right and may obscure diagnosis of right-sided injuries. Because of diaphragmatic movement, consider an injury for any penetrating trauma between fourth intercostal space anteriorly and the sixth intercostal space posterolaterally.

Diagnosis: CT scan. CXR may show an effusion, blurring of the diaphragm or herniated bowel.

Treatment: surgery.

7.5.5. Contusions

7.5.5.1. Cardiac

Occurs from high-speed trauma. In severe cases myocardial rupture can occur but is almost always immediately fatal.

Symptoms: tachycardia, dysrhythmias, shock, pain.

Diagnosis: difficult. ECG changes and cardiac enzymes nonspecific. 2D echo if highly suspicious.

Treatment: fluids and vasopressors for shock.

7.5.5.2. Pulmonary

Occurs from blunt chest trauma, commonly MVA. Can be insidious in onset, suspect due to mechanism or bony chest wall injury.

Diagnosis: chest X-ray shows patchy, irregular infiltrate or consolidation. Over time, patient develops an increasing A-a gradient.
Treatment: analgesics, pulmonary toilet, intubation.

7.5.6. Fractures

7.5.6.1. Rib fracture

Cause: direct trauma. Associated with hemothorax, pneumothorax, pulmonary contusion, post-traumatic pneumonia. Increased significance in children (more flexible chest), higher suspicion for underlying injury.

Ribs 1–3: require great force. Suspect great vessel injury, lung injury.
Ribs 4–9: most common. Associated hemothorax, pneumothorax, pulmonary contusion.
Ribs 9–12: More mobile. Associated intra-abdominal injury.
Flail chest: 3 or more adjacent ribs fractured in 2 or more places. Main problem is associated pulmonary contusion. Also poor ventilation due to pain leads to atelectasis, hypoxia.

Diagnosis: physical exam, X-ray, CT for evaluation of underlying injury.
Treatment: analgesia, intubation.

7.5.6.2. Sternal fracture

Cause: anterior blunt trauma. More common with seat belt. Associated myocardial contusion in 1–6%. No association with aortic injury.
Diagnosis: lateral CXR.
Treatment: analgesia. Rarely, operative fixation.

7.5.6.3. Clavicle fracture

Most common pediatric fracture.
Cause:

Medial third of clavicle (5%), blow to medial chest.
Middle third of clavicle (80%), blow to lateral shoulder.
Lateral third of clavicle (15%), blow to top of shoulder.

Diagnosis: X-ray.
Treatment: sling, analgesia.

7.5.7. Hemothorax

Blood in the pleural space.
Diagnosis: upright X-ray – 200–300 ml of blood blunts the costophrenic angles. Supine CXR shows diffuse haziness.

Treatment: chest tube (36 French or greater). Thoracotomy if initial drainage >1500 mL, continued output >200 mL/hr for 3 hours, persistent hypotension.

7.5.8. Pneumothorax

Air in the pleural space.

Signs: chest pain, dyspnea, decreased or absent breath sounds, subcutaneous emphysema.

7.5.8.1. Simple pneumothorax

Size: small <15%, moderate 15–60%, large >60%.

Treatment: small may be observed with serial CXR. Moderate and large require tube thoracostomy.

7.5.8.2. Tension pneumothorax

Injury is one-way valve, leads to increasing intrapleural pressure.

Signs: hypotension, tracheal deviation, jugular venous distension (JVD) (may be absent with large blood loss).

Treatment: needle decompress (14 gauge needle, second intercostal space, mid-clavicular line) then chest tube. Do not get CXR prior to needle decompression.

7.5.8.3. Open pneumothorax

Defect in chest wall equalizes intrapleural and atmospheric pressure. Affected lung becomes physiologic dead space.

Treatment: occlusive dressing taped on three sides. Chest tube at alternate site.

7.5.9. Pericardial tamponade

Pericardial effusion increases intrapericardial pressure. Impairs diastolic filling with as little as 60–100 mL. Associated with penetrating trauma, especially stab wounds.

Signs: hypotension, tachycardia, muffled heart sounds, JVD, pulsus paradoxus, electrical alternans.

Diagnosis: ultrasound. Pericardial fluid and diastolic right ventricular (RV) collapse. Distended inferior vena cava (IVC) in a hypotensive patient.

Treatment: fluid resuscitation. Pericardiocentesis (ultrasound guided if possible). Emergency department thoracotomy if patient meets criteria for procedure.

7.5.10. Penetrating cardiac injury

More anteriorly situated RV (43%) affected more than left ventricle (LV) (34%).

Two groups of patients. Exsanguinating hemorrhage communicates with pleural cavity and patient often dies prior to medical attention; or hemorrhage contained within pericardium, leading to tamponade.

7.6. Abdominal trauma [2–4]

7.6.1. General

Blunt trauma has greater mortality than penetrating because injuries can be difficult to diagnose and usually multisystem.

Indications for emergent laparotomy in abdominal trauma include: peritonitis, intraperitoneal free air, hypotension or hemodynamic instability and abdominal distension, diaphragmatic defect, hematochezia or hematemesis, evisceration, implement *in situ* (impaled object), clinical decision.

7.6.2. Hollow viscus injury

Involves hemorrhage and peritoneal contamination. Can occur by penetrating or blunt trauma. Symptoms may be delayed if injured viscus segment is retroperitoneal (such as classic "handle bar" injury in pediatrics with duodenal hematoma). Presents with abdominal pain, vomiting.

7.6.3. Solid organ

Hemorrhage is the main problem. Splenic injury is most common (40–55%) followed by liver (35–45%) and retroperitoneal hematoma (15%).

The liver is the most commonly injured organ in penetrating trauma.

The spleen is the most commonly injured organ in blunt trauma.

Pancreatic injuries occur from penetrating trauma or a direct blow to the epigastrium.

7.6.3.1. Splenic injuries [3, 4]

Table 7.5 Splenic injury grading and treatment

Grade	Description	Treatment
1	Subcapsular hematoma <10% surface area Laceration <1 cm parenchymal depth	Nonoperative management is 90% successful in proper patient population. Patient must be hemodynamically stable, have minimal free fluid or no significant peritoneal signs, and not anticoagulated. Reduces risk of infection due to retained splenic function
2	Subcapsular hematoma 10–50% surface area Laceration 1–3 cm parenchymal depth with no trabecular vessel involvement	
3	Subcapsular hematoma >50% or expanding Ruptured subcapsular or parenchymal hematoma Intraparenchymal hematoma 5 cm or expanding Laceration >3 cm or involving trabecular vessels	Operative management is splenectomy. Used for grade 5, and many grade 4.
4	Laceration involving segmental or hilar vessels producing major devascularization >25% of spleen	
5	Shattered spleen or hilar vascular injury which devascularizes spleen	

7.6.3.2. Liver injuries [3, 4]

Table 7.6 Liver injury grading and treatment

Grade	Description	Treatment
1	Subcapsular hematoma <10% surface area or capsular tear <1 cm parenchymal depth	Nonoperative management is 90% successful in proper patient population. Patient must be hemodynamically stable, low-grade injury, minimal free fluid or no significant peritoneal signs, no other significant injuries, and not anticoagulated.
2	Subcapsular hematoma 10–50% of surface area or capsular tear 1–3 cm parenchymal depth, <10 cm length	
3	Subcapsular hematoma >50% surface area or expanding	Grade of the laceration does not preclude nonoperative management however grade 4 and 5 account for 67% of failed nonoperative management
	Ruptured subcapsular or parenchymal hematoma	Operative management allows for hemostasis, debridement, and drainage.
	Intraparenchymal hematoma >10 cm or expanding	
	Capsular tear >3 cm parenchymal depth	
4	Parenchymal disruption 25–75% of hepatic lobe or 1 to 3 segments within a single lobe	
5	Parenchymal disruption 25–75% of hepatic lobe or 1 to 3 segments within a single lobe. Global destruction or devascularization of the liver	
6	Hepatic avulsion	

7.6.4. Imaging of abdominal trauma

Plain films of the abdomen are rarely indicated.

FAST exam is a screening exam and a negative study does not exclude intra-abdominal injury.

CT can be unreliable for hollow viscus, duodenal, diaphragmatic, and pancreatic injuries so persistent pain and symptoms in the setting of a negative CT should not be ignored.

CT does show retroperitoneal injury, solid organ injury and bony injury.

CT cystourethrogram is indicated for hematuria or blood at the urethral meatus.

Alternatively traditional cystourethrogram can be performed.

7.7. Genitourinary (GU) trauma [2–4]

80% of GU injuries involve the kidneys, 10% involve the bladder. The majority are due to blunt trauma. Degree of hematuria does NOT correlate with the severity of the injury. More than 50 RBCs per high-powered field (HPF) requires imaging in children with blunt trauma. Bedrest and observation is successful management in >90% of blunt renal injuries; however, all except the most minor of penetrating renal injuries require operative exploration. CT scan should be performed for: gross hematuria, microhematuria plus hypotension, rapid deceleration mechanism, penetrating injury in proximity to the kidney.

7.7.1. Renal trauma [4]

Table 7.7 Renal injury grading and treatment

Grade	Subtype	Description	Treatment
1	Contusion	Microscopic or gross hematuria, urologic studies normal	Discharge with close follow-up and repeat urinalysis to confirm resolution of hematuria
1	Hematoma	Subcapsular, nonexpanding without parenchymal laceration	
2	Hematoma	Nonexpanding perirenal hematoma confined to renal retroperitoneum	Admit for observation No need for operative management
2	Laceration	<1 cm parenchymal depth of renal cortex without urinary extravasation	Admit for observation
3	Laceration	>1 cm depth of renal cortex, without collecting system rupture or urinary extravasation	Possible need for operative management – controversial
4	Laceration	Parenchymal laceration extending through the renal cortex, medulla and collecting system	Admit Surgical repair required May necessitate nephrectomy
4	Vascular	Main renal artery or vein injury with contained hemorrhage	Admit
5	Laceration	Completely shattered kidney	Emergent surgical intervention <6 hours to prevent renal dysfunction
5	Vascular	Avulsion of renal hilum which devascularizes the kidney	35% salvageable with prompt surgery Up to 50% do not have hematuria

Causes: rapid deceleration, penetrating trauma, lower rib fractures and lumbar transverse process fractures.

7.7.2. Bladder trauma

Up to 10% of pelvic fractures have an associated bladder injury or rupture. Rupture may produce intraperitoneal or retroperitoneal extravasation of urine.

Diagnosis: contrast urethrogram, cystogram with CT.

Treatment: contusions and extraperitoneal ruptures can be successfully managed with Foley catheter drainage alone. Intraperitoneal rupture requires surgical repair.

7.7.3. Urethral trauma

A Foley catheter should never be placed if there is blood at the urethral meatus and concern for urethral injury. Virtually all urethral injuries are from blunt injuries and occur in males. Urethral injuries are rarely associated with fractures that do not involve the ischiopubic rami.

Diagnosis: contrast urethrogram, cystogram with CT.

Treatment: controversial and varies. Can include anything from stenting Foley to a suprapubic catheter. Consult urology.

Table 7.8 Urethral trauma

Location	Anterior	Posterior
Cause	Straddle injury, iatrogenic, fractured penis, fall, gunshot	Rapid deceleration, penetrating or compression trauma
Presentation	Hematuria	Blood at the meatus, dysuria, scrotal hematoma
Evaluation	Urethrogram	Urethrogram
Risks	Strictures, fistula	Incontinence

7.7.4. External genitalia

Cause: commonly a blunt or straddle injury.
Signs: edema, ecchymosis, hematuria.
Diagnosis: ultrasound.
Treatment: supportive care and urology consultation.

7.8. Skin trauma

7.8.1. Bite wounds

Bite wounds have a high risk for contamination. Closure should be avoided if possible, but weighed against long-term cosmetic effects (e.g. dog bites on the face).

Staphylococcus and Streptococcus are most common contaminants but there are some species specific bacteria to consider.

Human bite: *Eikenella corrodens*.
Cat bite: *Pasteurella multocida*.
Dog bite: *Capnocytophaga canimorsus*.

Treatment: consider rabies prophylaxis in high-risk animal bites (bat, raccoon, dog). X-rays are useful to check for retained tooth fragments.

7.8.2. Puncture wounds

High risk for infection with skin flora. Shoes and other rubber-containing objects may harbor pseudomonal species.
Treatment: do not close wound. Irrigate copiously.

7.8.3. High pressure injection

Most important factor is the type of material injected. Paint and paint thinner causes a large inflammatory response. Grease can lead to oleogranuloma, fistula formation, scarring.

Most frequently seen on the index finger of the non-dominant hand [2].

Presentation: may have an innocuous wound, fusiform swelling. Hours later the patient develops a painful, swollen, and pale digit.
Diagnosis: X-ray shows air or radio-opaque material dissecting along the tissue plane.

Treatment: splinting, elevation, pain control, tetanus prophylaxis, broad spectrum antibiotics, surgical consult for debridement. Avoid digital blocks as they can cause an increase in tissue pressure and neurovascular damage.

7.9. Extremity injuries

7.9.1. Amputation

Store the amputated portion in saline-moistened gauze placed in a dry plastic bag on ice. Ice should not come in direct contact with amputated portion. Update tetanus and give antibiotic prophylaxis (skin flora).

Stump care: irrigate with normal saline. Cover with saline-moistened dressing. No local antiseptics (hydrogen peroxide, alcohol) as they may damage tissue.

Indications for re-implantation: pediatric amputation, single digit with amputation between proximal and distal interphalangeal (IP) joints, thumb amputation, multiple digits, wrist, and forearm [2].

Contraindications: unstable patient, multiple level amputation, self-inflicted amputation, single-digit amputation proximal to flexor digitorum superficialis insertion, serious underlying disease (vascular, complicated diabetes mellitus [DM], congestive heart failure [CHF]), extremes of age.

7.9.2. Compartment syndrome

Develops when pressure increases in a closed fascial compartment.

Cause: crush injury or vascular injury with bleeding into the compartment, coagulopathy.

Signs (Ps): pain out of proportion to physical findings, pain on passive stretching of suspected compartment, pallor, paresthesias, poikilothermia, pulselessness, paresis, paralysis.

Common sites: most commonly occurs in lower leg after closed tib/fib fracture. Seen in forearm, associated with supracondylar humerus fracture (with subsequent Volkman's ischemic contracture) or compression injury associated with intoxication. Thigh is less common. Hand, foot also possible.

Diagnosis: check compartment pressure, >30 mmHg diagnostic.

Treatment: emergent fasciotomy.

Complications: rhabdomyolysis, myoglobinurina, acute renal injury, hyperkalemia.

7.10. Fractures

7.10.1. General principles

Evaluate for neurovascular compromise, deformity/displacement.

If no neurovascular compromise and minimal to no displacement, treat with splint and orthopedic follow-up.

If mild displacement, reduce, splint, orthopedic follow-up 24–48 hours.

If significant displacement, open fracture, or neurovascular compromise, get emergent orthopedic, possibly vascular, consult.

7.10.2. Lower extremity

7.10.2.1. Foot and ankle

7.10.2.1.1. Ottawa rules for obtaining ankle/foot radiographs

Apply to adults evaluated within 48 hours of injury.

Ankle radiographs are not needed in the absence of: bony tenderness along the posterior edge or tip of the distal 6 cm of either lower leg bone/malleoli, inability to bear weight for 4 steps at the time of injury or evaluation.

Foot radiographs are not needed in the absence of: bony tenderness of navicular bone or base of fifth metatarsal, inability to bear weight for 4 steps at the time of injury or evaluation.

7.10.2.1.2. Jones vs. pseudo-Jones

Jones fracture: fracture of the diaphysis of the fifth metatarsal. Treat with immobilization and non-weight bearing. May require surgery if non-union occurs.

Pseudo-Jones: avulsion fracture of proximal end of fifth metatarsal. Treat with walking boot.

7.10.2.1.3. Lisfranc fracture/dislocation

Cause: crush injury of the midfoot, or sudden rotational force on a plantar flexed foot.

Radiologic findings: dislocation of one or more metatarsal bones from the cuboid and cuneiform bones.

Treatment: immobilization, consult orthopedics.

7.10.2.2. Distal femur/knee

7.10.2.2.1. Tibial plateau fracture

Mechanism: axial loaded knee and valgus force.

Clinical appearance: effusion, patient refuses to bear weight, decreased range of motion (ROM), hemarthrosis.

Associated injury: popliteal artery, peroneal nerve, anterior cruciate ligament (ACL), medial collateral ligament (MCL) injury in 66% [2].

Treatment: immobilization, non-weight bearing, orthopedic follow-up.

7.10.2.3. Femur/hip

Hip and thigh can hold up to 3 units of blood. All hip/femur fractures should be typed and crossmatched for 2 units of blood.

7.10.2.3.1. Femur fractures

Femoral neck fracture: shortened, externally rotated, abducted leg. Associated avascular necrosis in 20% [2].

Intertrochanteric fracture: shortened, internally rotated leg.

Subtrochanteric: mostly cortical bone, often comminuted, risk for fat embolism. Traction prior to operative fixation not supported by literature [2].

Femoral shaft fracture: occurs with high-energy trauma, associated with hip and knee injury. Almost half have ligamentous knee damage [2].

7.10.3. Upper extremity

7.10.3.1. Elbow/humerus

7.10.3.1.1. Humeral shaft

Mechanism: blow to humerus or significant rotational force.
Associated injury: radial nerve.

7.10.3.1.2. Humeral intercondylar

Mechanism: blow to olecranon.
Difficult to treat, orthopedic follow-up.

7.10.3.1.3. Humeral lateral condyle

Second most common elbow fracture in children [2].
Mechanism: fall on outstretched arm with varus force. Less commonly has neurovascular injury.

7.10.3.1.4. Supracondylar humerus fracture

Most common elbow fracture in children, almost exclusively 5–10 year olds, 98% extension type [2].
Mechanism: fall on outstretched arm. Concern for associated median nerve and brachial artery injuries.
Treatment: only attempt reduction if neurovascular compromise already exists. Consult orthopedics.

7.10.3.1.5. Transcondylar humerus fracture

Seen primarily in elderly. Needs immediate orthopedic follow-up.

7.10.3.1.6. Radial head and neck

Caused by fall on outstretched arm.
Often associated with articular cartilage damage.

7.10.3.2. Forearm/wrist

7.10.3.2.1. Radial/ulnar shaft

Caused by fall on outstretched arm or direct blow.
Obtain films wrist and elbow to rule out dislocation, articular fracture.

7.10.3.2.2. Galeazzi's fracture

Fracture of mid to distal radius causing associated dislocation/subluxation of distal radial/ulnar joint.
Mechanism: axial load on hyperpronated forearm.
Treatment: open or closed reduction.

7.10.3.2.3. Monteggia fracture

Fracture of proximal third of ulna with radial head dislocation.

Occurs with fall on outstretched arm with excessive pronation or occurs from blunt trauma to back of upper forearm. Associated with radial nerve injury.

Treatment: typically needs open reduction with internal fixation.

7.10.3.2.4. Colles' fracture

Most common wrist fracture in adult.

Transverse fracture of distal radial metaphysis with dorsal displacement of radius.

Mechanism: fall on outstretched arm.

7.10.3.2.5. Scaphoid fracture

Most commonly fractured carpal bone, 62–87% of carpal bone fractures [2].

Mechanism: fall on outstretched hand, patient complains of dorsal wrist pain, tender in anatomic snuffbox.

Diagnosis: request scaphoid X-ray views. Risk for non-union, avascular necrosis.

Treatment: immobilize with thumb spica splint. Immobilize even if X-ray is negative if patient continues to complain of pain in the proper anatomic location.

7.10.4. Pelvic fractures

Often occur in MVA or MV versus pedestrian. Frequently associated with abdominal injury.

Associated injuries: urologic, gynecologic, neurologic (especially with sacral fractures, either vertical or transverse superior to S4), vascular (rich blood supply to pelvis along posterior pelvis can cause massive blood loss).

Stable fractures are far less likely to have associated neurovascular injury than partially stable or unstable fractures.

Open fractures: must inspect posterior pelvis and gluteal musculature, rectal exam, vaginal exam. Occult open fracture can lead to significant blood loss.

Diagnosis: X-ray anterior/posterior (AP) pelvis, can miss subtle posterior pelvis fracture. CT scan is definitive.

Treatment: stable fractures often treated conservatively. Unstable fractures need open fixation. If patient becomes unstable, consider surgery or interventional radiology with embolization as necessary to control bleeding.

7.10.5. Pediatric fractures

7.10.5.1. Epiphyseal fractures

In pediatrics, growth plate more likely to fracture than long bones.

Salter–Harris Classification [2]:

Type I: epiphyseal or metaphyseal separation. No fracture visible on radiograph.

Type II: fracture through metaphysis and physis. Most common type of Salter–Harris fracture.

Type III: fracture through epiphysis to physis. Alignment concerns, often displace while cast on.

Type IV: fracture from epiphysis through physis to metaphysis. Can lead to partial growth arrest.
Type V: epiphysis smashed into physis. May appear normal on initial radiographs. Severe growth arrest, progressive shortening, angulation deformity, premature physical fusion.
Type VI–IX (added classification): very rare, not tested.

7.10.5.2. Torus/buckle fracture

Common in distal radius with fall on outstretched hand. Soft cortex is longitudinally compressed, strong fibrous periosteum prevents displacement.
Treatment: splinting.

7.10.5.3. Greenstick fracture

Cortex disrupted on one side completely, bowing and angulation on other side.

7.11. Joint injury

7.11.1. Shoulder dislocation

7.11.1.1. Acromioclavicular (AC) separation

Graded 1–6 based on severity of separation.

1 – sprain of AC joint, no tearing.
2 – tearing of AC ligament.
3 – tearing of AC ligament and coracoclavicular ligament.
4 – type 3 injury plus avulsion of coracoclavicular ligament from the clavicle. May also have anterior dislocation of sternoclavicular joint.
5 – type 3 injury plus deltoid fascia is stripped from acromion and clavicle. Verticle displacement of clavicle from scapula is exaggerated.
6 – type 3 with inferior dislocation of clavicle below coracoid. Generally accompanied by paresthesias.

Mechanism: direct blow to lateral shoulder.
Treatment: sling, orthopedic referral if displacement on X-ray. Grades 4–6 generally require surgery.

7.11.1.2. Glenohumeral dislocation

Most common large joint dislocation, occurs most often in young men, older women [2].

7.11.1.2.1. Anterior dislocation

Much more common than posterior.

Mechanism for anterior dislocation: indirect anterior force applied to shoulder capsule via blow to extended, abducted, externally rotated arm.
Presentation: patient will hold arm abducted, externally rotated, supported by other arm. Acromial process prominent, anterior shoulder appears full. 50% will have associated fracture [2].

Hill–Sachs deformity: compression fracture of posterolateral humeral head.
Bankart fracture: fracture of anterior glenoid rim.
Associated brachial plexus, axillary nerve injury.

Treatment: reduction, immobilization, first time injuries need orthopedic referral.

7.11.1.2.2. Posterior dislocation

Less common, often missed on initial X-rays. Associated with seizures.

Presentation of posterior dislocation: patient holds arm across chest in adduction. X-ray show "lightbulb" or "drumstick" appearance of humeral head. Scapular Y view shows posterior displacement.

Treatment of posterior dislocation: same as for anterior dislocation.

7.11.2. Elbow dislocation

Second most commonly dislocated large joint [2].

7.11.2.1. Posterior dislocation

Most common.
Mechanism: fall on outstretched hand
Presentation: patient will hold elbow flexed ~45 degrees, prominent olecranon.
Concern: associated brachial artery and median nerve injury.
Treatment: reduce with direct traction on elbow flexed 30 degrees, supinated.

7.11.2.2. Anterior dislocation

Uncommon, much more likely to have neurovascular injury, frequently open.
Mechanism: posterior blow to elbow.
Presentation: patient holds elbow extended, upper arm appears short, forearm long.
Treatment: emergent orthopedic consult. Reduce by distal traction at wrist, posterior pressure on forearm.

7.11.2.3. Radial head subluxation/nursemaid's elbow

More than 20% of upper extremity injuries in young children [2]. Seen most in 1- to 4-year-old patients, seen in left arm more than right.
Mechanism: sudden pull on forearm while pronated.
Presentation: patient will hold arm pronated, slightly flexed.
Treatment: reduce by simultaneously supinating forearm with slight pressure on radial head and gentle traction. Also can be reduced by hyperpronation. Patient should start using arm shortly after successful reduction.

7.11.3. Hip dislocation

Requires significant force, often associated with major trauma. 80–90% posterior dislocation, often from MVA [2].
Posterior dislocation: hip adducted, flexed, internally rotated.
Anterior dislocation: hip abducted, flexed, externally rotated. More frequent femoral vessel and nerve injury.

10% have sciatic nerve palsy, often peroneal branch. Peroneal palsy presents as weakness of extensor hallucis longus, dorsiflexion, numbness over dorsum of foot.

Treatment: reduction within 6–12 hours, multiple methods otherwise patient has increased risk of avascular necrosis, joint instability. Apply post-reduction knee immobilizer.

7.11.4. Knee dislocation

Half will reduce spontaneously prior to evaluation [2]. Associated with popliteal artery injury and commonly has peroneal nerve injury. More than half are anterior dislocation, caused by hyperextension. Posterior dislocations are caused by direct trauma (e.g. dashboard in MVA).

Treatment: reduction (traction/countertraction), immobilize in posterior long leg splint with approximately 20 degrees flexion.

7.12. Sprains and strains

7.12.1. Sprains

Sprain degrees.

First: minor ligamentous tearing, mild hemorrhage and swelling.

Second: partial tear of a ligament, moderate hemorrhage and swelling, painful/abnormal motion, loss of function.

Third: complete tearing of ligament, similar signs as second degree but more pronounced, grossly abnormal joint motion.

Treatment: first and mild to moderate second degree need rest, ice, elevation, NSAIDs, possible non-emergent orthopedic follow-up. Moderate to severe second and third degree need immobilization, urgent orthopedic consultation.

Consideration: epiphyseal fractures more common in pediatrics than ligamentous strains as ligaments are stronger than epiphysis.

7.12.2. Strains

Strain degrees.

First: minor tearing of musculotendinous unit, swelling, local tenderness, minor loss of function.

Second: similar to first but more pronounced.

Third: complete disruption of muscle or tendon, may have associated avulsion fracture.

Treatment: first and second degrees need rest, ice, NSAIDs. Third degree needs same as first group plus orthopedic consult.

7.12.3. Specific tendon injury considerations

Achilles tendon: occurs usually during jumping. Diagnosed with Thompson's test: flexing knee and squeezing calf muscles causes foot to plantar flex if tendon is uninjured. Subtle difference left to right can indicate partial tear.

Biceps brachii: occurs trying to catch/lift person or object.

Gastrocnemius/plantaris: occurs from sudden acceleration.

Patellar tendon: patient unable to extend the knee, high-riding patella.

Hand/forearm tendons:
> **Extensor:** most commonly injured over dorsum of hand. Repair in the emergency department is possible. Splint and follow-up with orthopedics.
> **Flexor:** occult injury with laceration to palm or volar forearm. Requires hand specialist expertise for repair, splint and close follow-up.

7.13. Vascular injuries

Can occur from blunt or penetrating trauma.

Hard signs of arterial injury: absent distal pulses, arterial bleeding, expanding hematoma, audible bruit, palpable thrill, distal ischemia.

Soft signs of arterial injury: peripheral nerve deficit, history of moderate bleeding at the scene, reduced pulse or difference in ankle-brachial index (ABI) > 0.15 in the injured extremity, proximity to major vessel <1 cm.

Diagnosis: angiography can show the detail of injury, arterial Dopplers.

Treatment: operative repair for any hard signs. If equivocal or "soft signs" only admission with observation and serial arterial pressure index (ABI). A measurement > 0.9 is normal. < 0.9 is abnormal but cannot detect intimal flaps.

References

1. *ATLS, Advanced Trauma Life Support Program for Doctors.* Chicago, IL: American College of Surgeons, 2004.
2. Marx JA, Hockberger RS, Walls RM, Adams J, Rosen P, eds. *Rosen's Emergency Medicine: Concepts and Clinical Practice.* Philadelphia: Mosby Elsevier, 2010.
3. Asensio, JA, Trunkey DD. *Current Therapy of Trauma and Surgical Critical Care.* Philadelphia: Mosby Elsevier, 2008.
4. Scaletta T, Schaider J. *Emergent Management of Trauma.* Boston: McGraw-Hill, 2001.
5. MacCumber MW. *Management of Ocular Injuries and Emergencies.* Philadelphia: Lippincott-Raven, 1998.

Bibliography

Herndon, DN. *Total Burn Care.* Edinburgh: Saunders Elsevier, 2007.

Obstetrics and gynecology emergencies

Paul Matthews

8.1. Infectious disorders

8.1.1. Chlamydia

Most common sexually transmitted disease in the USA, co-infections common. Obligate intracellular bacteria.

Symptoms: vaginal itching and discharge, dysuria; may be asymptomatic.
Treatment: azithromycin 1 g PO or doxycycline 100 mg BID for 7 days. Alternatives include amoxicillin, erythromycin, fluoroquinolones.

8.1.2. Gonorrhea

Gram-negative diplococci.

Symptoms: purulent vaginal discharge, dysuria, abdominal pain; may be asymptomatic.
Treatment: 125 mg ceftriaxone IM, cefixime 400 mg PO, alternative spectinomycin 2 g IM, some strains resistant to fluoroquinolones.

8.1.3. Trichomoniasis

Pear-shaped flagellate.

Symptoms: vulvovaginal itching, discharge, malodorous.
Treatment: metronidazole 2 g PO or 500 mg BID for 7 days.

8.1.4. Syphilis

Gram-negative spirochete.

Symptoms: primary – painless genital ulcer that heals in 2–6 weeks. Secondary – disseminated with rash, adenopathy, condylomata lata. Tertiary onset after years of untreated disease. Can lead to aortic aneurysm, dementia, tabes dorsalis.
Treatment: depends on stage; penicillin, doxycycline.

Pocket Guide to the American Board of Emergency Medicine In-Training Exam, ed. Bob Cambridge.
Published by Cambridge University Press. © Cambridge University Press 2013.

8.1.5. Herpes simplex

Type II most common (80%), frequently genital. Type I can cause genital infection also.

Symptoms: painful grouped vesicles on an erythematous base. Recurrent; initial episode usually most severe.

Treatment: acyclovir, valacyclovir, famciclovir.

8.1.6. Pelvic inflammatory disease

Chlamydia and gonorrhea are common causes, may be polymicrobial.

Treatment: ceftriaxone 250 mg IM and doxycycline 100 mg PO BID x10 days, and metronidazole 500 mg PO BID x14 days. Inpatient cefotetan 2 g IV Q12 hours plus doxycycline 100 mg Q12 hours and gentamycin 2 mg/kg load plus 1.5 mg/kg IV Q8 hours. Complications include:

8.1.6.1. Fitz-Hugh-Curtis syndrome

Perihepatic inflammation due to direct or lymphatic spread of infection. Pain and tenderness right upper quadrant.

8.1.6.2. Tubo-ovarian abscess

Majority will resolve with antibiotics alone, may require surgical drainage.

8.1.7. Human papillomavirus

Symptoms: genital warts. Several types implicated in cervical cancer.

Treatment: can be treated with podofilox or imiquimod. Cryotherapy can also be used.

8.2. Ovarian pathology

8.2.1. Cyst

Higher risk for torsion if larger than 4 cm.

8.2.1.1. Functional cyst

Result from normal physiologic function. Usually resolve within 2–3 months.

8.2.1.2. Corpus luteum

Functional cyst during the luteal phase. Rupture may cause sharp pain; bleeding can be severe with peritoneal irritation.

8.2.1.3. Theca lutein cysts

Overstimulation from high beta human chorionic gonadotropin (β-HCG).

8.2.2. Hyperstimulation

Exogenous ovarian stimulation (i.e. infertility treatment), gestational trophoblastic disease, multiple gestation. Can result in massive ovarian enlargement.

8.2.3. Torsion

Torsion of ovary or fallopian tube.

Symptoms: acute-onset unilateral pain. Most often due to mass (tumors, cysts). May be intermittent. May occlude vascular supply.
Workup: pelvic sonogram study of choice.
Treatment: surgical emergency.

8.3. Uterine pathology

8.3.1. Dysfunctional bleeding

Diagnosis of exclusion. Most patients are anovulatory. Results from continuous estrogen production by ovary without progesterone induced-bleeding. Produces irregular sloughing of endometrium.

8.3.2. Endometriosis

Endometrial tissue outside the endometrial cavity. Degree of symptoms do not correlate with severity of disease. Causes inflammation, adhesions, and fibrosis.

Symptoms: typically cyclic pelvic pain before and during menses, may become more constant with progression of disease.
Workup: laparoscopy is diagnostic tool of choice.
Treatment: hormonal therapy use to induce pseudopregnancy or pseudomenopause. Surgical therapy may be used to remove endometriomas and endometrial implants. Pregnancy yields remission and is sometimes curative.

8.3.3. Prolapse

Results from failure of supporting ligaments, fascia, and pelvic floor musculature.

8.3.4. Tumors

8.3.4.1. Gestational trophoblastic disease

Abnormal proliferation of pre-placental tissue.

Benign: molar pregnancy treatment suction curettage (80% cure rate). Watch for hypertension and hyperthyroid symptoms.
Invasive: local and metastatic. Treatment involves chemotherapy (cure rate 85–90%).

8.3.4.2. Leiomyoma (fibroid)

Growth of smooth muscle cell of the myometrium. Problematic when they cause excessive bleeding, pain, or reproductive difficulty. Hysterectomy is definitive treatment. May be treated with hormones to decrease estrogen levels, uterine artery embolization, surgical resection.

8.4. Vaginal and vulvar pathology

8.4.1. Bartholin's abscess

Bartholin's glands are located at the 5 and 7 o'clock position of the vaginal orifice. Obstruction of the duct causes a cyst. Infection results in abscess. Abscess is polymicrobial, often sexually transmitted. Treated with incision and drainage and Word catheter placement. Sexually transmitted diseases and concurrent cellulitis need treatment with antibiotics.

8.4.2. Foreign body

May cause localized infection. Vaginal discharge, bleeding, foul odor are common findings. Treatment is removal of the foreign body.

8.4.3. Vaginitis/vulvovaginitis

Inflammation of the vulva and vaginal tissues.

8.4.3.1. *Candida albicans*

Most common candidal vaginitis. Treatment with PO or vaginal suppository antifungal medication.

8.4.3.2. Bacterial vaginosis

Can be polymicrobial. Malodorous discharge. May be asymptomatic. Implicated in premature labor. Treat with metronidazole.

8.4.3.3. Trichomonas

Treat with metronidazole

8.4.3.4. Contact vulvovaginitis

Chemical or allergenic (soaps, douches, tampons, feminine hygiene products, clothing, etc.) Most often removal of causative agent is curative.

8.5. Pregnancy

8.5.1. Normal changes during pregnancy

Uterine blood flow takes 15–20% of cardiac output at term. Heart rate increases 5–15%. Cardiac output increases 35–50%. Minute ventilation and tidal volume increase while functional residual capacity decreases. Plasma volume increases almost 50% while red cell numbers increase by about 30%, creating a relative anemia. White blood cell count increases to 10–14 thousand.

8.5.2. Complications of pregnancy

8.5.2.1. Abortion

8.5.2.1.1. Abortion types

Complete: expulsion of all products of conception.
Incomplete: expulsion of some but not all products of conception.

Inevitable: vaginal bleeding with cervical dilation.
Threatened: vaginal bleed without dilation of cervix.
Missed: death of the fetus with no expulsion of products of conception.

8.5.2.1.2. Abortion timeframes

First trimester: 60–80% associated with chromosomal abnormalities. Most present with vaginal bleeding. Abdominal pain/cramping is common. Stabilize as necessary. Pelvic exam to evaluate for bleeding site and possible infection. Consider pelvic sonogram to evaluate for ectopic pregnancy and retained products of conception, and to assess fetal viability. Measure be β-HCG. An intrauterine gestation should be visible (transvaginal view) if β-HCG is >2000 mIU/mL. Determine Rh factor and administer Rhogam if Rh negative.

Second trimester: multiple etiologies including infection, maternal uterine/cervical defects, maternal systemic disease, trauma, and fetal toxins.

8.5.2.2. Ectopic pregnancy

Implantation of the conceptus outside the uterus. 1–2% of all pregnancies. 99% of ectopic pregnancies are in fallopian tube.

Risk factors: including pelvic inflammatory disease, previous ectopic pregnancy, previous tubal surgery, intrauterine device (IUD), and exogenous fertility treatment.

Symptoms: rupture causes acute, sharp, severe unilateral pain. Unruptured ectopics may be pain-free.

Treatment: stabilize patient as necessary. Treatment dependent on patient's condition and study findings. Can have life-threatening bleeding. Laparotomy for ruptured unstable patients, although laparoscopy may be an alternative. Medical treatment (methotrexate most common) may be used in select stable cases. Sonogram evidence of intrauterine pregnancy (IUP) reduces risk of concurrent ectopic pregnancy to 1 in 3000.

8.5.2.3. Hypertension in pregnancy

Hypertension above 140/90 or an increase of 20 mmHg systolic or 10 mmHg diastolic from baseline. Differentiate between chronic hypertension and pregnancy related.

Preeclampsia: hypertension, proteinuria, nondependent edema in pregnancy >20 weeks. Treatment similar to HELLP syndrome. Antihypertensives (hydralazine, labetalol common).

Eclampsia: preeclampsia plus seizure. Treatment similar to preeclampsia.

8.5.2.4. HELLP syndrome

Hemolysis, elevated liver enzymes, low platelets.

Symptoms: patients may present with headache, abdominal pain, visual disturbance, and edema.

Risks: intracranial hemorrhage, renal failure, liver damage, abruptio placentae, fetal demise.

Treatment: definitive treatment is delivery of the fetus. Treatment includes magnesium sulfate 4–6 g IV, then 1–2 g/hr IV. Reflexes and magnesium level are monitored for neuromuscular depression. Calcium chloride for magnesium overdose.

8.5.2.5. Hemorrhage, antepartum

Abruptio placentae: abnormal separation of the placenta from the uterine wall resulting in bleeding. May result in fetal demise, hemorrhagic shock, disseminated intravascular coagulation (DIC), and maternal/fetal death. Vaginal bleeding is common, but may not occur if it is a concealed hemorrhage. Spontaneous cause most common. Risk factors include hypertension, previous abruption, cocaine use, advanced maternal age, trauma, and multiparity. Stabilize the patient as needed. Sonogram, CBC, coagulation profile, renal function, type and cross. Obstetric consultation emergently needed.

Placenta previa: complete previa occurs when the placenta covers the internal os, partial previa covers only a portion of the internal os. Small placental disruptions may cause profuse hemorrhage. Typical presentation is painless vaginal bleeding after 28 weeks' gestation. Vaginal exam may produce worsening bleeding and should be avoided. Ultrasound evaluation preferable. Stabilize patient as necessary. Blood work as in abruption. Emergent obstetric consultation may be needed.

8.5.2.6. Hyperemesis gravidarum

Excessive vomiting causes weight loss, electrolyte abnormalities, dehydration, ketonemia. Usually resolves around 16 weeks. May persist through entire pregnancy. Treatment with hydration, electrolyte replacement, antiemetics.

8.5.3. Infections in pregnancy

8.5.3.1. Asymptomatic bacteriuria

Much more readily progresses to cystitis and pyelonephritis in pregnant patients. Culture urine and treat with antibiotics.

8.5.3.2. Urinary tract infection (UTI)

Escherichia coli most common. Culture and consider 7 day treatment. Nitrofurantoin, amoxicillin, cephalexin.

8.5.3.3. Pyelonephritis

Risk for preterm labor and septic shock. Consider inpatient IV antibiotics and hydration.

8.5.3.4. Chorioamnionitis

Infection of the membranes and amniotic fluid around the fetus. Fever, uterine tenderness, elevated WBC. Broad spectrum IV antibiotics.

8.5.4. Rh isoimmunization

Exposure of Rh− mother to Rh+ fetal blood. Maternal IgG can cross the placenta, causing fetal hydrops. One 300 mcg dose of RhoGAM will treat 30 mL of fetal blood. Consider Kleihauer–Betke test to determine the amount of fetal blood in the maternal circulation for large bleeds as additional RhoGAM may be needed.

8.5.5. High-risk pregnancy

Seizure disorders: seizure frequency is increased during pregnancy. Treatment similar to non-pregnant patient.

Asthma: pregnant patients with acute asthma exacerbation are treated similar to non-pregnant patients.

Hyperthyroid: treatment with propylthiouracil. Thyroid storm treated with propylthiouracil, labetalol, IV fluids, cooling blanket, acetaminophen.

8.5.6. Normal labor and delivery terms

Rupture of membranes: amniotic fluid is alkaline, turning nitrazine paper blue. Ferning results from crystallization of amniotic fluid as it dries.

Station: position of the presenting part relative to the ischial spines. Zero at the ischial spines. Score becomes more negative when higher (closer to pelvic inlet), more positive when lower (+1 to +3) with +3 being at the vaginal introitus.

Six cardinal movements of delivery: engagement (fetal presenting part enters the pelvis); flexion (allows the smallest part of the head to present to the pelvis); descent (presenting part descends into the pelvis); internal rotation (rotation of the head so that the sagittal suture is aligned with the anterior-posterior vaginal dimension); extension (as the vertex passes the pubic symphysis, the neck will extend to deliver the head); external rotation (realigns the head with shoulders).

8.5.7. Complications of labor

8.5.7.1. Fetal distress

Presence of signs or symptoms indicating the fetus may not be well. Tachycardia or brady-cardia, decreased heart rate variability, late decelerations, meconium-stained amniotic fluid. Treatment is aimed at the cause, but rapid delivery by instruments or c-section may be advised.

8.5.7.2. Premature labor

Labor before 37 weeks. Causes include premature rupture of membranes, infection, sponta-neous, and iatrogenic. Potential contraindications to tocolytic therapy include uterine infec-tion, nonreassuring fetal testing, bleeding, premature rupture of membranes. Common treat-ment includes IV hydration and bedrest.

8.5.7.3. Preterm premature rupture of membranes (PPROM)

Rupture of membranes before 37 weeks' gestation and before onset of labor. Term prema-ture rupture of membranes is the rupture of membranes after 37 weeks' gestation, but before onset of labor. If there is concern for PPROM, carry out sterile speculum exam to con-firm. Nitrazine paper turns blue in alkaline fluid. Avoid bimanual exams. Risk for premature delivery, chorioamnionitis, endometritis, cord prolapse, fetal malposition, neonatal sepsis. Tocolytic is considered only to give premature fetus time for steroids to enhance lung matu-rity prior to delivery.

8.5.7.4. Rupture of uterus

Life-threatening to both mother and fetus. Emergency laparotomy with cesarean delivery. Symptoms include abdominal pain, ripping sensation, tachycardia, hypovolemic shock.

8.5.8. Complications of delivery

8.5.8.1. Malposition of fetus

Risk that the cervix will not be adequately dilated for delivery of the head, causing cord prolapse and/or fetal demise. Immediate obstetric consultation.

Breech presentation: longitudinal lie with head away from pelvis. Fetal buttocks presents in frank breech.

Incomplete breech: hips and knees are flexed with baby sitting with feet next to the buttocks.

Footling breech: feet first with buttocks superiorly located. Footling and incomplete breech are never safe for vaginal delivery.

8.5.8.2. Nuchal cord

Umbilical cord wrapped around neck of fetus. Attempt to manually reduce the cord over the fetus' head. It may be able to be reduced over the shoulders with the fetus delivered through the cord. If unable, clamp cord in two places and cut. Delivery must be immediate if cord is cut.

8.5.8.3. Prolapse of cord

Palpable pulsating cord on bimanual exam. Should not be replaced, instead apply pressure to the presenting part of the infant to relieve pressure on the cord. Do not remove hand – accompany patient to obstetrics for definitive c-section.

8.5.9. Post-partum complications

8.5.9.1. Endometritis

Infection of uterine lining.

Causes: delivery (especially c-section), premature rupture of membranes, medical instrumentation, retained products of conception, abortion.

Symptoms: fever, foul-smelling vaginal discharge and uterine tenderness on bimanual exam.

Treatment: IV antibiotics and admission for post-c-section patients and those with significant comorbidity or toxicity. Mild cases may be treated at home with oral antibiotics. Multiple antibiotic regimens, including ampicillin + gentamycin or cefoxitin/cefotetan/cefotaxime.

8.5.9.2. Hemorrhage

Causes: uterine atony, genital tract laceration, uterine rupture, retained products of conception, and uterine inversion.

Treatment: stabilize patient as necessary. Two large bore IVs for significant bleed.

8.5.9.3. Mastitis

Focal breast infection, usually normal skin flora or oral flora of a breastfeeding infant.

Symptoms: focal tenderness, difference in regional warmth, fever, and elevated white blood cell count. Abscess may complicate the infection.

Treatment: oral antibiotics and continued breast feeding or breast pumping. Incision and drainage if abscess present. Admission for toxic patients or those that do not respond to oral antibiotics.

Bibliography

Callahan T, Caughey A. *Obstetrics and Gynecology*. Wolters Philadelphia: Kluwer/Lippincott Williams & Wilkins, 2009.

CDC. Sexually transmitted diseases treatment guidelines [Internet]. 2010 [updated 2012; cited May 2012]. Available from: http://www.cdc.gov/std/treatment/2010.

D'Alton M, Norwitz E, McElrath T. *Maternal–Fetal Medicine*. Cambridge: Cambridge University Press, 2007.

Duff P, Edwards R, Davis J, Rhoton-Vlasak A. *Obstetrics and Gynecology*. New York: McGraw-Hill, 2004.

Marx JA, Hockberger RS, Walls RM, Adams J, Rosen P, eds. *Rosen's Emergency Medicine: Concepts and Clinical Practice*. Philadelphia: Mosby Elsevier, 2010.

Tintinalli JE, Stapczynski JS, Cline DM, *et al.* *Tintinalli's Emergency Medicine: A Comprehensive Study Guide*, 7th edn. New York: The McGraw-Hill Companies, Inc., 2011.

Chapter

9

Pediatric emergencies

Teresa Riech

9.1. Pediatric fever

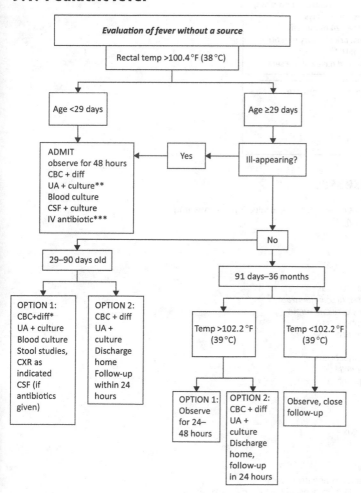

Figure 9.1. Workup of pediatric fever [1–8].

Pocket Guide to the American Board of Emergency Medicine In-Training Exam, ed. Bob Cambridge. Published by Cambridge University Press. © Cambridge University Press 2013.

Figure 9.1. (*cont.*)

*CBC in non-toxic children >29 days

If WBC count <15 000 and ANC <10 000: re-evaluate in 24 hours, follow-up culture results, consider Rocephin (ceftriaxone) 50 mg/kg IM or IV

If WBC count >15 000 or ANC >10 000, admit for observation, obtain blood culture, consider CSF studies if not already obtained

---

**UA/culture
- Circumcised males under 24 months if ≥2 risk factors: non-black, temp. ≥39 °C, duration of temp. ≥24 hours
- Uncircumcised males under 12 months
- Females under 24 months if ≥1 risk factor: non-black, temp. ≥39 °C, duration of temp. ≥2 days
- Consider in females older than 24 months if known urologic abnormality, prior history of febrile UTI, symptoms suggestive of UTI
- All children who have UA should have culture sent

***Antibiotic options for neonates

Ampicillin + gentamicin
Ampicillin + cefotaxime
+/– acyclovir

9.2. Infectious diseases

Table 9.1 Age-related causes of serious bacterial infection in very young children (in order of frequency)

Bacteremia/meningitis	
<1 month	GBBS
	Escherichia coli
	Listeria
	Pneumococcus
	Haemophilus influenzae
	Staphylococcus aureus
	Meningococcus
1–3 months	Pneumococcus
	GBBS
	Meningococcus
	Salmonella
	H. influenzae
	Listeria
Osteomyelitis/septic arthritis	
<1 month	GBBS
	S. aureus
1–3 months	*S.aureus*
UTI	
0–3 months	*E. coli*
	Other Gram-negative bacilli
	Group D streptococcus (including enterococcus)

GBBS, group B β-hemolytic streptococcus; UTI, urinary tract infection.

9.2.1. Desquamating rashes

9.2.1.1. Toxic shock syndrome (TSS) [9]

Defined by the Center for Disease Control (CDC) as body temperature over 38.9 °C (102.0 °F), systolic blood pressure <90 mmHg, diffuse rash, intense erythroderma, blanching with subsequent desquamation, especially of the palms and soles, involvement of three or more organ systems.

9.2.1.2. Streptococcal toxic shock syndrome

As above with isolation of group A streptococcus from a normally sterile site such as blood or cerebrospinal fluid (CSF) (definite case), or from a normally nonsterile site such as sputum or skin lesion (probable case).

Treatment: β-lactamase resistant antistaph antibiotic (oxacillin, nafcillin), or clindamycin. Aggressive supportive therapy. IVIG has been shown effective in neutralizing TSS toxin, aids in recovery. 1 g/kg should be given within 6 hours. IVIG has doubled 30-day survival.

9.2.1.3. Staphylococcal scalded skin syndrome (SSSS)

Usually seen in children <5 years old.

Presentation: red rash followed by diffuse epidermal exfoliation. Patient also often has malaise, fever, irritability, and skin tenderness prior to the rash. May have had a prodromal localized *S. aureus* infection of the skin, throat, nose, mouth, umbilicus, or gastrointestinal (GI) tract. Infection often is not apparent before the SSSS rash appears.

Rash description: sandpaper-like, progressing into a wrinkled appearance, accentuated in flexor creases; Nikolsky sign (gentle stroking of the skin causes the skin to separate at the epidermis); exfoliation of skin, may be patchy or sheetlike; facial edema; perioral crusting.

Note: on the exam think of SSSS if you see a screaming infant with desquamating rash. They almost always picture a baby.

9.2.1.4. Erythema multiforme (EM) spectrum

9.2.1.4.1. EM minor

Pruritic, non-blistering (fixed) urticaria-like lesions with little systemic reaction. Lesions fade slowly over a week. May be targetoid or flat-topped.

9.2.1.4.2. EM major (Steven–Johnson syndrome [SJS])

Involves mucous membranes and urogenital area. Systemic symptoms.

9.2.1.4.3. Toxic epidermal necrolysis (TEN)

Dramatic blisters develop rapidly all over body. High fever, severe mucous membrane involvement.

<10% body surface area involvement: SJS.
10–29%: SJS/TEN overlap.
≥30%: TEN.
Causes: "SOAP" (Sulfa, Oral hypoglycemics, Anticonvulsants, Penicillin). Other causes include malignancy, hormonal and lots of infectious causes. Herpes simplex virus (HSV) and *Mycoplasma* are "classic."

Note: SSSS differs from the more severe TEN, in that the cleavage site in SSSS is intraepidermal, as opposed to TEN, which involves necrosis of the full epidermal layer (at the level of the basement membrane).

9.2.1.5. Kawasaki disease

Leading cause-acquired heart disease in children in the USA. Occurrence peaks in at 18–24 months (85% <5 years old) – Asian more susceptible.

Diagnostic criteria: fever over 5 days and at least 4 of the following.

Bilateral, painless conjunctival injection.
Mucous membranes: injected, fissured lips, pharyngeal injection, "strawberry tongue".
Erythema/edema of hands and feet (acute) and periungual/generalized desquamation (convalescent).
Polymorphous truncal rash.
Cervical lymphadenopathy.

Lab abnormalities: high WBC count, very high platelet count, mild hemolytic anemia, elevated C-reactive protein (CRP) and erythrocyte sedimentation rate (ESR).

Treatment: IVIG (decrease aneurysms if <10 days from onset), high-dose aspirin (100 mg/kg/day), cardiac evaluation. Treatment is to prevent cardiac involvement; coronary aneurysms, valve insufficiency, congestive heart failure (CHF). MI is the most common cause of death. Some affected children develop gallbladder hydrops (self-limited).

Table 9.2 Comparison of desquamating rashes

	Kawasaki's	EM spectrum (SJS)	Streptococcal scarlet fever	Toxic shock syndrome
Age	<5 years old	Any	Usually 2–8 years old	10 years old
Eyes	Non-exudative conjunctivitis, limbal sparing	Exudative conjunctivitis, keratitis	Normal	Conjunctivitis
Fever	5 days	Prolonged	Varies (<10 days)	<10 days
Oral mucosa	Strawberry tongue, diffusely erythematous mucosa	Erythema, ulcers, pseudomembrane	Strawberry tongue, pharyngitis	Erythematous
Extremities	Palm/sole erythema, edema, induration, sheet-like desquamation (late)	Normal	Flaky desquamating	Swelling, no desquamation
Rash	Erythematous, polymorphous, targetoid, purpuric	Targetoid	Sandpaper, Pastia's lines, circumoral pallor	Erythroderma
Cervical lymphadenopathy	At least 1 node >1.5 cm	–	Tender LAD	–
Labs	Anemia, elevated ALT/AST, high platelets after day 7	Herpes-virus infection	+ throat culture	High platelets
Systemic	Arthritis	Arthritis, herpetic lesions		Mental status changes

LAD, left anterior descending.

9.2.2. Scarlet fever

Cause: streptococcal species.

Rash description: sandpaper rash (the rash you feel, not see), may be erythematous. Patient may have circumoral pallor, Pastia's lines, strawberry tongue.

Treatment: IM penicillin 25,000 U/kg. Azithromycin if allergic to penicillin.

9.2.3. Streptococcal pharyngitis [10]

Most common cause of pharyngitis is viral, but test and treat for streptococcus to avoid long-term complications such as glomerulonephritis.

Treatment: IM penicillin as for scarlet fever. Oral regimens: penicillin VK or amoxicillin for 10 days.

9.2.4. Impetigo

Caused by *S. aureus*, followed by groups A, C, and G streptococcus. Primary infections in children (ages 2–5), secondary in adults.

Rash: appears as bullous and non-bullous (more common) honey-crusted lesions occuring over 1 week.

Treatment: topical or topical and systemic (Bactroban ointment; clindamycin, dicloxacillin, cephalexin) for 7 days.

Note: glomerulonephritis is caused more often by strep skin infections than pharyngitis.

9.2.5. Viral infections

9.2.5.1. Fifth disease (erythema infectiosum)

Cause: human parvovirus (HPV) B19, which also is associated with polyarthropathy, aplastic anemia, and hydrops fetalis.
Patient is no longer infectious once rash appears.

Phase 1: a bright red, raised, slapped-cheek rash with circumoral pallor. Nasolabial folds usually spared.

Phase 2: 1–4 days later; erythematous maculopapular rash on proximal extremities (usually arms and extensor surfaces) and trunk, which fades into a classic lace-like reticular pattern as confluent areas clear. Palms/soles usually spared.

Phase 3: rash clears and recurrences for weeks/months due to stimuli like exercise, irritation, or overheating of skin from bathing or sunlight.

9.2.5.2. Roseola infantum

Seen in children 6 months to 3 years.

Cause: human herpesvirus-6 (HHV-6).

Presentation: several days of high fever. Rash appears when fever breaks.

9.2.5.3. Varicella

Presentation: incubation of 14–21 days. 1–2 day prodrome of respiratory symptoms and low-grade fever. Rash develops with papules becoming vesicles (dew drop) which then dry and crust (no longer infectious).

Complications: scarring, bacterial superinfection, pneumonia, arthritis, Reye's syndrome, encephalitis.

Treatment: symptomatic – antihistamines. Acyclovir if immune compromise (or if present within 24 hours of illness). For those at high risk for severe infection give varicella zoster immunoglobulin (VZIG).

9.2.5.4. Pityriasis rosea

Presentation: 50% are preceded by a herald patch. "Christmas tree" distribution of macular rash. No oral lesions.

Treatment: self-limited, lasts 8–12 weeks. Sunlight may help rash fade.

Mimic: secondary syphilis (check a rapid plasma regain [RPR] in sexually active patients on the boards and in real life).

9.2.5.5. HSV

Presentation: grouped vesicles arising on erythematous base on keratinized skin or mucous membranes. Regional lymphadenopathy during the primary outbreak. Patient may endorse a tingling sensation 24 hours prior to outbreak.

Diagnosis: Tzanck smear ("Tzanck goodness I don't have Herpes!").

Treatment: acyclovir QID or valacyclovir BID or famciclovir TID. Daily suppression can decrease frequency if >6 outbreaks/year.

9.2.5.5.1. Herpetic whitlow

Cause: HSV on the digits, usually HSV-1.

Presentation: painful, grouped, confluence of vesicles. Usually in children, sometimes in dental workers.

Treatment: oral antivirals as listed above. Can be misdiagnosed as paronychia; do not incise as it may cause spread and prolong course.

9.2.6. Pediatric rash wrap-up

9.2.6.1. Drug rashes

Most reactions occur within 1 week. Morbilliform rashes are common. Urticarial rashes are common. The reaction is usually IgE-mediated.

9.2.6.2. Common rash buzz words

Pityriasis rosea: herald patch (can be confused with nummular eczema or ringworm).
Smallpox: centripetal rash (starts peripherally, moves centrally).
Varicella: dew drop on a rose petal (centrifugal: starts centrally, moves peripherally).
Impetigo: honey-colored crusted lesions.

9.3. Infestations

9.3.1. Pinworms

Perianal itching worse at night, often has pets in the house.

Diagnosis: clinical suspicion. May be able to retrieve worm with tape applied to anus at nighttime.

Treatment: mebendazole if >2 years old; if < 2 years old, use pyrantel pamoate. Treat family. Repeat in 1 week.

9.3.2. Scabies

Symptoms: extremely itchy. Excoriations and papule with burrows (thin line with gray/red/brown appearance in webspaces, axillary folds, genital folds, wrists, buttocks, thighs, knees is pathognomonic).
Transmission: occurs by skin-to-skin contact, but may also occur through linens/clothing.
Treatment: 5% permetherin cream if >2 months old. Treat family and repeat in 1 week.

9.3.3. Head lice

Presentation: itchy scalp, nits seen on exam. Nits more than 1/4 inch from scalp are dead.
Treatment: permetherin 1–2% cream if > 2 months old. Malathion if > 6 years old.

9.3.4. Tinea capitus

Treatment: topicals are not very effective. Microsize griseofulvin 10–20 mg/kg/day or ultramicrosize griseofulvin 5–15 mg/kg/day (max 750 mg) orally once a day. Give with a fatty meal. Treat 4–6 weeks (2 weeks beyond clinical resolution). Healthy children do not need LFTs.

9.3.4.1. Kerion

Tinea capitus that has become secondarily infected with bacteria. Erythematous boggy appearance.

Treatment: griseofulvin, prednisone (1.5–2 mg/kg/day, max 20 mg – taper over 2 weeks).
Note: On the exam, scalp problem in an African American child is tinea capitus until proven otherwise and in a white child is head lice until proven otherwise.

9.4. Non-accidental trauma [11, 12]

Red-flag injury patterns: symmetric wounds (especially burns), wounds/bruises with unusual shape (i.e. loops), bucket-handle fractures and corner fractures (from limb jerking), trunk bruises, injuries inconsistent with developmental age or described mechanism, rib fractures (especially posterior ribs), wounds, or fractures in different stages of healing
Mimics of abuse: "toddler's fracture" (spiral tibia fracture), birth trauma (especially clavicles), metabolic bone disease (rickets), neoplasm, osteogenesis imperfect, infection, osteomyelitis, congenital syphilis, drug toxicity.
Note: for an apparent life-threatening event (ALTE) in a child >1 year old think medical child abuse. All ALTEs should have a retinal exam.
Workup:
> **<12 months old:** skeletal survey, head CT, trauma screening labs (can include; coags, LFTs, CBC, amylase, lipase, creatinine phosphokinase [CPK] if lots of bruises, urinalysis [UA]), abdominal CT (if trauma labs positive, if bilious vomiting, or if truncal bruising), formal retinal exam.

13–24 months old: skeletal survey is required, the rest of the workup as above is recommended.

2–4 years old: skeletal survey if developmental delay, severe or life-threatening trauma or failure to thrive. The rest of the workup as above is recommended.

9.5. Rheumatologic diseases

9.5.1. Juvenile idiopathic/rheumatoid arthritis

Presentation: refusal to walk or limping ("happy limpers"). May complain of chest pain (pericarditis at onset). As disease progresses joint flexion contractures can develop. Seen commonly in age <16.

9.5.2. Henoch–Schönlein purpura

Presentation: severe abdominal pain. Purpura on extremities, usually over buttocks, lower legs, and elbows.

Diagnosis: hypertension, persistent proteinuria (10–20%), thrombocytosis (platelet count always normal or high; if thrombocytopenia present, consider idiopathic thrombocytopenic purpura [ITP], hemolytic uremic syndrome [HUS], systemic lupus erythematosus [SLE], other vasculidities).

Treatment: can be managed as outpatient. Treat arthralgias with acetaminophen or NSAIDs, need follow-up, urine and blood pressure monitoring. Glomerulonephritis develops within 1 month of rash. Recurrences common.

9.5.3. Acute rheumatic fever

Diagnosis: modified Jones criteria of 1992: requires evidence of antecedent streptococcal infection (elevated/rising anti-streptolysin antibody [ASO] titer, or positive rapid streptococcal test or streptococcal culture).

> **Major Jones criteria of rheumatic fever:** polyarthritis, carditis, subcutaneous nodules, erythema marginatum, Sydenham's chorea.
>
> **Minor criteria:** fever, arthralgias (cannot use if you count polyarthritis as a major criteria), elevated acute phase reactants (CRP or ESR), prolonged PR interval.
>
> **High probability of acute rheumatic fever:** 2 major or 1 major and 2 minor.

9.5.4. Synovial fluid analysis [13]

Table 9.3 Synovial fluid analysis

Gross exam	Normal	Non-inflammatory	Inflammatory	Septic
Color	Colorless or straw	Straw/yellow	Yellow	Variable
WBCs (mm³)	<200	50–1000	1000–75 000	Usually >100 000
PMNs	<25%	<25%	50%	75% (less if partially treated)
Culture, Gram stain	Negative	Negative	Negative	Often positive

PMNs, polymorphonuclear neutrophils. [12]

9.6. Gastroenterology and abdominal emergencies

Most are covered in Chapter 3.

9.6.1. Meconium ileus

Diagnosis: dilated small bowel loops, air–fluid levels, bubbly appearance on X-ray.
Associated with: cystic fibrosis, Hirschsprung's, ileal stenosis, meconium plug syndrome, ileal atresia.

9.6.2. Pyloric stenosis

Presentation: non-bilious projectile vomiting in the first month of life.
Diagnosis: hypochloremic metabolic alkalosis, exaggerated peristalsis, pyloric wall >3 mm, canal elongation >14 mm diagnostic on ultrasound.
Treatment: surgery.

9.6.3. Midgut volvulus

Presentation: bilious vomiting in first week of life.
Diagnosis: corkscrew appearance or double-bubble sign on plain films.
Treatment: surgery.

9.7. Toxic ingestions

9.7.1. Button batteries [14]

Found in hearing aid, calculator, watch, camera. Usually contain metal salt (mercury or lithium) plus alkali. Concern over caustic injury if leaks. 86% pass within 4 days.
Diagnosis: chest X-ray and /or soft tissue neck films to localize.
Treatment: batteries in the esophagus must be removed by endoscopy. Batteries in the stomach/intestines; recommend mild cathartic, check stools until it passes; if not passed in 5–7 days, repeat films. Repeat films sooner if abdominal pain, tenderness, diarrhea/constipation. Surgery consult if symptomatic.

9.7.2. Hydrocarbon inhalation/ingestion

Deliberate inhalation of volatile hydrocarbons for mood-altering effects in adolescents ("huffing"). Volatile hydrocarbons are contained in glues, solvents, lighter fluid, gasoline, paints, and propellants in pressurized aerosol products. Pulmonary toxicity results from hydrocarbon aspiration.

Pathophysiology: direct injury to respiratory epithelium leading to inflammation/bronchospasm. Direct contact with alveolar membranes leads to hemorrhage, hyperemia, edema, surfactant inactivation, leukocyte infiltration, vascular thrombosis, poor oxygen exchange, atelectasis, pneumonitis.
Diagnosis: obtain chest X-ray in all symptomatic patients, although initial chest X-ray may be normal. Findings (atelectasis, perihilar opacities, bibasilar infiltrates) may develop over the first few hours. Labs, blood gas can be drawn.
Treatment: GI decontamination (consider for CHAMP: Camphor, Halogenated hydrocarbons, Aromatic Hydrocarbons, hydrocarbons with heavy Metals or Pesticides).

Decontaminate skin, oxygen as needed, inhaled β2-agonists for bronchospasm. Respiratory support as needed. If discharge is considered for asymptomatic patient, chest X-ray should be obtained 6 hours after the ingestion to document the negative findings.

9.8. Pediatric miscellany

9.8.1. Ossification centers of the elbow

Mnemonic: "CRITOE".

Table 9.4 Ossification centers of the elbow

	Appear	Disappear
Capitellum	2	4
Radial head	4	6
Internal (medial) epicondyle	6	8
Trochlea	8	10
Olecranon	10	12
External (lateral) epicondyle	12	14

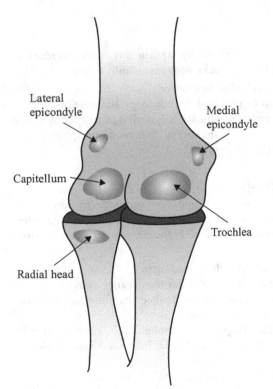

Figure 9.2. Ossification centers of the elbow.

Lateral epicondyle

Medial epicondyle

Capitellum

Trochlea

Radial head

9.8.2. Radiographic clues to necrotizing enterocolitis (NEC)

Abdominal distention, pneumatosis intestinalis, hepatic portal venous gas.

9.8.3. Causes of neonatal jaundice (in order 24 hours to 2 weeks)

"Babies Hate Pediatricians Because Pain is Inevitable"
Breast milk jaundice.
Hemolysis.
Physiologic.
Bruising (i.e. cephalohematoma or caput succedaneum).
Polycythemia.
Infection (i.e. UTI).

9.8.4. Endotracheal tube size calculations

Endotracheal tube size (3 options to calculate):
   (age+16)/4.
   (age/4)+4 for uncuffed.
   (age/4)+3 for cuffed.
Depth of insertion: tube size x3 is desired depth at the gum.

9.8.5. General growth rules

Infants double birthweight by 4–5 months and triple by 12–14 months.
Children double their birth length by 3–4 years old.

References

1. Byington CL, Enriquez FR, Hoff C, *et al.* Serious bacterial infections in febrile infants 1 to 90 days old with and without viral infections. *Pediatrics.* 2004; **113**(6): 1662–6.
2. Baraff LJ, Bass JW, Fleisher GR, *et al.* Practice guideline for the management of infants and children 0 to 36 months of age with fever without source. Agency for Health Care Policy and Research. *Ann Emerg Med.* 1993; **22**(7): 1198–210.
3. Jaskiewicz JA, McCarthy CA, Richardson AC, *et al.* Febrile infants at low risk for serious bacterial infection: an appraisal of the Rochester criteria and implications for management. Febrile Infant Collaborative Study Group. *Pediatrics.* 1994; **94**(3): 390–6.
4. Bachur RG, Harper MB. Predictive model for serious bacterial infections among infants younger than 3 months of age. *Pediatrics.* 2001; **108**(2): 311–16.
5. Bleeker SE, Derksen-Lubsen G, Grobbee DE, *et al.* Validating and updating a prediction rule for serious bacterial infection in patients with fever without source. *Acta Paediatr.* 2007; **96**(1): 100–4.
6. Isaacman DJ, Shults J, Gross TK, Davis PH, Harper M. Predictors of bacteremia in febrile children 3 to 36 months of age. *Pediatrics.* 2000; **106**(5): 977–82.
7. Lacour AG, Zamora SA, Gervaix A. A score identifying serious bacterial infections in children with fever without source. *Pediatr Infect Dis J.* 2008; **27**(7): 654–6.
8. AAP Clinical Practice Guideline. Urinary tract infection: clinical practice guideline for the diagnosis and management of the initial UTI in febrile infants and children 2 to 24 months. *Pediatrics.* 2011; **128**(3): 595–610.
9. CDC. National notifiable diseases surveillance system [Internet]. 2011 [updated 2012 Jun; cited 2012 Jun]. Available from:

http://www.cdc.gov/osels/ph_surveillance/nndss/casedef/toxicsscurrent.htm.

10. Pickering, LK, ed. *Red Book: 2012 Report of the Committee on Infectious Diseases*, 29th edn. Elk Grove Village: American Academy of Pediatrics, 2012.

11. Kaczor K, Pierce MC, Makoroff K, Corey TS. Bruising and physical child abuse. *Clin Ped Emerg Med*. 2006; **7**: 153–60.

12. Pierce, MC. Appendix 2: Physical child abuse workup for children 4 years of age and younger in the emergency department setting. *Clin Ped Emerg Med*. 2006; **7**(3).

13. Pickering, LK, edr. *Red Book: 2012 Report of the Committee on Infectious Diseases*, 29th edn. Elk Grove Village: American Academy of Pediatrics 2012. Table 3.67, p. 673

14. Litovitz T, Whitaker N, Clark L, White NC, Marsolek M. Emerging battery ingestion hazard: clinical implications. *Pediatrics* 2010; **125**(6): 1168–77.

Chapter

10

Psychobehavioral emergencies

Paul Matthews

10.1. Addictive behavior

10.1.1. Drug dependence

Compulsive need to use drugs to function normally. Withdrawal symptoms occur when drugs are unavailable. May exhibit tolerance despite larger doses. Continued use despite unwanted social/physical outcomes. Reduction in normal activities and excessive time spent seeking substance.

10.1.2. Alcohol

Alcohol dependence is common – patient develops tolerance to alcohol and withdrawal symptoms occur when intake is stopped.

Withdrawal: symptoms may begin as little as 6 hours after last drink. Blood alcohol level at symptom onset varies from patient to patient. Autonomic instability – hypertension, tachycardia, sweating; nausea, vomiting, diarrhea, anxiety, tremor, hallucination, seizure.

Delirium tremens: may occur in 5% of patients during withdrawal. Manifests with hallucination, delirium, severe autonomic instability. Delirium tremens is lethal in 20–35% without treatment, 5–10% with treatment. Lorazepam first-line treatment.

Wernicke–Korsakoff syndrome: caused by thiamine deficiency likely due to malnutrition in alcoholics. Wernicke encephalopathy – confusion, nystagmus, ataxia, coma. Korsakoff psychosis – anterograde and retrograde amnesia, hallucination, confabulation.

10.1.3. Eating disorders

10.1.3.1. Anorexia nervosa

Abnormal eating behavior associated with low body weight, directed at achieving a specific body image.

10.1.3.2. Bulimia nervosa

Abnormal eating behavior associated with normal body weight, directed at achieving a specific body image.

Pocket Guide to the American Board of Emergency Medicine In-Training Exam, ed. Bob Cambridge.
Published by Cambridge University Press. © Cambridge University Press 2013.

10.1.4. Substance abuse

Maladaptive substance use that leads to failure to fulfill expected obligations, to recurrent legal and social problems, and recurrent physical dangers.

10.2. Mood disorders and thought disorders

10.2.1. Acute psychosis

Acute loss of contact with reality. Delusions, hallucination, speech disturbance, disorganized/catatonic behavior. Often accompanied by cognitive disability and emotional lability, resulting in inability to function.

10.2.2. Bipolar disorder

Bipolar I has at least one episode of mania and major depressive episodes. Bipolar II is a milder form with at least one episode of hypomania and major depressive episodes.

Criteria for manic episode: include grandiosity/highly inflated self-esteem, decreased need for sleep, pressured speech, flight of ideas, poor attention span, increased activity, excessive involvement in pleasurable activities with potential for poor outcomes such as excessive spending and promiscuous sexual activity.

10.2.3. Depression

Most common major psychiatric disorder.

Mnemonic: CASE PIGS.

<u>C</u>oncentration – inability to concentrate.
<u>A</u>ppetite – increased or decreased.
<u>S</u>leep – insomnia or hypersomnia.
<u>E</u>nergy – low energy/fatigue.
<u>P</u>sychomotor – agitation or depression.
<u>I</u>nterest – decreased interest in activities.
<u>G</u>uilt – inappropriate guilt or worthlessness.
<u>S</u>uicidiality – ideation, plan, attempt.

Suicide risk: factors associated with higher risk include male sex, widowed/divorced/separated, unemployed, legal/disciplinary trouble, drug/alcohol abuse, acute/chronic medical illness, depression/bipolar or schizophrenia, panic disorder, previous suicide attempts with realistic, high-risk suicide plan, unsupportive family, and social isolation. Lower risk associated with female sex, married, employed, good health without drug/alcohol abuse, no previous suicide attempts or low-risk suicide plans, strong family and social support.

10.2.4. Grief reaction

Normal response to significant loss. Restlessness, disorganization, sadness, apathy. May last days to months. Somatic symptoms may include generalized weakness, headache, palpitation, shortness of breath.

10.2.5. Schizophrenia

Break from reality. Hallucination, delusion, disorganized speech and thinking. Can cause significant social and occupational dysfunction.

10.3. Factitious disorders

10.3.1. Drug-seeking behavior

Common complaints include back pain, headache, extremity pain, and dental pain. May also complain of withdrawal symptoms. May cite lost prescription or state their regular doctor is unavailable. May add blood to urine specimen to mimic kidney stone. Often difficult to truly make "drug-seeking" diagnosis. Be careful to chart factual/objective findings.

10.3.2. Munchausen syndrome/Munchausen by proxy

Exaggeration or creation of symptoms of illness to get attention, sympathy, evaluation, and treatment from medical profession. Munchausen by proxy is rare form of child abuse where others create symptoms or inflict harm on others for the same purpose. May be unusually happy with abnormal test results. Rule out true medical disease as a cause of symptoms then treat the underlying psychiatric disorder.

10.4. Psychosomatic disorder

10.4.1. Hypochondriasis

Occurs in 1–5%. Patient is certain of serious, unrecognized illness. Seeks medical attention, doctor shops, insists on testing. Seems pleased with diagnosis of illness. May be temporarily consoled with reassurance, but symptoms and concerns typically return within days to weeks.

10.4.2. Hysteria/conversion

Pattern of loss of function incompatible with known physiology, without organic pathologic explanation. Paralysis, paresthesia, globus hystericus, seizure, blindness, deafness, unconsciousness. Primary gain is in hiding an unconscious mental conflict.

10.5. Neurotic disorders

10.5.1. Anxiety/panic

As many as 1 in 4 in the general population may be affected by anxiety disorder. Occurs more often in women than men; also more common in lower socioeconomic groups. Panic disorder lifetime prevalence 1.5–5%. Additional psychiatric disorder found in 91% of panic patients. Evaluate with a calm and confident demeanor. Attention to slow breathing. Benzodiazepines may be helpful in short term.

10.5.2. Obsessive–compulsive

1 in 50 adults. Obsession is the intrusive thoughts leading to fear, apprehension, or worry. Compulsion is the repetitive behaviors patients use to reduce anxiety. Patients generally recognize their behaviors as irrational.

10.5.3. Phobia

Most common mental illness in women and second in men >25 years old. Persistent fear of a situation or object inappropriate for the true danger it poses. Patients will go to great lengths to avoid encounters which may cause marked distress and social/occupational difficulty.

10.5.4. Post-traumatic stress disorder (PTSD)

Anxiety disorder caused by exposure to a situation resulting in psychological trauma. Flashbacks, nightmares, hypervigilance, avoidance of stimuli related to the sensitizing event. Approximately 8% of those exposed to trauma will develop PTSD.

10.6. Organic psychoses

10.6.1. Chronic organic psychotic conditions

10.6.1.1. Alcoholic psychoses

Common cause of acute psychosis, but can become chronic. Alcohol abuse associated with 8 times increase in psychotic disorders in men and 3 times in women.

10.6.1.2. Drug psychoses

Many drugs can cause acute psychosis. Drugs of abuse include alcohol, cannabinoid (plant based and synthetic analogs), barbiturate, benzodiazepine, cocaine, LSD, amphetamine, MDMA, mephedrone ("bath salts"). Other over-the-counter and prescription drugs include dextromethorphan, antihistamines, prednisone, antidepressants, and antiepileptics. Inhalant abuse (toluene, butane, gasoline). Plants (jimson weed, deadly nightshade, morning glory).

10.6.2. Delirium

Acute onset, with fluctuating course of level of consciousness and alertness. Other findings include disorganized behavior, cognitive deficits, altered sleep cycle, and hallucination. Delirium is a symptom and treatment is based on the cause – infection, metabolic disorder, drugs/medications/toxins, central nervous system (CNS) injury/lesion.

10.6.3. Dementia

Globally impaired cognitive function that is progressive, but does not affect level of consciousness. Affects memory, attention, language, orientation, problem solving. Usually irreversible, but reversible metabolic, endocrine, and medication induced causes should be ruled out.

10.7. Personality disorder

10.7.1. Cluster A (odd/eccentric)

Paranoid: lifetime prevalence of 0.5–2.5%. Suspicious, distrustful, anticipate harm.
Schizoid: up to 7.5%. Emotional detachment; like to be left alone.
Schizotypal: 3%. Odd affect. Strange thoughts, perception, and beliefs.

10.7.2. Cluster B (dramatic/emotional)

Antisocial: 3% men, 1% women. Remorseless and repetitive disregard for rules and laws of society.

Borderline: 1–2%. Poor impulse control. Unstable relationships and self-image.

Histrionic: 2–3%. Attention craving. Excessive emotionality.

Narcissistic: 1%. Extreme low self-esteem but appears arrogant and entitled.

10.7.3. Cluster C (anxious/fearful)

Avoidant: 0.5–1%. Strong desire to have relationships, but avoid due to feelings of inadequacy.

Dependent: 15–20%. Needy. Reliant on others for emotional support. Need help in decision making.

Obsessive–Compulsive: 1%. Need for order and control.

10.8. Patterns of violence/abuse/neglect

10.8.1. Interpersonal violence

Between 4% and 15% of women in the emergency department are there because of domestic violence; going to the emergency department may be a de-escalating strategy.

10.8.2. Child, intimate partner, elder

Lifetime prevalence of 29% for women and 22% for men for intimate partner violence. Women are victims in 85% of non-lethal cases.

Homicidal risk: approx. 3/4 victims are women. Women threatened or assaulted with a gun or other weapon are 20 times more likely to be murdered. Women who are threatened are 15 times more likely to be murdered. A gun in the house increases an abused woman's chances of being murdered by 6 times. Drug and alcohol abuse where the abuser is drunk every day or almost every day also increases risk.

10.8.3. Elder abuse

Estimated 3–10% of all elders (>65 years) have been abused. Mortality is 3 times that of non-abused. Includes physical, emotional, financial exploitation, neglect, sexual, and abandonment.

10.8.4. Sexual assault

Lifetime prevalence of 1 in 6 women, 1 in 33 men. Perform complete physical exam with evidence collection. Offer sexually transmitted disease, hepatitis, HIV prophylaxis. Determine pregnancy status and potential for unwanted pregnancy.

Sexually transmitted disease prophylaxis: common sexually transmitted disease regimen includes ceftriaxone 125 mg IM, metronidazole, 2 g PO, and azithromycin 1 g PO.

Bibliography

Marx JA, Hockberger RS, Walls RM, Adams J, Rosen P, eds. *Rosen's Emergency Medicine: Concepts and Clinical Practice*. Philadelphia: Mosby Elsevier, 2010.

Murphy M, Cowan R, Sederer L. *Psychiatry*. Philadelphia: Wolters Kluwer-Lippincott Williams & Wilkins, 2009.

Riba M, Ravindranath D. *Clinical Manual of Emergency Psychiatry*. Arlington: American Psychiatric Publishing, 2010.

Tintinalli JE, Stapczynski JS, Cline DM, *et al. Tintinalli's Emergency Medicine: A Comprehensive Study Guide*, 7th edn. New York: The McGraw-Hill Companies, Inc., 2011.

Tomb D. *Psychiatry*. Philadelphia: Wolters-Kluwer/Lippincott Williams & Wilkins 2008.

Chapter 11

Infectious emergencies

Mari B. Baker and Alex Koyfman

11.1. Sepsis and SIRS (systemic inflammatory response syndrome)

SIRS: 2 or more of the following: tachycardia, tachypnea, hyper/hypothermia.
Sepsis: combination of SIRS plus infection.
Severe sepsis: sepsis plus organ dysfunction.
Septic shock: severe sepsis plus hypotension (systolic blood pressure [SBP] <90 mmHg) not responsive to fluid challenges.

Bacteremia is common, but is not required in the diagnosis [1].
Common causes: pneumonia, abdominal abscess with perforated viscus, pyelonephritis. Risk factors include elderly, multiple comorbidities, chemotherapy-induced neutropenia, AIDS, steroid dependency, and presence of indwelling devices [1].
Pathophysiology: inflammatory cells are released to the site of infection. Cytokines trigger release of inflammatory mediators. Clotting cascade becomes activated, increased D-dimer levels, decreased protein C. Unchecked proinflammatory and procoagulant activity leads to altered hemostasis. Ongoing cascade of cellular hypoxia, tissue injury, shock, multiorgan failure, and potential death [1].

Table 11.1 Surviving sepsis campaign

Initial resuscitation – first 6 hour goals	CVP 8–12 mmHg MAP ≥65 mmHg Urine output ≥0.5 mL/kg/hr Central venous (≥70%) or mixed venous (≥65%) oxygen saturation; if not achieved with fluid resuscitation to CVP target:[1] 1. Supplemental oxygen 2. Transfuse PRBCs to HCT ≥30% 3. Administer dobutamine infusion (max 20 mcg/kg/min)
Diagnosis	Minimum 2 sets of blood cultures (one from EACH lumen of central catheter if present), urine, CSF, wounds, respiratory, body fluids. Imaging studies as appropriate to confirm potential source.
Antibiotic therapy	Administer antibiotics within 1 hour of recognizing septic shock and severe sepsis.
Fluid therapy	At least 1000 mL over 30 minutes to target CVP 8–12 mmHg (12 mmHg in ventilated patients). Reduce rates if CVP increases without hemodynamic response. *(cont.)*

Pocket Guide to the American Board of Emergency Medicine In-Training Exam, ed. Bob Cambridge. Published by Cambridge University Press. © Cambridge University Press 2013.

Table 11.1 (cont.)

Vasopressors	NE and dopamine are first line, to maintain MAP >65 mmHg. Epinephrine as alternative to poor response with NE or dopamine. Vasopressin 0.03 units/min may be added to NE.
Inotropic therapy	Dobutamine infusion 2–20 mcg/kg/min in presence of myocardial dysfunction[2]
Corticosteroids	Hydrocortisone with shock poorly responsive to fluids and vasopressors. Wean when pressors no longer required.
Recombinant human activated protein C	Adult patients with sepsis-induced organ dysfunction with clinical assessment of high risk of death[3]
Blood products	Transfuse to target HGB 7–9 g/dL[4]. Do not use FFP in absence of bleeding/planned invasive procedures.

[1] <70% indicates metabolic active tissues extracting high percentage of available oxygen, hypoxemia, diminished oxygen carrying capacity, low cardiac output [3].
[2] Elevated filling pressure with low cardiac output.
[3] Contraindications: active internal bleeding, recent hemorrhage stroke (3 months), recent intracranial or intraspinal surgery or severe head trauma (2 months), trauma with increased risk of bleeding, presence of epidural catheter, intracranial neoplasm or mass lesion/evidence of herniation, known hypersensitivity to medication.
[4] If no evidence of MI, severe hypoxemia, acute hemorrhage, cyanotic heart disease, lactic acidosis.
　CSF, cerebrospinal fluid; CVP, central venous pressure; FFP, fresh frozen plasma; HCT, hematocrit; MAP, mean arterial pressure; NE, norepinephrine; PRBCs, packed red blood cells. [2]

Supportive therapy strategies of severe sepsis [2]:

Tidal volume 6 mL/kg with acute lung injury/ARDS, upper limit plateau pressure <30 cm H_2O

Permissive hypercapnea in acute respiratory distress syndrome (ARDS) to minimize plateau pressures and tidal volume. Positive end expiratory pressure (PEEP) to avoid lung collapse at end expiration.

Elevate head of bed to limit aspiration and development of ventilator-associated pneumonia.

Noninvasive ventilation only for mild to moderate symptoms in patients with stable hemodynamics, able to protect their airway, appear comfortable, able to clear secretions, and are expected to rapidly recover.

Insulin infusion for target glucose <150 mg/dL.

Empiric antibiotics in sepsis:

Table 11.2 Empiric antibiotics in sepsis

Source/location	Treatment option	Alternative	Alternative
Unknown	Carbapenem	Ceftazidime	Piperacillin/tazobactam
Community acquired pneumonia	Ceftriaxone plus moxifloxacin/levofloxacin	Ceftriaxone plus azithromycin	(If PCN allergic) aztreonam plus moxifloxacin/levofloxacin
Healthcare associated pneumonia	Ceftazidime	Carbapenem	Piperacillin/tazobactam plus levofloxacin/aminoglycoside
Abdominal	Carbapenem	Tigecycline	
Skin/soft tissue	Piperacillin/tazobactam	Cephalexin	
MRSA	Vancomycin	Linezolid	
Fungal	Fluconazole	Caspofungin	

MRSA, methicillin-resistant *Staphylococcus aureus*; PCN, penicillin. [3]

11.2. Neutropenic fevers

Definitions:

Fever: single oral temperature ≥38.3 °C (101 °F), or sustained temperature ≥38 °C (100.4 °F) for 1 hour or greater.

Neutropenia: Absolute neutrophil count (ANC) <500 cells/mm^3 or ANC expected to decrease to <500 cells/mm^3 during the next 48 hours (lowest value generally 7–10 days after chemotherapy) [4].

Pathophysiology:

Neutropenic fevers may result from insults to bone marrow, either due to malignancy, irradiation, or chemotherapy. The high cell turnover of normal mucosa that occurs with chemotherapy allows for endogenous bacteria to translocate across the damaged mucosal barrier. Endogenous flora accounts for 80% of infections. Gram-positive infections are common due to permanent IV access. Other commons [5]:

Gastrointestinal (GI): *Escherichia coli, Enterobacter*, anaerobes.

Skin: *Staphylococcus, Streptococcus.*

Respiratory: *Streptococcus pneumoniae, Klebsiella, Corynebacterium, Pseudomonas.*

Others: *Clostridium difficile, Mycobacterium, Candida, Aspergillus.*

Viruses: herpes simplex/zoster and influenza potentially lethal.

Clinical: clinical manifestions of disease may not be evident due to immune status. Rectal temperatures should be avoided due to risk of mucosal tearing and increased bacterial seeding. Significant history to obtain should include: comorbidities, current medications, time since last chemotherapy, chemotherapeutic regimen, recent antibiotic usage, recent exposure to infections [5].

Testing: CBC with differential, serum chemistries with hepatic transaminases and bilirubin, at least 2 sets of blood cultures (one from each lumen of central venous catheter, if present). Cultures from other body sites, as indicated (CSF, sputum, wound, urine, stool). Imaging to consider chest X-ray (CXR), CT sinuses, chest, abdomen/pelvis [4].

Treatment:

High risk: anticipated prolonged (>7 days) and profound neutropenia (ANC ≤100 cells/mm^3 following cytoxic chemotherapy) and/or significant medical comorbidities (hypotension, pneumonia, new-onset abdominal pain, neurologic changes) should be ADMITTED for IV antibiotics.

Low risk: anticipated brief (≤7 days) neutropenic periods with no/few comorbidities may be considered candidates for oral therapy [4].

Recommended empiric antibiotic therapy [4]:

High risk: IV antibiotics

Third- or fourth-generation cephalosporin (cefepime or ceftazidime) OR

carbapenem OR

piperacillin-tazobactam

Note: vancomycin is not given routinely unless: hypotension, preliminary culture with Gram-positive flora, known history of MRSA, prior prophylaxis with fluoroquinolone or trimethoprim-sulfamethoxazole (TMP-SMX), or probable catheter-related infection.

Low risk: candidates for oral therapy

ciprofloxacin + amoxicillin-clavulanate
ciprofloxacin or levofloxacin monotherapy (should not be used if already on prophylactic fluoroquinolones)
ciprofloxacin + clindamycin

Special high-risk infections [5]:

Neutropenic enterocolitis (typhlitis) – bacterial invasion and necrosis of the bowel wall.

Typically involves the cecum. Generally occurs 10–14 days after cytotoxic chemotherapy.

Symptoms include fever, right lower quadrant (RLQ) pain, nausea, vomiting, abdominal distension.

Diagnosis is preferentially by CT demonstrating cecal distension and wall thickening.

Treatment includes bowel rest, nasogastric (NG) suction, IV fluids, broad spectrum antibiotics (piperacillin-tazobactam or imipenem-cilastin good initial choice), and surgical consultation in event right hemicolectomy is required.

Zygomycosis (mucormycosis) – fungal hyphae invades the vasculature, leading to tissue necrosis and destruction.

Infection most commonly involves the paranasal sinuses, but may also occur in the lungs, GI tract, and central nervous system (CNS).

Symptoms may mimic bacterial sinusitis, but there is more rapid expansion to the surrounding anatomy.

Treatment is with amphotericin B and immediate surgical consultation for debridement.

11.3. Meningitis/meningococcemia

Life-threatening bacteremia or inflammation of the meninges surrounding the brain and spinal cord. Up to 1/3 have long-term neurologic sequelae, and an overall mortality of 10–30% [6].

Risk factors: age >50 years, upper respiratory infection (URI), otitis media (OM), sinusitis, mastoiditis, head trauma, recent neurosurgery, immunocompromised state, crowded living conditions, male gender, socioeconomic status, diabetes, alcoholism, cirrhosis/liver disease, asplenia [6, 7].

Pathophysiology: encapsulated bacteria from nasal or oral pharynx invade the intravascular space and enter the bloodstream or subarachnoid space. Bacteria replicate, consume glucose, and liberate proteins. An inflammatory reaction is initiated from released proinflammatory cytokines, allowing for an increased permeability of the blood–brain barrier. Bacteremia may cause signs/symptoms of localized infection, sepsis, or fulminant infection [6, 8].

Signs/symptoms:

Cardinal: headache, fever, neck stiffness, and altered mental status (only approximately 1/4 demonstrate).

Children and elderly may have nonspecific signs/symptoms: fever, nausea, vomiting, lethargy, irritability, ill appearance, refusal to eat/drink, respiratory symptoms [9].

Kernig: hips flexed to 90 degrees, pain develops in back/legs with extension of knee.
Brudzinski: passive flexion of neck causes flexion in hips.
Presentation of those with meningococcemia can vary widely from mild viral symptoms to fulminant disease/death.

Labs/workup for meningitis/meningococcemia: CBC, C-reactive protein (CRP), coagulation screen, blood culture, PCR for *Neisseria meningitides*, lumbar puncture.

Treatment:

Empiric antibiotics should be initiated once acute bacterial meningitis is suspected, especially if the lumbar puncture is to be delayed (i.e. – CT scan). CSF sterilization can occur 2–4 hours after parenteral antibiotics are administered [9].

Table 11.3 Antibiotics by age and organism: [8]

Most isolated bacteria	
Neonates: group B streptococcus, Gram-negative enterics (*Escherichia coli, Klebsiella*), *Listeria monocytogenes*	
1–23 months: *Streptococcus pneumoniae, Neisseria meningitides*, group B streptococcus, *Haemophilus influenzae, E. coli*	
2–50 years: *S. pneumoniae, N. meningitides*	
>50 years: *S. pneumoniae, N. meningitides, L. monocytogenes*	
Neonates	ampicillin + cefotaxime; OR ampicillin + aminoglycoside
1 month to 50 years	vancomycin + third-generation cephalosporin[1]
50 years	vancomycin + third-generation cephalosporin[1] + ampicillin

[1] Ceftriaxone or cefotaxime.
True PCN allergy: substitue meropenem for cephalosporin.
Special considerations [7]: *H. influenzae*.

Isolated bacteria	
Impaired immunity: *S. pneumoniae*, Gram-negative bacilli, *L. monocytogenes*	
Neurosurgery: *S. aureus*, coagulase negative staphylococci, *Pseudomonas aeruginosa*	
CSF leak: *S. pneumoniae*, streptococci, *H. influenzae*	
CSF shunt: Coagulase negative staphylococci, *S. aureus, P. aeruginosa*	
Immunocompromised	Third-generation cephalosporin[1] + vancomycin + ampicillin; OR meropenem + vancomycin + TMP-SMX
Neurosurgery	Fourth-generation cephalosporin[2] + vancomycin; OR third-generation cephalosporin[1] + vancomycin; OR meropenem + vancomycin
CSF leak	Third-generation cephalosporin[3] + vancomycin; OR meropenem + vancomycin
CSF shunt	Fourth-generation cephalosporin[2] + vancomycin; OR third-generation cephalosporin[1] + vancomycin

[1] Ceftazidime.
[2] Cefepime.
[3] Cefotaxime or ceftriaxone.

Steroids should be given before/with the first dose of antibiotics in suspected acute bacterial meningitis. Dexamethasone 0.15 mg/kg (max 10 mg) QID for 4 days helps suppress the inflammatory response that occurs with bacterial cell lysis. Guidelines support the use in children 3 months of age and older to help decrease rates of complications (i.e. hearing loss) [10].

Treatment considerations:
Patient with a fever and petechial rash should receive IV ceftriaxone immediately if they display any of the following: spreading petechiae, purpuric rash, signs of bacterial meningitis, signs of meningococcal septicemia, ill appearance [11].
Infectious Diseases Society of America (IDSA) recommends CT prior to lumbar puncture in the following conditions: immunocompromised state, history of CNS disease, new-onset seizure, papilledema, abnormal level of consciousness, focal neurologic deficit. However a normal CT does not exclude possibility of neurologic catastrophe following lumbar puncture [9].

Complications: myocarditis, conduction abnormalities, electrolyte derangements, acute respiratory failure, seizures, focal neurologic deficits, shock, disseminated intravascular coagulation (DIC), altered mental status, coma, Waterhouse–Friderichsen syndrome, death [7, 8, 10].

Chemoprophylaxis for *N. meningitides* (not required for *S. pneumoniae*): household contacts, intimate nonhousehold contacts, healthcare workers having direct exposure to secretions, schoolmates, daycare exposure in previous 7 days [6].
Treat with single-dose ciprofloxacin (500 mg PO), OR single-dose ceftriaxone (250 mg IM), OR rifampin 10 mg/kg (max 600 mg) orally every 12 hours for 4 doses.

11.4. Toxic shock syndrome (TSS)

Sudden onset of fever, chills, vomiting, diarrhea, muscle aches, rash – quickly progresses to multiorgan system failure and death [10].

Etiology:
S. aureus – primarily affects women. May be associated with tampon use, intravaginal contraceptives, nasal packing, infection of skin lesions (burns, surgical sites, dialysis catheters), staph respiratory infections or colonization without infection [10].
Group A streptococcus – affects all ages/genders. May be associated with severe soft tissues infections (necrotizing fasciitis and myositis), pneumonia, peritonitis, myometritis, osteomyelitis [8].

Pathophysiology: *S. aureus* and group A streptococcus both release exotoxins. A large number of T cells are activated with cytokines; tumor necrosis factor (TNF) and interleukins released. Subsequently, a systemic vasculitis and multisystem manifestations result.

Clinical:
Temperature ≥ 38.9 °C (102 °F).
Rash: nonpruritic, diffuse, blanching, macular erythroderma.
Desquamation 1–2 weeks after onset, particularly palms and soles.
Hypotension.

Multisystem involvement (3 or more of the following):

GI: vomiting, diarrhea.

Muscular: severe myalgia or CK twice normal.

Mucous membranes: vaginal, oropharyngeal or conjunctival hyperemia.

Renal: BUN/creatinine twice normal, or urine with ≥5 WBC/hpf without urinary tract infection (UTI).

Hepatic: twice normal or higher total bilirubin, AST, and ALT.

Hematologic: platelets ≤100 000/μL.

CNS: disorientation or altered level of consciousness without focal neurologic signs (in absence of hyptension and fever).

Blood cultures may be negative with *S. aureus*, group A streptococcus causes more invasive infection [8].

Complications: ARDS, shock, gangrene, DIC, renal failure. Complication rates are higher with streptococcal TSS than with staphylococcal TSS. Rhabdomyolysis is frequently seen in streptococcal TSS [8].

Treatment [10]:

Hypotension often requires aggressive large volumes of IV fluids. Vasopressors may/may not be beneficial.

The source of bacteria should be removed (tampon, nasal packing, foreign body). Surgical consultation for deep infections requiring debridement, fasciotomy, amputation, aspiration.

Antibiotics – clindamycin generally accepted as first line for both staphylococcal and streptococcal infection. May be changed to nafcillin/oxacillin based on culture results.

11.5. Food-borne illnesses

11.5.1. *Staphylococcus aureus* [12]

One of the most common food-borne illnesses.

Clinical: nausea, crampy abdominal pain, vomiting usually within 1–6 hours of eating contaminated foods.

Foods: meat, poultry, egg products, egg/tuna/potato/macaroni salads, foods handled directly, cream-filled pastries, casseroles.

Treatment: supportive, antiemetics and IV fluids.

11.5.2. *Salmonella* [12]

US serotypes: Typhimurium and Enteritidis.

Clinical: fever, abdominal pain, diarrhea (may be bloody) 12–72 hours after eating contaminated foods.

Treatment: most recover 5–7 days with supportive therapy, TMP-SMX or ciprofloxacin.

Complications: septic arthritis, sepsis, more severe infections noted in elderly and immunocompromised.

11.5.3. *Clostridium perfringens* [12]

Anaerobic spore-forming bacterium.

Clinical: profuse, watery diarrhea, severe abdominal cramping, gas usually 8–16 hours after eating contaminated foods.

Foods: poor temperature control of cooked/reheated foods.

Treatment: self-limited, supportive therapy, resolves 12–24 hours.

11.5.4. *Campylobacter jejuni* [12]

Gram-negative curved, rod-shaped enteric bacterium.

Clinical: fever, abdominal cramps, diarrhea (may be bloody).

Foods: poultry, contact with infected animals.

Treatment: resolves without therapy in 1 week, may be fatal in immunocompromised patients. 5–7 days erythromycin, azithromycin, or ciprofloxacin.

11.5.5. *Shigella sonnei* [12]

Gram-negative, rod-shaped bacterium.

Clinical: invasive gastroenteritis, fever, abdominal pain, diarrhea (may be bloody), seizures in children.

Treatment: 5–7 days TMP-SMX, ciprofloxacin, or ampicillin can shorten duration of symptoms. Reiter's syndrome, rare.

11.5.6. *E. coli* O157:H7 [12]

Gram-negative rod-shaped bacteria, shiga toxin-producing strain of *E. coli*.

Clinical: bloody diarrhea, abdominal pain, fevers, infectious colitis.

Foods: fresh spinach, fast food restaurants, ground beef patties.

Complications: can develop hemolytic uremic syndrome (HUS) – microangiopathic hemolytic anemia, acute renal failure, and thrombocytopenia.

Treatment: use of antibiotics is associated with development of HUS. Supportive therapy with close monitoring for HUS. Most recover 5–10 days.

11.5.7. Enterotoxigenic *E. coli* (traveler's diarrhea) [12]

Non-shiga toxin-producing strain of *E. coli*.

Clinical: water diarrhea (may be bloody).

Treatment: supportive therapy, TMP-SMX or fluoroquinolones, lactobacillus.

11.5.8. *Vibrio* [12]

Gram-negative curved rod-shaped bacteria.

Clinical: gastroenteritis in healthy individuals, sepsis syndrome in elderly/ immunocompromised.

Treatment: inpatient admission, rapid administration of antibiotics (doxycycline with third-generation cephalosporin).

11.5.9. Scombroid fish poisoning [12]

Consumption of fish with high levels of histadine.

Clinical: facial flushing, rash, itching, abdominal pain, diarrhea, facial or tongue swelling, blurry vision, and respiratory distress; metallic taste in mouth.

Foods: tuna, mackerel, mahi-mahi, bluefish, anchovies, sardines, swordfish.

Treatment: clinical diagnosis with supportive therapy, treat similar to acute hypersensitivity reaction (H1 and H2 blockers, epinephrine, fluids, airway management) but DO NOT label as allergic reaction.

11.5.10. Ciguatera fish poisoning [12]

Consumption of fish with high concentrations of "ciguatoxin," causing prolonged opening of sodium channels.

Clinical: GI, neurologic, and cardiac manifestations: nausea, vomiting, abdominal pain, diarrhea, severe weakness, paresthesias, pain, pruritis, tooth pain, loosened tooth sensation, hot/cold reversal, hypotension, bradycardia, dysrhythmia.

Foods: barracuda, grouper, snapper, shark, sea bass.

Treatment: clinical diagnosis, supportive therapy, IV fluids for dehydration, atropine for bradycardia, antihistamines for pruritis. Most recover in weeks, persistent neurologic symptoms may last weeks to months.

11.6. Assorted commonly tested bacterial diseases [13–15]

11.6.1. Botulism

Organism: *Clostridium botulinum* (anaerobic Gram-positive rod). Neurotoxin blocks release of acetylcholine (Ach).

3 forms: infant, wound, food-borne.

Infant: most common form; 2–4 months; ingestion of spores (honey) – limited intestinal flora; constipation as presenting symptom; ptosis, weak suck, poor feeding, failure to thrive, hypotonia ("floppy child").

Wound: open wound, IV drug abuse (black tar heroin).

Food-borne: home-canned food; diplopia, ptosis, dysarthria, dysphagia; symmetric, descending flaccid paralysis; parasympathetic blockade (increased temperature, dilated pupils, dry skin, constipation, urinary retention).

Diagnosis: clinical; can isolate toxin from blood, wound, stool, ingested food.

Treatment: airway management + supportive care (most common cause of death is respiratory failure). Antitoxin is available. Antibiotics not effective and possibly cause toxin release.

11.6.2. Gas gangrene

Most common organism: *Clostridium*; other organisms: *E. coli*, *Bacteroides fragilis*, *Klebsiella*, *Peptostreptococcus*, *Enterobacter*; infection in damaged skin (trauma).

Presentation: pain (earliest symptom), fever, tachycardia; tense wound leads to dark fluid-filled vesicles/bullae.

Diagnosis: clinical.

Treatment: supportive care (ABCs, IV fluids, pressors PRN), surgical debridement, antibiotics (PCN + clindamycin). Consider hyperbaric oxygen.

11.6.3. Syphilis

Organism: *Treponema pallidum*.
Primary: painless, indurated chancre with demarcated edges and inguinal lymphadenopathy; resolves spontaneously after several weeks.
Secondary: constitutional symptoms; truncal maculopapular rash that spreads to extremities involving palms and soles; rash resolves even if not treated; condyloma lata.
Tertiary: several years after untreated infection; dementia, meningitis, thoracic artery aneurysm (syphilitic aortitis), peripheral neuropathies, tabes dorsalis, gummas.
Diagnosis: darkfield microscopy, venereal disease research laboratory test (VDRL), and rapid plasma regain (RPR; nonspecific)/fluorescent treponemal antibody absorption (FTA-ABS; confirmatory).
Treatment: benzathine penicillin G 2.4 million units IM, need 3 doses for tertiary syphilis/doxycycline alternative; desensitization for allergic patients; Jarisch-Herxheimer reaction transiently following antibiotics (fever, headache, myalgias).

11.6.4. Malaria

Organism: *Plasmodium vivax* (relapse possible), *P. ovale* (relapse possible), *P. falciparum* (most severe), *P. malariae*.
Vector: *Anopheles* mosquito; Central and South America, Africa, Asia.
Presentation: initial flu-like symptoms + travel to tropics; *P. falciparum* can present with severe anemia, renal failure, DIC, cerebral malaria, pulmonary edema.
Diagnosis: thick/thin peripheral blood smears.
Treatment:
  P. ovale/vivax/malariae: chloroquine; primaquine to eradicate hepatic phase.
  P. falciparum: mefloquine; quinine + doxycycline/clindamycin.

11.6.5. Toxoplasmosis

Most common cause of focal intracranial lesions in AIDS patient. Found most often when CD4 <100/μL.
Presentation: fever, headache, seizures, focal neuro deficit, altered mental status.
Diagnosis: multiple subcortical ring-enhancing lesions.
Treatment: pyrimethamine + sulfadiazine + folinic acid; if significant mass effect, add steroid.

11.6.6. Ehrlichiosis

Two forms: human monocytic (*Ehrlicia chaffeensis*) and human granulocytic (*E. equi* and *E. phagocytophila*); intracellular coccobacillus; peak June–August.
Vector: *Ixodes, Dermacentor, Amblyomma* ticks.
Presentation: nonspecific; can progress to renal failure, meningitis, DIC, pancarditis.
Diagnosis: clinical; labs with leukopenia, thrombocytopenia, elevated LFTs.
Treatment: immediate; doxycycline 1–2 weeks.

11.6.7. Rocky Mountain spotted fever

Organism: *Rickettsia rickettsii*; obligate intracellular; vector (*Dermacentor* tick); southeastern USA.

Presentation: fever, headache, myalgias; erythematous, irregular macules on forearms, wrists, soles, ankles, palms (begins 3 days after fever) => centripetal spread; palpable, non-blanching.

> Cardiac effects: tachycardia; first-degree AV block; atrial fibrillation; paroxysmal atrial tachycardia.
> GI effects: abdominal pain; nausea and vomiting.
> Neurologic effects: ataxia; aphasia; seizure; meningitis.
> Pulmonary effects: pleural effusion; pulmonary edema; interstitial pneumonitis.

Diagnosis: clinical; labs with anemia, thrombocytopenia, hyponatremia; punch biopsy (most rapid); serologic test not useful acutely.

Treatment: immediate; doxycycline, tetracycline, chloramphenicol ×7–10 days; start once suspect diagnosis.

11.7. HIV/AIDS [16]

HIV is the human retrovirus, causing immune deficiency. AIDS is lab evidence of HIV infection with an associated AIDS-defining illness (recurrent bacterial infections, candidiasis, coccidioidomycosis, cryptococcosis, cryptosporidiosis, cytomegalovirus [CMV], histoplasmosis, Kaposi's sarcoma, lymphoma, *Mycobacterium avium* or tuberculosis, *Pneumocystis jiroveci*, toxoplasmosis, CD4 count <200/μL).

Risk factors: men having sex with men, IV drug use, heterosexual encounter with infected partner, maternal–neonatal transmission.

Routes of transmission: semen, vaginal secretions, blood products, breast milk, transplacental.

Diagnosis: enzymes-linked immunoassay and Western blot (confirmatory); false negatives may occur in first few months.

Clinical signs of HIV: fever, weight loss, fatigue, malaise. Seroconversion commonly occurs 2–6 weeks after initial exposure.

11.7.1. AIDS illnesses

Neurologic:

> *Cryptococcus*: positive CSF cryptococcal antigen, India ink, fungal culture, serum cryptococcal antigen; Treat with amphotericin.
> *Toxoplasma gondii*: most common focal intracranial lesion; differential includes lymphoma, cerebral tuberculosis, fungi, progressive multifocal leukoencephalopathy, CMV, Kaposi's sarcoma; Treat with pyrimethamine plus sulfadiazine with folinic acid.
> Primary CNS lymphoma: hyper/isodense round or multiple enhancing lesions, poor prognosis; Treat with brain irradiation, steroids, and chemotherapy.
> HIV encephalopathy: progressive memory impairment, cognitive deficits.

Ophthalmologic:

> **CMV retinitis:** most common cause of blindness, blurred vision, floaters, flashes of light, photophobia, scotoma; Treat with ganciclovir.
>
> **Retinal cotton wool spots:** no treatment needed.
>
> Kaposi's sarcoma or eyelid of conjunctiva.

Pulmonary:

> *Pneumocystis* **pneumonia (PCP):** caused by *P. jiroveci*, nonproductive cough with dyspnea, hypoxia. CXR with diffuse interstitial infiltrate; Treat with TMP-SMX (alternatives pentamidine, dapsone).
>
> *Mycobacterium* **tuberculosis:** fever, cough, hemoptysis, CXR with upper lobe infiltrates/cavitary lesions. Treat with 4 drug therapy: isoniazid, rifampin, pyrazinamide, and ethambutol for 6 months.

Dermatologic:

> **Kaposi's sarcoma:** typically skin nodules, lymph node involvement or GI tract. Treat with cryotherapy, radiotherapy, intralesional/systemic chemotherapy.
>
> **Varicella zoster:** may involve multiple dermatomes. Treat with oral acyclovir, famciclovir, penciclovir or valacyclovir. IV acyclovir is indicated for systemic involvement or multidermatomal involvement.
>
> **Herpes simplex virus (HSV):** common to oral mucosa, genitalia, and rectum. Treat with acyclovir, famciclovir, penciclovir, or valacyclovir.

Gastrointestinal:

> **Oral disease:** fungal infections, viral lesions, bacterial lesions, neoplasms.
>
> **Esophageal disorders:** esophagitis from *Candida*, HSV, CMV, Kaposi's sarcoma, *M. avium* complex, reflux esophagitis.

Diarrhea:

> **Parasites:** *Cryptosporidium, Enterocytozoon, Isospora, Giardia, Entamoeba.*
>
> **Bacteria:** *Salmonella, Shigella, Campylobacter, M. tuberculosis, Clostridium difficile.*
>
> **Viruses:** CMV, HSV, HIV.
>
> **Fungi:** *Histoplasma, Cryptococcus.*

11.7.2. Antiretroviral therapy

Four classes: nucleoside reverse transcriptase inhibitors, non-nucleoside reverse transcriptase inhibitors, protease inhibitors, fusion inhibitors. Treatment recommended for patients with low CD4 counts or high viral loads.

Postexposure prophylaxis (PEP): risk of HIV transmission 0.3% for significant percutaneous exposure, 0.09% for mucocutaneous exposure.

No PEP for HIV negative sources.

PEP with 4 weeks of 2 drug regimen for known HIV + percutaneous or mucous membrane exposure; 3 drug regimen for higher-risk exposure.

Higher-risk exposure: deep percutaneous injuries, visible blood on device, injury sustained while placing catheter in artery/vein.

Lower-risk exposure: superficial injuries, solid needles.

High-risk sources: patient with acute seroconversion, high viral load, AIDS.
Low-risk sources: asymptomatic HIV infection, viral load <1500 copies/mL.

11.8. Rabies [17]

Caused by neurotropic rhabdovirus, animals are natural reservoir. Bats considered the most important, but others include raccoons, skunks, foxes. Low-risk rodents include squirrels, gophers, rats, chipmunks, guinea pigs, rabbits, hares. Domestic animals also considered low risk unless in underdeveloped nations or along borders.

Infected animals generally die 3–9 days after secreting the virus in their saliva. May display aggressive behavior, ataxia, irritability, lethargy, or excessive salivation.

Pathophysiology: virus replicates near the bite, enters the peripheral nerve and rapidly ascends by retrograde conduction to the CNS. The virus has affinity to the thalamus, basal ganglia, and brainstem. Creates Negri bodies in the nuclei of neurons.

Clinical stages:
Incubation – bite to first symptoms.
Prodrome – numbness/pain at bite site, flu-like symptoms, fever, nausea, vomiting, headache, myalgias, sore throat, rhinorrhea, malaise.
Acute neurologic illness.
Encephalitic form – agitation, hydrophobia, fluctuating consciousness, extreme irritability.
Paralytic form – limb weakness, fevers, can be confused with Guillain–Barré.
Coma – generally 7–10 days after onset of acute neurologic phase, seizures, respiratory and vascular collapse.
Death.

Postexposure prophylaxis: recommended for direct contact between human and bat; or bat found in room with sleeping individual, unattended child or mentally disabled. Contact state/local health department for low-risk rodents or domestic animals that cannot be observed. Treatment includes 1 dose immune globulin (day 0) and 4 doses of rabies vaccine (day 0, 3, 7, and 14).
For healthy-appearing domestic animals (dogs, cats, ferrets) that can be observed, prophylaxis should be withheld. Initiate treatment if animal displays signs/symptoms of illness.

11.9. Assorted commonly tested viral diseases [13–15]

11.9.1. Infectious mononucleosis

Organism: Epstein–Barr virus (EBV)/CMV; infects B lymphocytes.
Most common among high school/college students; "kissing disease"; rash after amoxicillin.
Presentation: fatigue, fever, exudative pharyngitis, posterior cervical adenopathy, abdominal pain, splenomegaly, hepatitis.

Diagnosis: clinical; labs with lymphocytosis (atypical lymphocytes); + heterophile antibodies (monospot).
Treatment: supportive care; steroids; avoid contact sports for 4 weeks.

11.9.2. Hantavirus

Deer mouse urine or feces; inhalation; southwestern USA.

Presentation: nonspecific => pulmonary symptoms (tachypnea, hypoxia, ARDS).
Diagnosis: clinical; CXR with bilateral interstitial infiltrates.
Treatment: supportive care, particularly respiratory system. Death occurs secondary to worsening cardiac output, circulatory failure.

11.9.3. Roseola

Organism: human herpesvirus-6 (HHV-6); children 6 months to 2 years; spring/fall.
Presentation: high fever (3–5 days) => maculopapular rash after defervescence (1–2 days).
Treatment: fever control; reassurance.

11.9.4. Rubella

Spread via respiratory secretions (1 week before and 4 days after rash presence).

Congenital presentation: mental retardation, retinopathy, cataracts, hearing loss, cardiac abnormalities, prematurity.
Presentation: headache, fever, malaise, tender lymphadenopathy (sub-occipital, post-auricular), rash (pink maculopapular; face => trunk).
Diagnosis: clinical.
Treatment: supportive; do not expose women of childbearing age.

References

1. Shapiro N, Zimmer G, Barkin A. Sepsis syndromes. In: Marx JA, Hockberger RS, Walls RM, Adams J, Rosen P, eds. *Rosen's Emergency Medicine: Concepts and Clinical Practice*. Philadelphia: Mosby Elsevier, 2010; 1848–58.

2. Dellinger RP, Levy MM, Carlet JM, *et al.* Surviving Sepsis Campaign. International guidelines for management of severe sepsis and septic shock: 2008. *Intensive Care Med.* 2008; **34**(1): 17–60.

3. Booker E. Sepsis, severe sepsis and septic shock: current evidence for emergency department management. *Emergency Medicine Practice.* 2011; **13**(5).

4. Freifeld AG, Bow EJ, Sepkowitz KA, *et al.* Clinical practice guideline for the use of antimicrobial agents in neutropenic patients with cancer: 2010 update by the Infectious Diseases Society of America. *Clin Infect Dis.* 2011; **52**(4): e56–93.

5. McCurdy MT, Mitarae T, Perkins J. Oncologic emergencies, part II: neutropenic fevers, tumor lysis syndrome, and hypercalcemia of malignancy. *Emergency Medicine Practice.* 2010; **12**(3).

6. Sadoun T, Singh A. Adult acute bacterial meningitis in the United States: 2009 Update. *Emergency Medicine Practice.* 2009; **11**(9).

7. Mace SE. Bacterial meningitis. *Emerg Med Clin N Am.* 2008; **38**: 281–317.

8. Fernandez-Frackelton M. Bacteria. In: Marx JA, Hockberger RS, Walls RM, Adams J, Rosen P, eds. *Rosen's Emergency Medicine: Concepts and Clinical Practice*. Philadelphia: Mosby Elsevier, 2010; 1676–99.

9. Laurich VM. Current guidelines for management of acute bacterial meningitis in the emergency department. *EM Practice Guidelines.* 2011; **3**(2).

10. Hans D, Kelly E, Wilhelmson K, Katz E. Rapidly fatal infections. *Emerg Med Clin N Am.* 2008; **26**: 259–79.

11. National Collaborating Centre for Women's and Children's Health. *Bacterial Meningitis and Meningococcal Septicaemia: Management of Bacterial Meningitis and Meningococcal Septicaemia in Children and Young People Younger than 16 Years in Primary and Secondary Care.* London: National Institute for Health and Clinical Excellence (NICE); 2010.

12. Pigott DC. Foodborne illnesses. *Emerg Med Clin N Am.* 2008; **26**: 475–97.

13. Marx JA, Hockberger RS, Walls RM, Adams J, Rosen P, eds. *Rosen's Emergency Medicine: Concepts and Clinical Practice.* Philadelphia: Mosby Elsevier, 2010.

14. Tintinalli JE, Stapczynski JS, Cline DM, *et al. Tintinalli's Emergency Medicine: A Comprehensive Study Guide,* 7th edn. New York: The McGraw-Hill Companies, Inc., 2011.

15. Wolfson AB, Hendey GW, Ling LJ, *et al. Harwood-Nuss' Clinical Practice of Emergency Medicine.* 5th edn. Philadelphia: Lippincott Williams & Wilkins, 2009.

16. Marco, CA, Rothman RE. HIV infection and complications in emergency medicine. *Emerg Med Clin N Am.* 2008; **26**: 367–87.

17. Weber E, Ramanujam P. Rabies. In: Marx JA, Hockberger RS, Walls RM, Adams J, Rosen P, eds. *Rosen's Emergency Medicine: Concepts and Clinical Practice.* Philadelphia: Mosby Elsevier, 2010; 1723–31.

Toxicologic emergencies

12

Robert Schwaner and Joshua Zavitz

12.1. Toxidromes [1]

12.1.1. Anticholinergic

Component of numerous agents: antihistamines, antipsychotics, tricyclic antidepressants (TCAs), muscle relaxants, antispasmodics.

Clinical: "dry as bone, blind as bat, mad as hatter, red as beet, hot as hades" for dry skin, mydriasis, altered mental status, urinary retention/ileus, hyperthermia.

Treatment: supportive care. Physostigmine given slowly IV for severe symptoms and only without suspicion for TCA or antipsychotics exposure.

12.1.2. Benzodiazepines (sedative-hypnotic)

Mechanism: indirect central nervous system (CNS) GABA agonist, leads to CNS depression, which leads to coma.

Treatment: supportive. Flumazenil (0.5–1 mg IV) is reversal agent, but give slowly with caution as seizures/arrhythmia risk with co-ingestants or chronic use (only to be used in a patient with known lack of chronic use).

12.1.3. Cholinesterase inhibitors (cholinergic)

Found in: insecticides, carbamates, and nerve gases.

Mechanism: binds acetylcholinesterase (AChE) to prevent breakdown of acetylcholine (ACh) at muscarinic (M) and nicotinic (N) receptors.

Clinical: SLUDGE (Salivation, Lacrimation, Urination, Defecation, Gastrointestinal symptoms, Emesis) and killer B-s (Bradycardia, Bronchorrhea, Bronchoconstriction) (alternative mnemonic: "DUMBELS," Diarrhea, Urination, Miosis, Muscle weakness, Bradycardia, Bronchospasm, Emesis, Lacrimation, Salivation).

Treatment: supportive; atropine, a competitive antagonist of ACh at M receptors (titrate dose by doubling every time until bronchorrhea controlled), glycopyrrolate may be substituted; Pralidoxime (2-PAM) binds organophosphate-inactivated acetylcholinesterase allowing enzyme regeneration – early treatment essential to decrease "aging" (covalent bonding); benzodiazepines.

Pocket Guide to the American Board of Emergency Medicine In-Training Exam, ed. Bob Cambridge. Published by Cambridge University Press. © Cambridge University Press 2013.

12.1.4. Cocaine (sympathomimetic)

Clinical: sympathomimetic (agitation, hyperthermia, rhabdomyolysis, mydriasis), vasoconstrictor (myocardial ischemia, placental abruption leading to low birthweight infant), sodium channel blockade (prolonged QRS, seizures).

Treatment: benzodiazepines, cooling, sodium bicarbonate or lidocaine for widened QRS or dysrhythmias, nitroglycerin/prusside or phentolamine for hypertension (HTN). Do not give selective β-blockers due to risk of unopposed α action.

12.1.5. Opioids

Clinical: respiratory depression/pulmonary edema, CNS depression, miosis, hypotension, rhabdomyolysis. Tolerance does not develop to respiratory depression.

Treatment: supportive care, naloxone 0.1–2 mg IV/IM/SQ slowly every 2–3 minutes. For long-acting opioids, give naloxone infusion.

Note: Fentanyl rapid IV administration may lead to "stone chest." Continued adsorption/toxicity possible hours after patch removal as skin "reservoir" formed with normal transdermal delivery.

12.2. Gastrointestinal (GI) decontamination [2]

12.2.1. Gastric lavage

Indications: within 1 hour, rapid deterioration expected, lethal agent, intubated.

Contraindications: caustic, foreign body, airway protection, delayed presentation.

Treatment: airway protection, left lateral position, place 36–40 French tube (22–24 French tube in children) and lavage/suction until clear.

12.2.2. Activated charcoal (AC)

Large surface area adsorbs toxins. Some toxins benefit from multidose AC (enterohepatic or "gut" dialysis).

Contraindications: unprotected airway, caustic ingestions, bowel obstruction/perforation.

Substances not significantly absorbed : PHAILS (pesticides, hydrocarbons, acids/alkaki/alcohol/arsenic, iron/iodide, lithium, solvents).

12.2.3. Whole bowel irrigation

Catharsis to clear GI tract rapidly.

Indications: agents not adsorbed by AC, sustained release (SR), body packers/stuffers.

Contraindications : bowel obstruction/perforation, unprotected airway, hemodynamic instability, anticholinergics.

Dose: Golytely 1.5–2.0 L/hr (500 mL/hr) until effluent is clear; via NG tube, charcoal before and after whole bowel irrigation, antiemetics.

12.3. Toxins (alphabetical) [3]

12.3.1. Acetaminophen

Most common cause of acute liver failure in the USA. 150 mg/kg is potential toxic dose in adult. 90% is metabolized by liver via glucoronidation/sulfation. In overdose, cell saturation leads to glutathione depletion and increased NAPQI$^+$ formation. Cells are damaged via free radicals, which leads to elevation of transaminases. Alcoholics, CYP450 inducers (isoniazid), malnourished are at increased risk.

Clinical: 0–18 hours post ingestion patient may have GI symptoms. At 18–48 hours elevated LFTs/PT/international normalized ratio (INR) develops. At 48–96 hours hepatic dysfunction, coagulopathy, acidosis, renal dysfunction, jaundice, and cerebral edema can develop.

Treatment: measure acetaminophen 4 hours after ingestion and plot on Rumack-Matthew nomogram, if >4 hours or unknown obtain immediate level. Use *N*-acetylcysteine (NAC) if level is greater than treatment line in acute (>140 mg/dL at 4 hours) and use with signs of toxicity (elevated transaminases, coagulopathy, renal dysfunction, acidosis) in chronic/repeated ingestions/late presentations. Continue NAC if repeat LFTs are elevated and acetaminophen level is measurable, or with continued liver/renal dysfunction in severe intoxications.

12.3.2. Amphetamines

Source: decongestants, methylphenidate, MDMA, methamphetamine.

Clinical: sympathomimetic signs, agitation, autonomic instability, ischemia, CNS depression/hemorrhage, rhabdomyolysis, organ failure; hallucinations greatest with MDMA.

Treatment: benzodiazepines, supportive, cooling.

12.3.3. Anticoagulants

Source: warfarin (inhibits factors II, VII, IX, X) and dicoumarol rodenticides (toxicity lasts months), heparin (stimulates antithrombin III), low molecular weight heparin (LMWH; inhibits factor X), lepirudin (inhibits thrombin).

Clinical: signs are dose dependent and may go from asymptomatic to spontaneous bleeding.

Treatment: charcoal, observe if asymptomatic. Hold next warfarin dose for INR 5–9 without active bleeding. Fresh frozen plasma (FFP)/vitamin K for INR over 9, or active bleeding. Consider protamine for heparin. PT/INR/PTT checks for at least 2–3 days.

12.3.4. Antipsychotics

Clinical: monoamine oxidase inhibitor (MAOI) potential depends on effect on antagonism of 5HT, dopamine.

Positive symptoms: (hallucinations, delusions) respond more to D2, more typical agents.
Negative symptoms: (blunted affect, apathy) respond more to 5HT2, more atypical agents.

Table 12.1 Antipsychotic drug receptor effects and treatment

Receptor affected	Clinical presentation	Treatment
Dopamine.	Dystonia, akathisia, dyskinesia.	Diphenhydramine, benzodiazepine.
α-adrenergic.	Hypotension, tachycardia.	Fluids, α-agonist.
Muscarinic.	Seizures, anticholinergic symptoms.	Benzodiazepines, supportive care.
Histamine.	Sedation.	Supportive.
Sodium channel.	Wide QRS, dysrhythmia.	Sodium bicarbonate, lidocaine.
Potassium channel.	Wide QT, torsades.	Magnesium.

12.3.5. Beta-blockers

Types: β1 and β2 selective; α-receptor (carvedilol, labetalol), potassium channel blocker (sotalol), sodium channel blocker/high lipid solubility (propranolol).

Clinical: hypotension, bradycardia, AV blocks, CNS depression, hypoglycemia.

Treatment: charcoal, consider gastric lavage or whole bowel irrigation; fluids, atropine, glucagon (bypasses β-receptor; 3–5 mg IV followed by infusion of effective dose per hour), calcium chloride 1 g or calcium gluconate 3 g and repeat if positive response; pressors; intraaortic balloon pump and extracorporeal membrane oxygenation (ECMO) for severe cases.

12.3.6. Calcium channel blockers

Toxicity: diphenylalkylamines (verapamil) > benzothiazepines (diltiazem) > dihydropyridines (nifedipine, amlodipine).

Clinical: inhibits myocardial contractility (cardiovascular collapse, hypotension), AV conduction, and vascular tone (hypotension, reflex tachycardia), can cause hyperglycemia.

Treatment: multidose charcoal or whole bowel irrigation for sustained release, consider atropine; Ca^{2+} boluses followed by infusion; consider glucagon 2–10 mg IV followed by drip if clinical response; pressors.

12.3.7. Carbon monoxide (CO)

Exposure to incomplete combustion of organics (exhaust, fires) which produces odorless/colorless gas. Binds and alters hemoglobin (HGB). CO has a >200× affinity for HGB than oxygen. Patient develops cellular hypoxia.

Clinical: headache, dizzy progressing to syncope; seizures, dysrhythmia, ischemia, coma.

Workup: diagnosed with co-oximeter (readings up to 10% can be normal in smokers). Measurable level confirms exposure and not degree of toxicity. CO binds HGB but exerts majority of toxicity as a mitochondrial toxin. Binds cytochrome oxidase.

Treatment: 100% oxygen reduces half-life to 90 minutes, hyperbaric oxygen (for patients with syncope, ischemia, pregnancy) decreases half-life further and increases dissolved oxygen, which may decrease cognitive impairments.

12.3.8. Cardiac glycosides

Sources: medicine/foxglove (digoxin/digitalis), lily of the valley, oleander.

Mechanism: increases vagal tone, inhibits Na^+/K^+-ATPase, leading to decreased sodium–calcium exchange. Intracellular calcium rises and contractility rises.

Toxicity: excess intracellular calcium lowers resting membrane potential, leading to dysrhythmias. Premature ventricular contractions (PVCs) most common. Risk increases with renal insufficiency, hypokalemia, dehydration.

Clinical: nausea and vomiting, lethargy/confusion, visual changes, hyperkalemia (acute)/ hypokalemia (chronic). ECG can show arrhythmias, AV blocks; scooped ST segments.

Treatment: charcoal (acute ingestion), electrolyte replacement, atropine/external pacing as needed (never internal pacing due to increased irritability of myocardium), lidocaine for ventricular dysrhythmias, digoxin-specific Fab is definitive.

Digibind indications and dosing: symptomatic bradycardia or ventricular dysrhythmias, potassium above 5 mEq/L, digoxin concentration over 10 ng/mL or ingestion of more than 10 mg (4 mg in child). Empiric dosing: acute overdose 10 vials; chronic overdose 5 vials adult and 2 vials child. Serum concentrations are not clinically helpful after Fab given.

12.3.9. Cyanide

Sources: jewelry production, metal refining, labs, nitroprusside, illegal drugs, *Prunus* plants (apricots/almonds pits), cassava, smoke inhalation. Cyanide inhibits cytochrome oxidase, which halts electron transport chain, leading to rapid death.

Clinical: acute headache, confusion, seizures, vascular instability, tachypnea/bradypnea, pulmonary edema, cherry red skin color. Suspect in patient with almond scent, coma, acidosis, and lactic acid >8 mmol/L.

Treatment: decontamination, bicarbonate, antidote kit (amyl nitrite should be inhaled first, followed by sodium nitrite IV to induce a methemoglobinemia as cyanide preferentially binds methemoglobin); then give sodium thiosulfate 12.5 g to produce thiocyanate for excretion. Hydroxocobalamin chelates cyanide; repeat over 6–8 hours unless unstable (causes red skin discoloration).

12.3.10. Ethylene glycol

Source: found in de-icing/antifreeze solutions. Metabolized by alcohol dehydrogenase to toxic oxylate, glycolate, glyoxylic acid.

Lab findings: osmolar gap low and anion gap high as metabolites produced. Hypocalcemia can lead to prolonged QT.

Clinical: inebriated state → hypotension, tachypnea, dysrhythmia, (acute respiratory distress syndrome [ARDS]) → acute renal failure (ARF).

Treatment: fomepizole – competes for alcohol dehydrogenase (alcohol works just as well, cheaper but difficult to titrate alcohol drips). Hemodialysis indications: severe acidosis, organ dysfunction, large ingestion.

12.3.11. Hydrogen sulfide

Source: decay of sulfur products (rotten egg odor) – industry (well workers) and nature (manure). Highly lipid soluble but typically inhaled. Binds cytochrome a3, which terminates electron transport chain, leading to death.

Clinical: nausea and vomiting, CNS depression, cardiovascular collapse. Suspect with rapid loss of consciousness in an enclosed space, blackening of coins/jewelry.

Treatment: remove from source, give oxygen, consider hyperbaric oxygen and/or sodium nitrite.

12.3.12. Hypoglycemics

Mechanism: .

Sulfonylureas (glipizide) stimulates insulin secretion, can last up to 24 hours.

Meglitinides (repaglinide) stimulates insulin secretion.

Biguanides (metformin) increases peripheral glucose uptake and decreases hepatic gluconeogenesis. Increased risk of lactic acidosis especially with renal/liver dysfunction.

Alpha-glucosidase inhibitors (acarbose) delay carbohydrate digestion.
Thiazolidinediones (pioglitazone) enhance insulin production, risk of liver toxicity.

Clinical: lightheaded, diaphoresis, altered mental status, seizure, syncope.
Treatment: PO glucose source when able. IV D50 (adults) 1–2 mL/kg, D25 (children) 2–4 mL/kg, D10 (neonates) at 2.5–5 mL/kg bolus. Glucagon if persistent hypoglycemia or no IV. Octreotide – inhibits insulin release (50 mcg every 6 hours). Bicarbonate and possible hemodialysis in severe metformin overdose.

12.3.13. Iron

Elemental Fe^{2+} varies with form (i.e. ferrous gluconate 12% vs. sulfate 20%). Toxic effects at >20 mg/kg of elemental Fe^{2+}.

Clinical: latent period up to 24 hours followed by multisystem organ failure starting up to 2 days after ingestion. Liver failure and GI strictures/obstruction (caustic) can occur.
Treatment: supportive; consider whole bowel irrigation if visible on X-ray; IV fluids. Deferoxamine to chelate Fe^{2+} if patient has serum Fe^{2+} >500 mcg/dL or signs of toxicity.

12.3.14. Isoniazid

Used for treatment of tuberculosis, can lead to pyridoxine and GABA deficiency.

Clinical: acutely altered mental status or seizures. Chronic: hepatotoxicity.
Treatment: pyridoxine 5 g adults (70 mg/kg child up to 5 g) – repeat if needed, benzodiazepines.

12.3.15. Lead

Sources: paint, gasoline, battery, pottery, contaminated drugs, mining. Acceptable whole blood lead is <10 mcg/dL, treatment >25 mcg/dL in children.
Clinical: various CNS (mental status change), hematologic, renal, GI, cardiovascular, and developmental effects in children. Obtain X-ray, CBC, blood lead level.
Treatment: whole bowel irrigation if radio-opacities on X-ray, chelation for lead encephalopathy or levels >70 mcg/dL children or >100 mcg/dL adult. Chelation strategies include DMSA/succimer (10 mg/kg TID × 5 days) or BAL/Dimercaprol ($75mg/m^2$ IM Q4 hours ×5 days if encephalopathy or unable to take PO). Replete iron.

12.3.16. Lithium

Element similar to sodium, stabilizes membranes. Excreted primarily by kidneys. Chronic exposure: high total body burden and small increase can cause symptoms. Acute ingestions tolerate higher lithium level before symptoms occur because lithium has not distributed to other compartments.

Risk for toxicity: dehydration, renal dysfunction (decreases clearance), medications, stress.
Clinical: chronic – CNS symptoms (tremor, hyperreflexic, ataxia, lethargy, seizures) hypothyroid. Acute – GI symptoms, prolonged QT then CNS symptoms, diabetes insipidus, serotonin syndrome, neuroleptic malignant syndrome.

Treatment: consider whole bowel irrigation. Give IV fluids 2× maintenance. Consider hemodialysis for the following: neuro symptoms, renal failure, fluid overload, lithium level >4 mEq/L (acute), >2.5 mEq/L (chronic).

12.3.17. Methanol

Source: found in windshield washer fluid, glass cleaner, antifreeze, paint remover. The toxic metabolite (formic acid) leads to acidosis and retinal toxicity.

Clinical: nausea, vomiting, abdominal pain followed by a latent period. After that visual disturbance, respiratory issues, seizure, coma can develop.

Treatment: give bicarbonate to enhance elimination. Treat with IV ethanol or fomepizole. Folic acid can be given to convert formic acid to carbon dioxide. Hemodialysis indications: severe acidosis, organ dysfunction, large ingestion.

12.3.18. Monoamine oxidase inhibitors (MAOIs)

Selective and non-selective, acting mostly on CNS and GI tract. Exacerbated by tyramine, which is indirect sympathomimetic found in aged cheese, meats, wines.

Clinical: latent phase up to 24 hours. Sympathetic excitation symptoms, CNS depression with risk of serotonin syndrome, rhabdomyolysis, ARDS, organ failure.

Treatment: supportive, cooling, pressors for hypotension.

12.3.19. Phenytoin

Sodium channel blocker, fosphenytoin is prodrug. Highly protein bound; increased toxicity at lower level in setting of hypoalbuminemia.

Clinical: nausea, vomiting, lethargy, ataxia, nystagmus, hypotension/dysrhythmias can occur secondary to propylene glycol diluent from rapid IV administration.

Treatment: charcoal, supportive.

12.3.20. Salicylates

Source: acetylsalicylic acid (aspirin), methyl salicylate (oil of wintergreen), mixed preparations (Pepto Bismol). Absorption is rapid in stomach, delayed with salicylate-induced pylorospasm/outlet obstruction, concretion formation.

Pathophysiology: stimulation of medulla causes initial respiratory alkalosis. Impaired renal function and uncoupling of oxidative phosphorylation leads to anion gap metabolic acidosis.

Clinical: nausea, vomiting, tinnitus, CNS effects, hyperthermia, tachypnea/acute lung injury, acute renal failure, coagulopathy, hepatitis, Reye's syndrome.

Treatment: multiple dose activated charcoal, IV fluids. Give bicarbonate infusion at 2× maintenance to alkalinize urine and trap ions in urine. Urine pH goal 7.5–8.0. Hemodialysis indications – altered mental status, acute lung injury, coagulopathy, severe academia, unable to tolerate fluids or bicarbonate, renal failure, serum concentration >100 mg/dL acute or >60 mg/dL chronic. For airway concerns intubate if necessary but be sure to hyperventilate to keep serum pCO_2 low otherwise pH will drop.

12.3.21. Tricyclic antidepressants

Clinical: tachycardia, mydriasis, hyperthermia, hypotension, seizures, altered mental status.
ECG: large R in aVR, right axis deviation, QRS widening.
Treatment: GI decontamination/lavage if <1 hour, benzodiazepines for seizures, sodium bicarbonate boluses for wide QRS or dysrhythmias.

12.4. Miscellaneous toxic effects [1]

12.4.1. Methemoglobinemia

Occurs with increased oxidative stress of HGB causing Fe^{2+} to convert to Fe^{3+}, which is unable to release oxygen to tissues, leading to central cyanosis.

Causes: dapsone, topical anesthetics, nitrites, phenazopyridine, sulfonamides, anti-malarials, well water (nitrate contamination), analine dyes (shoe polish).
Clinical: typical pulse oximetry is unable to read methemoglobinemia so reads 85%; need co-oximeter. Patient often has nonspecific symptoms. >50% methemoglobinemia causes CNS/cardiac hypoxia. >70% methemoglobinemia leads to coma/death.
Treatment: if >20% methemoglobinemia in symptomatic or >30% in asymptomatic use methylene blue as a cofactor of NADPH reduction. Methylene blue may induce hemolysis in G6PD deficient patients.

12.4.2. Neuroleptic malignant syndrome

May occur after first dose or years of taking neuroleptic, atypical antipsychotics, and antiemetics. Higher risk with typical antipsychotics, high potency agents, severe agitation, increasing dose, IV dosing, concomitant lithium use, concomitant psychotropic drug use, substance abuse, or acute medical illness.

Clinical: hyperthermia, altered mental status, muscle rigidity (lead pipe), autonomic instability; consider when offending agent plus at least 2 of 4 criteria: hyperthermia, autonomic instability, muscle rigidity, altered mental status.
Treatment: stop agent, supportive care, cooling, benzodiazepines, dantrolene, bromocriptine.

12.4.3. Serotonin syndrome

Occurs with MAOIs, selective serotonin reuptake inhibitors (SSRIs), cocaine, meperidine, dextromethorphan, MDMA, lithium, tryptophan, LSD.

Clinical: mental status changes, autonomic instability, neuromuscular abnormalities, hyperthermia within minutes to hours after exposure.
Treatment: stop offending agent, cooling, benzodiazepines, cyproheptadine.

12.5. Assorted toxicologic mnemonics and lists [3, 4]

12.5.1. Radio-opaque substances on chest X-ray

CHIPES (Chloral hydrate; Heavy metals; Iron/Iodides, Potassium, Enteric coated tabs, Solvents).

12.5.2. Substances cleared by hemodialysis

Salicylates, methanol, bromide, chloral hydrate, lithium, isopropyl alcohol, ethylene glycol.

12.5.3. Substances cleared by hemoperfusion

Barbituates, phenytoin, theophylline, digoxin.

12.5.4. Causes of anion gap acidosis

MUDPILERS (Methanol, Uremia, DKA, Paraldehyde, Iron/Isoniazid, Lactic acidosis, Ethanol/Ethylene glycol, Rhabdomyolysis, Salicylates).

12.5.5. Causes of non-anion gap acidosis

USED CARP (Ureterostomy, Small bowel fistula, Extra chloride, Diarrhea, Carbonic anhydrase inhibitors, Adrenal insufficiency, Renal tubular acidosis, Pancreatic fistula).

References

1. Marx JA, Hockberger RS, Walls RM, Adams J, Rosen P, eds. *Rosen's Emergency Medicine: Concepts and Clinical Practice*. Philadelphia: Mosby Elsevier, 2010.

2. Nelson LS, Goldfrank L, Hoffman R, *et al. An Intensive Review Course in Clinical Toxicology*. New York: New York City Poison Control Center and Bellevue Hospital Center, 2012.

3. Nelson LS, Lewin NA, Howland MA, *et al. Goldfrank's Toxicologic Emergencies*, 9th edn. New York: McGraw-Hill, 2012.

4. Kazzi Z, Shih R. *AAEM Resident and Student Association Toxicology Handbook*, 2nd edn. Milwaukee: AAEM/RSA/BTG International, 2011.

Chapter 13

Environmental emergencies

Timothy Schaefer and Vivian Lau

13.1. Bites and envenomation

13.1.1. Arthropods

13.1.1.1. Black widow spider bite

Black body, red hourglass marking on underside.

Clinical features: bite lesion appears blanched in the middle with a red surrounding ring. Dull crampy pain begins at site, spreads to body, leading to severe crampy pain; abdomen can become rigid. Dizziness, nausea and vomiting, headache, dyspnea, weakness, hypertension, respiratory/cardiac arrest can develop. With care, symptoms usually resolve after 2–3 days in adults; more severe in children, may lead to death.

Indications for antivenin/admission: age >65, pregnancy, pediatrics, respiratory distress, cardiac arrest, history of hypertension or heart disease, severe pain despite adequate benzodiazepines and narcotics.

Treatment: antihistamines especially if giving antivenin, benzodiazepines and analgesics. Antivenin: 1–2 vials.

13.1.1.2. Brown recluse spider bite

Tan/dark-brown body, violin-shaped dark area.

Clinical features: burning pain and blanching around the bite. Bleb and erythematous ring forms. Necrotic center then spreads. Fever, rash, nausea and vomiting, weakness can develop. Can have hemolysis, hemorrhage, renal failure, shock.

Treatment: analgesics and antibiotics. No antivenin on market. Dapsone (50–200 mg/day), hyperbaric oxygen with questionable efficacy [1]. Excision may be detrimental.

13.1.2. Snake bites

Pit vipers (e.g. rattlesnakes, copperheads) cause 98% of envenomed bites in the USA.

Treatment: ABCs, immobilize affected area, supportive care, antivenin.

Antivenin CroFab: Ovine based. Pretreat as desired with antihistamine or epinephrine to reduce anaphylactoid reaction. Additional doses may be needed based on serial exams.

Distal bites have better prognosis. Bites can be evaluated using grading system. Assists in dosing of antivenin.

Pocket Guide to the American Board of Emergency Medicine In-Training Exam, ed. Bob Cambridge. Published by Cambridge University Press. © Cambridge University Press 2013.

Table 13.1 Snake bite grading system and treatment

Grade	Envenomation signs and symptoms	Antivenin CroFab
Grade 0 "dry bite"	± Fang marks, minimal pain, erythema, no systemic symptoms	0 vials
Grade I *Minimal*	Fang marks, moderate pain/edema, no systemic symptoms	4 vials
Grade II *Moderate*	Fang marks, severe pain, moderate edema in first 12 hours, mild symptoms (nausea and vomiting, paresthesias), coagulopathy without bleeding	4–6 vials
Grade III *Severe*	Fang marks, severe pain/edema, systemic symptoms (hypotension, dyspnea), coagulopathy with bleeding, lab abnormalities, initially low grade but rapidly progresses	8+ vials
Grade IV *Severe*	Fang marks, severe pain/edema, systemic symptoms (nausea and vomiting, paresthesias, tachycardia), rapid progression, necrosis of wound, could arrest early on	8+ vials

[1]

13.1.3. Mammal bites

Majority are caused by dogs; also caused by cats, rodents, other wild animals, humans.

Clinical features: depends on nature of bite. Can be a crush wound, puncture, avulsion, laceration, or have other appearance. Hand and feet bites have higher risk of infection.

Treatment: standard wound care, imaging as indicated, update tetanus.

Table 13.2 Mammalian bite source and treatment option

Bite	Suture	Antibiotics
Dogs	Most (± hands/feet)	High-risk wounds
Cats	Face	All wounds
Rodents	Most	No
Human	Most (no hand wounds)	Hand wounds

[2]

13.1.4. Marine organisms

13.1.4.1. Octopi bites

Supportive treatment.

13.1.4.2. Nematocysts (jellyfish, corals, anemones)

Toxin may cause sting, respiratory or cardiovascular collapse, death. May have anaphylactic reaction, can be fatal.

Treatment: carefully remove offender if attached, tetanus prophylaxis, antivenin if applicable, supportive treatment, immerse in hot water for analgesia.

13.1.4.3. Stings: sea urchins, catfish, stingrays, cone shells

Treatment: wound care, imaging for foreign body, may require surgical removal of stingers/spines, immerse in hot water for analgesia.

13.2. Dysbarism

Most common in scuba diving.
Conditions caused by changes in ambient pressure.
Each foot below sea level = additional 23 mmHg.

13.2.1. Barotrauma

Damage to tissue due to differences in pressure between an air space in the body and surrounding environment.
Middle ear barotrauma/barotitis: most common injury.
Recompression therapy not required.

13.2.2. Air embolism

Severe form of pulmonary barotrauma, air bubbles forced across alveolar-capillary membrane into pulmonary venous circulation which then flows into the arterial system.

Clinical presentation: headache, dizziness, blurred vision, altered mental status, weakness, ataxia, chest pain, dyspnea. Can cause cardiac ischemia, MI, cardiac arrest, loss of consciousness (LOC), cerebrovascular accident (CVA).

Treatment: 100% oxygen, recompression therapy.

13.2.3. Decompression syndrome

Divers breathe gas which dissolves in the body at varying pressures. On rapid ascent, pressures drop and dissolved gases come out of solution forming bubbles in the body. Nitrogen bubbles accumulate in various locations.

Type I (bends): musculoskeletal and skin.
  Symptoms: pruritus, erythema, articular pain, skin marbling.

Type II: various organ systems.
  Spinal: paralysis, paresthesia, weakness, numbness, bladder/bowel dysfunction, symptoms are often dermatomal.
  Cerebral: headache, blurred vision, dysarthria, fatigue, consciousness intact (compared to air embolism).
  Pulmonary: dyspnea, cough, pain, may progress to respiratory arrest.

Treatment: 100% oxygen, recompression therapy.

13.3. High-altitude illness

13.3.1. Acute mountain sickness

Recent travel to new altitude with development of headache, dizziness, anorexia, nausea and vomiting, fatigue, difficulty sleeping.
  Onset occurs within few hours, lasts several days.

Treatment:
  Mild symptoms: restrict further ascent until acclimatized, rest, NSAIDs, aspirin.
  Continued/worsening symptoms: descent (definitive treatment), supplemental oxygen, acetazolamide, dexamethasone.

13.3.2. Barotrauma of ascent

See dysbarism.

13.3.3. High-altitude cerebral edema

Uncommon, but most severe.

Onset typically 1–3 days, but can last up to 9 days; typically above 12 000 ft.

Symptoms: headache, nausea and vomiting, fatigue, cough, dyspnea, seizures, dysarthria, ataxia, altered mental status, can lead to coma or death.

Treatment: ABCs, immediate descent, oxygen, steroids, decrease elevated intracranial pressure (ICP) (hyperventilation, mannitol).

13.3.4. High-altitude pulmonary edema

Most common fatality of high-altitude illness.

Onset typically 2–4 days; typically above 14 500 ft.

Symptoms: cough, worsening dyspnea, hemoptysis, along with symptoms of acute mountain sickness.

Diagnosis: chest X-ray (CXR) shows patchy infiltrates, ECG shows right heart strain.

Treatment: immediate descent or hyperbaric therapy, oxygen, rest, lasix, nifedipine.

13.4. Submersion incidents

13.4.1. Cold water immersion syndrome

Cardiac dysrhythmias causing syncope due to sudden contact with cold water at least 5 °C less than body temperature [3].

Possible increased risk of dysrhythmia with prolonged QT.

Hypothermia shunts blood to heart and brain, may be neuroprotective, leading to survival of some extended submersions [4].

Warm to >35 °C to declare death.

13.4.2. Near drowning

Survivor of submersion.

More common in toddlers and males aged 16–20 (usually due to recklessness, alcohol, trauma).

Poor prognostic factors: <3 years old, submerged >5 minutes, CPR >10 minutes, trauma.

Workup: ECG, ABG, monitor, CXR, toxicology screen PRN.

Treatment: ABCs, antibiotics PRN infection.

13.5. Temperature-related injuries

13.5.1. Heat injuries

13.5.1.1. Heat exhaustion

Vague symptoms: weakness, headache, nausea and vomiting, muscle cramps, sweaty. Mental status will be normal. Core temperature typically normal or mildly elevated.

Pathophysiology: water or salt depletion typically caused by profuse sweating and intense physical activity with inadequate fluid intake or replacement with hypotonic fluids.

Treatment: cool environment, IV fluids with electrolyte replacement. Healthy young patients may be discharged home.

13.5.1.2. Heatstroke

CNS dysfunction is hallmark, temperature usually >40.5 °C.

Sweating typically absent in classic heatstroke, may have sweating initially in exertional heatstroke.

Vague prodrome: weakness, dizziness, nausea and vomiting, headache, confusion, drowsy, irritability.

Risk factors: extremes of age, comorbidities, medications (anticholinergics, neuroleptics, diuretics).

Treatment: rapid cooling to <39 °C, remove from heat source, tepid water spray with fan (prevents vasoconstriction of vessels, maximizing radiant/convection heat loss), ice packs to axilla/groin, IV fluid normal saline, cardiac monitor for tachydysrhythmias, which respond to cooling (attempt to cool first before cardioversion).

13.5.2. Cold injuries

Vasoconstriction limits blood flow, causing capillary leakage, extravasation of plasma, increased blood viscosity, increased platelet affinity; stasis promotes thrombosis. Intracellular ice destroys cell architecture and extracellular ice further intensifies damage.

Reperfusion injury: rewarming with subsequent return of blood flow allows damaged cells to release large amounts of thromboxane and prostaglandins, leading to vasoconstriction, platelet clumping, and further tissue damage.

Refreezing of thawed extremity causes extensive tissue damage. DO NOT thaw until refreezing risk has passed.

Exposed appendages at greatest risk (hands, feet, face, nose, ears).

13.5.2.1. Trench foot (immersion foot)

Prolonged exposure (hours to days) to cool, wet, non-freezing temperatures.

Symptoms: numbness, pallor, leg cramps, then cyanotic and edematous tissue.

Treatment: hyperemic phase occurs after rewarming becomes painful. Analgesics as necessary. Tissue loss is uncommon, but infection can be a concern. Clean and dry feet, apply sterile dressings, debride/aspirate clear blisters.

13.5.2.2. Chilblains (pernio)

Prolonged exposure to cool, air (dry) non-freezing temperatures.

Features: develops on exposed areas, typically face, ears, hands, feet: erythema, pruritus, burning paresthesias.

Women with Raynaud's phenomenon at highest risk. Tissue loss uncommon; can have plaques, nodules, ulcers.

Treatment: supportive. Calcium channel blockers for severe/recurrent cases.

13.5.2.3. Frostbite [5]

Local cold injury can occur above or below freezing temperatures.

First degree: erythema, hyperemia, no blisters.

Second degree: erythema, edema, clear vesicles, blisters desquamate, forming black eschar.

Third degree: full thickness and subcutaneous tissue, violaceous/hemorrhagic blisters, blue-gray discoloration.

Fourth degree: involves muscle and bone; mottled, dry, deep red/cyanotic, mummified, black.

Treatment: rapid rewarming important. Rewarm with wet heat at 40–42 °C, gentle motion, no direct massage. Analgesia, tetanus, hypothermia treatment. Elevate, debride/aspirate clear blisters (reduce ischemic mediators). Apply sterile dressings.

13.5.2.4. Hypothermia

Defined as core body temperature less than or equal to 35 °C.

Mild: 33–35 °C.

Moderate: 29–32 °C.

Severe: less than or equal to 28 °C.

Immersion hypothermia has quicker onset than non-immersion. Shivering response disappears at 30–32 °C, metabolic activity slows, decreased oxygen consumption and carbon dioxide production.

High-risk patients: extremes of age, intoxication, sepsis.

ECG findings in hypothermia: T wave inversions; prolonged PR, QRS, and QT intervals; J waves (Osborne waves – distinct upright deflection after QRS complex; commonly in leads II and V6 at <32 °C, then V3 and V4 at <25 °C). Under 30 °C dysrhythmias occur. Sinus bradycardia progresses to slow atrial fibrillation which progresses to ventricular fibrillation (V-fib) then asystole. Spontaneous V-fib/asystole can occur at <25 °C.

Treatment: ABCs. Handle with care. Risk of V-fib increases with "rough" handling of patient. Active core rewarming preferred for severely hypothermic or cardiac instability/dysrhythmia. Most cardiovascular medications are inactive during hypothermia and should be given once core body temperature >35 °C.

Rewarming techniques

Passive external: place in warm environment, remove wet clothes, insulate.

Active external: Bair Hugger, warming blanket, radiant heat, warm water immersion.

Active core noninvasive: inhaling warm humidified oxygen or warm IV fluids.

Active core invasive: bladder, gastric/colonic, thoracic or peritoneal lavage; extracorporeal rewarming (cardiopulmonary bypass, dialysis).

Beware of core temperature after-drop and rewarming shock. Risk reduced by applying heat only to trunk and including active core rewarming modality.

"No one is dead, until they are warm and dead." Warm to >35 °C before declaring death.

13.6. Burns

13.6.1. General burn information

Severity based on: type (thermal, chemical, electrical, radiation), depth (superficial, partial thickness, full thickness), extent (total percent body surface area (BSA) covered with second- and third-degree burns), body part, and other factors (e.g. age <10 or >50, medical conditions or multiple trauma, associated inhalation injury).

Table 13.3 Burn degrees

Burn depth	Example	Sign/symptoms	Prognosis
Superficial (first degree), epidermis	Sunburn	Red/pink, dry, painful, no blister	Heals in 7 days, no scar
Superficial partial (second degree), superficial dermis	Hot liquid	Red, moist, blanches, painful, clear blisters	Heals in 2–3 weeks
Deep partial (second degree), deep dermis	Hot liquid, oil, steam	Red/pink/white, dry, poor cap refill, painful, blisters	Heals 3–6 weeks, scarring, +/− skin grafts
Full thickness (third and fourth degree), through dermis into deep structures	Flame, hot liquid, hot oil, electrical	White/brown/charred, dry, leathery feel, painless, no blisters	Surgical repair, skin grafts

[6]

Table 13.4 Rule of nines – used to estimate total body surface area affected

	Adult	Child
Head	9%	18%
Arms (each)	9%	9%
Legs (each)	18%	13.5%
Trunk (front)	18%	18%
Trunk (back)	18%	18%
Perineum	1%	1%

13.6.1.1. Assessment of burn

Rule of palms: Patient's palm = 1% BSA. Helpful for irregular, small burns.

Severity based on total body surface area (TBSA) [6].

Mild: partial thickness: <10% (<5% if age <10 or >50 years old) or full thickness: <2%.

Moderate (consider transfer to burn center): partial thickness: 10–20% (5–10% if age <10 or >50 years old), or full thickness: 2–5%.

Severe (transfer to burn center): partial thickness: >20% (>10% if age <10 or >50 years old), or full thickness >5%.

Additional reasons for transfer to burn center: Involvement of face, hands, major joints, feet, perineum; Immunocompromised; Burns + trauma and/or inhalational injury;

High-voltage electrical burns; Caustic chemical burns; Circumferential burns of extremities, chest, neck.

13.6.1.2. Management

IV fluid resuscitation: used for all types of burns.

Burns >20% BSA require fluid resuscitation. Lactated Ringers or normal saline may be used.
Parkland formula: 4 mL/kg x BSA burned (partial and full-thickness). Give half over 8 hours (from time of burn), give second half over next 16 hours.
Monitor urinary output (>50 mL/hr in adults, 0.5–1.0 mL/kg/hr in children), vitals, cap refill and sensorium to determine adequacy of fluid resuscitation.

Minor: cool compresses, debride loose tissue or ruptured blisters, cleanse with mild soap and water. Topical antibiotic: bacitracin, polymyxin B, silver sulfadiazine.
Contraindications to silver sulfadiazine include third trimester pregnancy (can cause kernicterus), sulfa allergies, use on face (silver staining).
Major: apply dry sterile sheet and call burn center to coordinate further treatment.
Escharotomy – incision down to fat layer if leathery eschar is causing circulatory or respiratory compromise.
Note: Burns are tetanus prone wounds and treat patient's pain.

13.6.2. Chemical burns

Chemicals cause damage by reaction with skin and protein denaturation. Key factors: type of chemical, concentration and duration of contact.

13.6.2.1. Alkali burns

Causes liquefaction necrosis, no eschar formed, leads to deeper injury. Tissue damage is ongoing until decontaminated.

13.6.2.2. Acidic burns

Causes coagulation necrosis, forms eschar, which limits penetration.

Management: rapid removal of chemical agent. Decontamination procedures, personnel wear protective clothing. Copious irrigation using normal saline or water. Brush off dry particles before irrigating.

13.6.3. Special burns and management

13.6.3.1. Ocular injury

Immediate irrigation at scene, 2 L over 30 minutes in the emergency department then check tears for normalization of pH, continue irrigation if necessary; alkali require longer treatment than acid [7].

13.6.3.2. Hydrofluoric acid

Penetrates like strong alkali. Can cause systemic hypocalcemia and hypomagnesemia. After irrigation, may need to treat with calcium gluconate.

13.6.3.3. Electrical burns

See electrical injury section.

13.6.3.4. Inhalation injury

Injury can result from thermal, chemical, or inhaled toxins (e.g. carbon monoxide, cyanide).

Suspect if: enclosed space, respiratory symptoms (dyspnea, wheezing, cough, stridor). Early intubation may be indicated if patient is unconscious, had the history of enclosed-space fire, respiratory distress, or has minor respiratory distress with facial burn, sooty sputum, singed facial hairs, pharyngeal erythema or swelling, hypoxia.

13.7. Electrical injury

13.7.1. Artificial source electrical burns

13.7.1.1. Alternating current

Explosive exit wounds. Effects usually worse than DC current. V-fib is common dysrhythmia.

13.7.1.2. Direct current

Discrete exit wounds. Asystole is common dysrhythmia.

13.7.1.3. Electrical burn injury patterns

Usually the higher the voltage, the more severe the injury. High voltage considered >1000 V.

Wound appearance: electrical wounds have a "bull's eye" appearance: central charred area surrounded by grayish white area (coagulation necrosis) adjacent to red, edematous area. Internal injuries can occur at any organ or structure between entry and exit wounds.

Workup and treatment: rhabdomyolysis needs to be excluded as do other traumatic injuries. Important not to debride wounds as the eschar aids in controlling hemostasis. Take caution with lip electric burns at corners of mouth: significant delayed hemorrhage from labial artery can occur between 3–14 days post injury when eschar falls off.

Disposition: Admit all high-voltage injuries or low-voltage injuries with symptoms such as chest pain, arrhythmia, myoglobulinuria. Asymptomatic low-voltage burns can be discharged home after brief emergency department observation.

Delayed complications of major electrical burns: myoglobulinuric renal failure, compartment syndrome, dysrhythmias, cataracts.

13.7.2. Natural source electrical burns

13.7.2.1. Lightning

General: ~70% are non-fatal but most suffer sequelae. Injuries can be mechanical (blunt trauma), thermal (burns) or electrical.

Three types of strikes

Direct strike – current flows through patient – highest mortality.

"Splash-over" or "side flash" – current jumps from a nearby object or person.

Ground strike – current radiates out from impact point.

Skin findings:

Flashover effect – current flow over body, vaporized skin moisture, blasts apart clothing.
Feathering (also called fern-like, Lichtenberg figures, or spider-like) cutaneous patterns –
pathognomonic for lightning strike, resolve in less than 24 hours.
Linear burns – in areas of moisture or across flexion areas– groin, axillae.
Punctate burns – small, discrete, clusters of full-thickness burns (about the size of a
cigarette burn).

Clinical presentation: may be in asystolic cardiac arrest or respiratory arrest due to
paralysis. Other signs include loss of consciousness, confusion, amnesia, transient
partial paralysis. Vasospasm and autonomic dysfunctions. Dilated, non-reactive pupils
seen in up to 50%. Tympanic membrane (TM) ruptures in up to 50% (barotraumas).

Management: ABCs, secondary survey, wide variety of organ systems can be affected.
Reverse triage: treat apneic and pulseless first when there are multiple victims. Extensive
burns should go to burn center.

13.8. Radiation emergencies

Alpha particles → Beta particles → Gamma rays → X-rays → Neutron (least to most body
penetrating form of radiation).

Exposure types [4]:

Irradiated: exposed to ionizing radiation (no risk to staff).
Contaminated (risk to staff).

External: radioactive material on surfaces.
Internal: material ingested, inhaled, etc.

Incorporation: radioactive material absorbed into tissues/organs (risk to staff).
Tissues/organs with high rate of cell division more sensitive – bone marrow,
gastrointestinal (GI) tract, reproductive system, skin, also pediatric and developing fetus
very sensitive to radiation. Among blood cell lines, lymphocyte count drops first.

Acute radiation syndrome: usually seen with whole body irradiation.

Table 13.5 Stages of acute radiation syndrome

Acute radiation syndrome stages	Time from exposure	Symptoms and signs
Prodromal	0–72 hours	Nausea and vomiting, diarrhea, nonspecific constitutional symptoms (cephalgia, diaphoresis, fatigue)
Latent	1–3 weeks	Lack of clinical symptoms, apparent recovery
Manifest illness	0–4 weeks	*Subsyndromes* – dose-dependent with significant overlap –Hematopoietic → 150–200 rad – Pancytopenia, immunosuppression –GI → 600–700 rad – loss of mucosal barrier, profound fluid and electrolyte disruptions, bleeding, bacterial invasion –Pulmonary syndrome – 800–900 rad – pneumonitis, respiratory failure, pulmonary fibrosis –Cerebrovascular syndrome – 2000–3000 rad – headache, ataxia, convulsions, altered mental status
Recovery (or death)	3–6 weeks	

[8]

Management: designate receiving area and decontamination area. Remove patient's contaminated clothing (eliminates 80–90% of external contamination), cleansing with soap and tepid water for 3 minutes, assess for further contamination [9]. Therapy generally supportive with IV fluids, antiemetics, analgesics [8]. Long-term therapy may include IV fluids, blood products, total parenteral nutrition (TPN), reverse isolation, antibiotics, etc. If exposure is due to ingestion or inhalation it may warrant administration of blocking (e.g. iodine) or chelating agents. Give potassium iodide to prevent thyroid uptake if exposed to radioiodine (iodine-131).

References

1. Otten EJ. Venomous animal injuries. In: Marx JA, Hockberger RS, Walls RM, Adams J, Rosen P, eds. *Rosen's Emergency Medicine: Concepts and Clinical Practice.* Philadelphia: Mosby Elsevier, 2010; 743–57.
2. Weber EJ, West HH. Mammalian bites. In: Marx JA, Hockberger RS, Walls RM, Adams J, Rosen P, eds. *Rosen's Emergency Medicine: Concepts and Clinical Practice.* Philadelphia: Mosby Elsevier, 2010; 733–42.
3. Richards DB, Knaut AL. Drowning. In: Marx, JA Hockberger RS, Walls RM, Adams J, Rosen P, eds. *Rosen's Emergency Medicine: Concepts and Clinical Practice.* Philadelphia: Mosby Elsevier, 2010; 1929–32.
4. Danzl DF. Frostbite. In: Marx, JA, Hockberger RS, Walls RM, Adams J, Rosen P, eds. *Rosen's Emergency Medicine: Concepts and Clinical Practice.* Philadelphia: Mosby Elsevier, 2010; 1861–7.
5. Geeting GK. Environmental disorders. In: Schofer JM, Mattu A, Colletti JE, *et al.*, eds. *Emergency Medicine: A Focus Review of the Core Curriculum.* Milwaukee: AAEM/RSA Inc., 2008; 369–80.
6. Singer AJ, Taira BR, Lee CC, Soroff HC. Thermal burns. In: Marx JA, Hockberger RS, Walls RM, Adams J, Rosen P, eds. *Rosen's Emergency Medicine: Concepts and Clinical Practice.* Philadelphia: Mosby Elsevier, 2010; 758–66.
7. Levine M, Zane R. Chemical injuries. In: Marx JA, Hockberger RS, Walls RM, Adams J, Rosen P, eds. *Rosen's Emergency Medicine: Concepts and Clinical Practice.* Philadelphia: Mosby Elsevier, 2010; 767–77.
8. Catlett CL, Piggott PL. Radiation injuries. In Tintinalli JE, Stapczynski JS, Cline DM, *et al. Tintinalli's Emergency Medicine: a Comprehensive Study Guide,* 6th edn. New York: The McGraw-Hill Companies, Inc., 2004; 50–9.
9. Suyama J, Sztajnkrycer MD. Radiation injuries. In: Wolfson Hendey GW, Ling LJ, *et al. Harwood-Nuss' Clinical Practice of Emergency Medicine,* 4th edn. Philadelphia: Lippincott Williams & Wilkins, 2005; 1775–80.

14

Procedures in emergency medicine

E. John Wipfler, III

This section will discuss clinical procedures in emergency medicine, with a focus on the indications, contraindications, and potential complications. Elsewhere there have been entire textbooks written on the topic of clinical procedures that discuss the exact step-by-step directions, equipment, and materials involved and therefore one should use these sources as appropriate for detailed learning. The knowledge of when and when not to perform a medical procedure, as well as potential complications that may result from performing an emergency medical procedure, is of high importance and is the objective of this chapter.

The following procedures will be discussed with a focus on the following:

- Name of the procedure and basic description.
- Indications – when to perform the procedure.
- Contraindications – when to not perform the procedure.
- Complications – what to watch out for during and after the procedure.

14.1. Airway techniques and respiratory procedures

14.1.1. Pulse oximetry

- Noninvasive method allowing the monitoring of the oxygen saturation of a patient's hemoglobin (HGB).
- Measure oxygenation, and not ventilation (caution).
- May be abnormal if HGB is bound to something else (carbon monoxide, cyanide, etc.).

Indications: "fifth vital sign," very important in children; used to help assess patient's respiratory status and adequacy of oxygenation before and after airway procedure; evaluation of stable and exacerbation of respiratory disease (chronic obstructive pulmonary disease [COPD], asthma, pneumonia, etc.), breathlessness in adults and children, and toxicology; provide early warning of ventilator dysfunction; monitor during medical procedure/operation.

Contraindications: none.

Limitations: darkly pigmented skin and nail polish and dirt can overestimate oxygen saturation, poor perfusion may result in difficulty obtaining a reading (shock, hypothermia, cardiac failure); anemia may result in normal readings until less than

Pocket Guide to the American Board of Emergency Medicine In-Training Exam, ed. Bob Cambridge.
Published by Cambridge University Press. © Cambridge University Press 2013.

5 mg/dL; carbon monoxide and cyanide poisoning results in inadequate oxygen transport despite normal pulse oximeter readings.

Complications: none.

14.1.2. Carbon dioxide monitoring = capnometry

Noninvasive determination of the carbon dioxide concentration of expired air, assess ventilation adequacy.

Carbon dioxide is a better, more sensitive and more rapid indicator of ventilation problems than SpO_2.

Indications: confirm proper location and function of endotracheal tubes, s/p intubation; predictive value when determining the efficacy of CPR and survival prediction; monitor and guide ventilation parameters and patient ventilation (during transport too); monitor patients during sedation and procedural sedation; determine if patients are responding to medical care (trends).

Contraindications: none.

Complications: device should be routinely maintained and tested to be accurate.

14.1.3. Airway adjuncts/artificial airways

14.1.3.1. Oxygen supplementation (nasal, facemask, other)

Oxygen considered a type of 'therapy' or treatment and should be used appropriately.

Indications: patients with hypoxia or severe medical/traumatic condition who will benefit from supplemental oxygen; generally indicated when hypoxia is present: P_aO_2 less than 60 mmHg, or SaO_2 less than 90– 95%; other indications are carbon monoxide poisoning and other toxic exposures; high altitude (airplane) may require supplementation for some patients.

Contraindications: use caution in patients with COPD/chronic lung disease who may have their respiratory drive mostly from oxygen, in which the use of oxygen may suppress their ventilatory drive and lead to an excess buildup of carbon dioxide with mental status changes and deterioration.

Complications: use caution in some patients with chronic lung disease that may be at risk for respiratory and subsequent mental dysfunction if oxygen is used at too high an amount; avoid unnecessary use of high oxygen levels, due to cytotoxic injury and chronic effects of hyperoxygenation (oxidation, radical formation, etc.); physical hazards include increased threat of fire and explosions near patients who use oxygen in large amounts.

14.1.3.2. Nasopharyngeal airway (also called an "NPA" or nasal trumpet)

Tube with a flared end, an airway adjunct, is designed to be inserted into the nasal passageway to secure an open airway.

Indications: an NPA may be used to keep an open airway in patients in situations where an artificial form of airway maintenance is necessary but it is impossible or inadvisable to use an oropharyngeal airway or more invasive device.

Contraindications: avoid use in patients with severe head or facial injuries, or basilar skull fracture (Battle's sign), due to risks of inadvertent placement inside the head or brain.

Complications: nasal bleeding, pain, nausea and vomiting, potential plugging/obstruction of airway.

14.1.3.3. Oropharyngeal airway (OPA)

Artificial airway that is placed in the mouth/oropharynx with a goal of preventing the tongue from obstructing the airway by falling back against the posterior pharyngeal wall.

Indications: use to prevent the tongue and oral airway structures from closing off the airway; use when patient has unresponsiveness and lack of a gag reflex; provides relief from fatigue that is caused by the continuous application of chin-lift or jaw-thrust maneuvers.

Contraindications: if patient is actively vomiting and gagging when the OPA is placed in the mouth then stop attempts to place the OPA, and consider NPA or other technique.

Complications: may cause obstruction if not properly sized; also do not use this as a definitive airway in the comatose patient with lack of a gag reflex (this patient needs to be intubated soon); may cause bleeding, aspiration.

14.1.3.4. Bag-valve-mask (BVM) mechanical ventilation

BVM ventilation is simple and effective, but requires skill and experience to do well.

Adequate tidal volume with BVM ventilation requires a tight mask seal and adequate compression of the bag, and often use of NPA or OPA to maintain airway.

Indications: requirement to assist ventilations or completely ventilate a patient.

Contraindications: relative contraindication is inexperience; it is difficult to perform.

Complications: emesis, aspiration, inadequate tidal volumes, inadequate oxygen delivery, gastric distention.

14.1.4. Intermediate airways

Esophageal obturator airway, Combitube, dual-lumen airways (King LT, other). Laryngeal-mask airway (LMA).

Indications: need for airway and BVM is not adequate or is difficult to use, and esophageal intubation would be too difficult or impossible given conditions. Speed and simplicity are advantages over tracheal intubation; can be placed blindly.

Contraindications: active oropharyngeal bleeding and excessive secretions are relative contraindications; ingestion of caustic agent, known esophageal stricture or injury, or conditions predisposing to perforation.

Complications: improper insertion angle causing inadequate seal with insufficient ventilation, hypoxia, oropharyngeal trauma, bleeding, emesis/aspiration.

14.1.5. Noninvasive ventilatory management

BiPAP (bilevel positive airway pressure), CPAP (continuous positive airway pressure).

Indications: treatment of impending ventilatory failure in an attempt to avoid intubation and standard mechanical ventilation, with their associated higher morbidity and mortality; most useful in patients whose respiratory failure is expected to quickly respond to medical therapy (congestive heart failure [CHF] with pulmonary edema, volume overload in a hemodialysis patient, etc.).

Contraindications: BiPAP and CPAP require an alert patient who can protect their airway; in cases where the patient has an altered mental status and/or is not cooperative with the mask, or a good seal is not obtained, then intubation will likely be preferred.

Complications: facial irritation, abrasion, facial necrosis, conjunctivitis, aspiration, and gastric distention.

14.1.6. Foreign body removal (upper airway obstruction)

Patients who present with airway obstruction due to a foreign body impairing or preventing air flow to their lungs are at risk for death, and the foreign body should be removed as soon as practically possible.

Indications: obstruction or partial obstruction of airway from a foreign body.

Contraindications: the most ideal and available methods should be considered; there are no contraindications other than seeking the most qualified persons to deal with the critical airway issue at hand.

Complications: iatrogenic injury to the teeth, gums, lips, oropharynx, or neck tissues; trauma or injury to the airway from the foreign body, possible retained foreign body, airway obstruction, inhalation of the foreign body into the lung or stomach.

14.1.7. Endotracheal intubation

Nasotracheal intubation.
Guided digital intubation.
Lighted stylet intubation.
Fiberoptic intubation.
Direct laryngoscopy.
Indirect laryngoscopy.
Intubating LMA.
RSI – rapid sequence intubation.

Indications: patients who need definitive airway protection with a cuffed endotracheal tube but will need to have this tube inserted in a manner which ideally is less stressful and least damaging to the body.

Contraindications: if a better alternate method of respiratory support can be introduced and utilized (BiPAP, treatment of underlying medical cause, etc.), then intubation may not be indicated.

Complications: hypoxia, cardiac decompensation from prolonged efforts, bradycardia (vagal-mediated), teeth trauma, oropharyngeal and larynx trauma, neck movement may exacerbate underlying fracture/spinal cord injury, vomiting, aspiration, unrecognized esophageal intubation, air lead, endotracheal tube cuff leak, tracheal stricture (long-term complication), vocal cord damage.

14.1.8. Surgical airways

Retrograde intubation.
Needle cricothyrotomy (percutaneous translaryngeal jet ventilation).
Open cricothyrotomy.

Indications: need for a definitive airway and other intubation techniques failed or are not possible, including: massive oral, nasal, or pharyngeal hemorrhage, emesis, masseter spasm, clenched teeth, structural deformities, stenosis of upper airway, mass effect, oropharyngeal edema, traumatic injuries making oral or nasal intubation difficult, need for definitive airway during procedures on face/neck/upper airway.

Contraindications: relatively few; should not be done in patients who can be quickly, easily, and safely intubated; transection of trachea with retraction of distal end is a contraindication; a fractured larynx or cricoid cartilage is another contraindication.

Complications: bleeding, hematoma, incorrect tube placement, prolonged procedure time, subcutaneous emphysema, vocal cord injury, aspiration, pneumothorax; late complications include obstructive problems, voice changes, infections, persistent stoma.

14.1.9. Mechanical ventilation

Bag ventilation – see BVM above.
Ventilator use (multiple types of devices).

After intubation, patients will generally need to have their ventilations "breathing" function continued, which will require either a hand-held bag or a mechanical ventilator to maintain.

Types of ventilators: Flow generators, pressure generators; pressure-cycled, volume-cycled, or time-cycled; volume-cycled is generally used most often; use proper ventilator settings: rate and tidal volume, F_iO_2, and mode of ventilation (controlled ventilation, Assist-Control, Intermittent mandatory ventilation (IMV), and synchronized IMV (SIMV); PEEP (positive end expiratory pressure).

Indications: patients who are unable to breathe/ventilate themselves.
Contraindications: none.
Complications: pressure phenomena (nasal and tongue necrosis, laryngeal ulceration, tracheal stenosis and lamacia, fistulas; failure to deliver adequate ventilation, alarm failure, inadequate humidification, accidentally disconnected, direct effects of positive pressure ventilation (pneumothorax, tension pneumothorax, decreased venous return, pneumonia, oxygen toxicity).

14.2. Anesthesia

14.2.1. Local

Topical anesthetics used in emergency medicine include lidocaine, bupivacaine, with and without epinephrine; other types may be used as well.

Indications: topical anesthetics may be applied topically to mucous membranes, skin, and lacerations; they may also be injected directly into tissue (infiltration anesthesia) or in a field block, to decrease pain and sensation and thus allow relief of pain and allow surgical procedures to be performed (laceration repair, incision and drainage, etc.).

Contraindications: patients with allergies to some anesthetics should be identified and use of these agents avoided; avoid too large a dose of anesthetic, especially in children; other anesthesia may be considered (regional/nerve block, general anesthesia).

Complications: systemic toxic effects, especially if allergic or if a significant amount of epinephrine is used; methemoglobinemia (rare, some SQ use of benzocaine).

14.2.2. Regional nerve block

Injection of local anesthetic medication near regional nerves is used to cause regional loss of pain perception. This has the advantages as below:

Indications: use when anesthesia is required over a large area and multiple injections would be painful, or the large amount of anesthetic needed exceeds the recommended dose; use when distortion from local infiltration hampers closure or blood flow; some nerve blocks (rib fracture in a patient with COPD) will aid in appropriate therapy.

Contraindications: none; consider use of ultrasound to guide needle placement and confirm injection of anesthetic agent at the appropriate location.

Complications: ischemia of nearby skin, permanent nerve damage if not done properly, bleeding, infection, abscess.

14.2.3. Sedation: for procedures

Indications: use of procedural sedation is individualized to the existing medical condition and length and type of surgical or diagnostic procedure required, with a goal of decreasing or eliminating pain and anxiety during the procedure.

Contraindications: allergies to sedation medications; difficult airway that would make resuscitation or airway support difficult if hypoxia or decreased ventilation occurs; medical conditions too complicated for sedation in the emergency department or office location.

Complications: hypoxia, aspiration, emesis, hypotension, medication reaction, re-emergence reaction (nightmares/hallucinations with scary dreams), allergic reaction, delayed medication side effects (dystonic reaction).

Table 14.1 American Association of Anesthesiologists (ASA) classification

Classification	Physical condition of the patient
1	Healthy
2	Discrete systemic disease
3	Serious non-incapacitating systemic disease
4	Life-threatening incapacitating systemic disease
5	Moribund with death expected within 24 hours

14.2.3.1. Levels of sedation

Minimal sedation (anxiolysis): a drug-induced state during which patients respond normally to verbal commands. Although cognitive function and coordination may be impaired, ventilatory and cardiovascular functions are unaffected.

Moderate sedation (usual state for most procedural sedation): A drug-induced depression of consciousness during which patients respond purposefully to verbal commands, either alone or accompanied by light tactile stimulation. Reflex withdrawal from a painful stimulus is not considered a purposeful response. No interventions are required to maintain a patent airway, and spontaneous ventilation is adequate. Cardiovascular function is usually maintained.

Dissociative sedation: a trance-like cataleptic state induced by the dissociative agent ketamine characterized by profound analgesia and amnesia, with retention of protective airway reflexes, spontaneous respirations, and cardiopulmonary stability.

Deep sedation: a drug-induced depression of consciousness during which patients cannot be easily aroused but respond purposefully after repeated or painful stimulation. The ability to independently maintain ventilatory function may be impaired. Patients may require assistance in maintaining a patent airway and spontaneous ventilation may be inadequate. Cardiovascular function is usually maintained.

General anesthesia: a drug-induced loss of consciousness during which patients are not arousable, even by painful stimulation. The ability to independently maintain ventilatory function is often impaired. Patients often require assistance in maintaining a patent airway, and positive pressure ventilation may be required because of depressed spontaneous ventilation or drug-induced depression of neuromuscular function. Cardiovascular function may be impaired.

14.3. Blood and fluid administration

14.3.1. Blood, fluid, and component therapy administration

Resuscitation of critically ill or injured patients may involve IV blood and fluid resuscitation.

Indications: shock, hypovolemia.

Contraindications: suspected volume overload or CHF with excessive fluids.

Complications: infiltration of fluid or blood products, allergic or transfusion reaction, chills/hypothermia, hypomagnesemia, hypocalcemia, overload of fluid, pulmonary edema/CHF.

14.3.2. Transfusion of blood products (packed red blood cells, fresh frozen platelets, specific blood components)

Indications: treat anemia/acute or chronic blood loss, or treat abnormal coagulation.

Contraindications: known chronic anemia due to known cause and stable HGB level.

Complications: infection of small virus particles (hepatitis, HIV, others), transfusion reactions, hypothermia, electrolyte disturbances, fluid overload, pulmonary edema, CHF.

14.4. Diagnostic procedures

14.4.1. Anoscopy

Examination of the anorectal tract using an anoscope.

Indications: rectal bleeding, diagnose foreign bodies, infections, anal tears, or internal hemorrhoids or masses, evaluation of rectal pain, discharge, pruritis.

Contraindications: imperforate anus, anal stenosis, severe rectal pain.

Complications: anoscopy is a safe procedure, unusual to have complications; may include irritation of local tissues, abrasion, increased bleeding; use of sterilized instruments is imperative, due to transmission of viruses and warts and other infectious diseases.

14.4.2. Arthrocentesis

Arthrocentesis is the puncture and aspiration of a joint.

Indications: diagnosis of nontraumatic joint disease by analyzing synovial fluid, diagnose ligament and bony injury by confirming blood in the joint; if fat globules are present this indicates high likelihood of a fracture.

Contraindications: overlying skin infection.

Complications: bleeding, infection, pain, tendon inflammation.

14.4.3. Bedside ultrasonography

The use of bedside sonography is considered the "stethoscope of the twenty-first century".
There are multiple uses of bedside sonography, and the below is a partial listing of the many potential uses.

Indications: diagnostic applications throughout the body, and assistance with multiple procedures including peripheral and central vascular access, lumbar puncture, incision and drainage, detorsion, foreign body localization/removal, and many others.

Contraindications: there are no radiation risks or tissue toxicity, and no contraindications exist.

Complications: none.

14.4.3.1. Type of bedside sonography in emergency medicine

FAST = Focused Assessment with Sonography for Trauma.

Is there free intraperitoneal fluid?

Is there free fluid in the thorax? Pericardial tamponade?

Cannot show: solid organ injury reliably; source of free fluid, nature of fluid, presence of retroperitoneal injury, or perforation of viscous organ.

Abdomen – rule out abdominal aortic aneurysm, cholecystitis, renal stone (hydronephrosis).

Genitourinary (GU) – rule out testicular torsion.

OB/GYN – rule out ectopic pregnancy.

Cardiac – evaluate cardiac contractility and presence/absence of pericardial tamponade.

Procedure assistance: foreign body removal, identify abscess location and size, vascular access, evaluate central venous pressure (CVP), intraocular pressure (IOP), retinal detachment, others.

14.4.4. Cystourethrogram

Retrograde urethrogram and/or cystogram is performed any time a urethral or bladder injury is suspected (i.e. blood in urine or pelvic trauma with suspicion for this injury).

Indications: document/look for disruption or abnormal urethra or bladder.
Contraindications: none.
Complications: extravasation of contrast material, radiation exposure, pain.

14.4.5. Lumbar puncture

Placement of a small hollow needle (with stylet) into the lower spine with a goal of obtaining cerebrospinal fluid (CSF) for diagnostic purposes (and sometimes therapeutic).

Indications: suspected subarachnoid hemorrhage (SAH) or central nervous system (CNS) infection/sepsis workup (children); meningitis; therapeutic reduction in CSF pressure (i.e. pseudotumor cerebri).
Contraindications: evidence of cellulitis, infection, burn at desired insertion site; raised intracranial pressure (ICP) (except pseudotumor cerebri); suspected spinal cord or intracranial mass or brain abscess; coagulopathy (or severe thrombocytopenia).
Complications: post lumbar puncture headache (most common; may be treated with a "blood patch"); infection; bleeding (i.e. spinal epidural or subdural hematoma).

14.4.6. Nasogastric tube (diagnostic and/or therapeutic)

Placement of a hollow tube into the stomach for treatment or diagnosis.

Indications: aspirate the stomach contents, and remove excess fluid and air from patients who have a bowel obstruction or other medical condition causing decreased bowel activity.
Contraindications: facial fractures, history of esophageal strictures, history alkali ingestion, comatose patients (at risk for aspiration/gagging if airway is not protected).
Complications: nausea, vomiting, aspiration, cough, sinus infection (if in nose), bleeding, perforation of the stomach or esophagus.

14.4.7. Paracentesis

Insertion of a needle or catheter into the peritoneal cavity to drain the peritoneal fluid in order to decrease the abdominal pressure and allow improved breathing, as well as help diagnose any bleeding or infections or pancreatitis.

Indications: abdomen distention from ascites, difficulty breathing due to increased abdominal pressure and size.
Contraindications: known scar tissue in abdomen, bowel obstruction with high pressure, contaminated skin nearby.
Complications: contaminated or infected skin.

14.4.8. Pericardiocentesis

Placement of a hollow needle or catheter inside the pericardiac sac in order to drain/remove the fluid or blood that is causing cardiac compromise due to the high pressure and large amount of fluid present. Two categories of pericardial fluid: acute hemopericardium (mostly trauma and post-procedure), and pericardial effusion from other causes (CHF, malignancy, HIV, infection), slowly accumulates, may be as large as 2000 cc of fluid.

Indications: diagnose the cause or presence of pericardial effusion; to relieve tamponade.

Contraindications: none; should not be performed when better treatment modalities are available (surgery for trauma patients, hemodialysis for renal failure patients).

Complications: "dry tap" (failure), injuries to thoracic organs, abdominal organs; venous air embolism, pneumothorax, cardiac arrhythmias, cardiac arrest and death, infection, bleeding.

14.4.9. Slit lamp examination

Use of a special magnifying scope/lens system that allows one to more accurately see up close and identify and diagnose and treat a particular problem with the patient's eyes.

Indications: diagnosis of cornea and other eye structures.

Contraindications: none.

Complications: eye pain, minor abrasions.

14.4.10. Thoracentesis

Temporary insertion of a needle or small catheter into the pleural space.

Indications: treat suspected tension pneumothorax, treat and diagnose pleural effusion, sometimes treat small stable pneumothoraces.

Contraindications: inserting needle through area of infection; bleeding problems or patients taking anticoagulants.

Complications: creation of a pneumothorax, tension pneumothorax (if on ventilator especially); cough, chest pain, unilateral pulmonary edema, re-expansion hypotension, hypoxia/V-Q mismatch, infection, shearing of plastic catheter.

14.5. Genital/urinary

14.5.1. Urinary bladder catheterization (Foley catheter; suprapubic aspiration)

Indications: acute urinary retention, urethral or prostatic obstruction leading to compromised renal function, urine output monitoring in any critically ill or injured patient; collection of a sterile urine specimen for diagnostic purposes (need to determine if there is a urinary tract infection [UTI] or bleeding in the GU system); intermittent bladder catheterization in patients with neurogenic bladder dysfunction.

Contraindications: avoid catheterization when other less invasive procedures will be as informative; trauma patients with suspected urethral injury as evidenced by blood at the urethral meatus, an abnormal feeling of high-riding prostate on rectal examination, or penile, scrotal, or perineal hematoma.

Complications: iatrogenic UTI, trauma, urethral stricture, bleeding, prostate infection, latex allergy, hematuria, bladder obstruction, retained urethral catheters due to catheter knotting.

14.5.2. Testicular detorsion

Goal of manual detorsion is to reestablish or increase blood flow to a previously ischemic testis; it should never delay operative intervention.

Indications: suspected or proven testicular torsion.

Contraindications: none if true testicular torsion is present.

Complications: possible re-torsion, loss of testicle (if done too late), pain, swelling.

14.6. Head and neck

14.6.1. Control of epistaxis

Nosebleeds should be evaluated, the patient treated, bleeding stopped, and any anemia or blood problems identified or known prior. Nosebleeds are mostly anterior in location (90%) and the rest are posterior nosebleeds.

Indications: epistaxis/nosebleed.

Contraindications: none.

Complications: airway compromise with significant bleeding, dizziness, syncope, bradycardia (due to manipulation of airway, nasal/sinus tissues), anemia, sinusitis, infection (if nasal packing used), pain, burns (from silver nitrate on mucosa), nausea and vomiting (from blood swallowed/in patient's stomach).

14.7. Hemodynamic techniques

14.7.1. Arterial catheter insertion

Indications: critically ill patients who need an accurate blood pressure continuous measurement via an "art line" for arterial intravascular line. This also allows routine serious testing of arterial blood gas.

Contraindications: none; an appropriate artery should be used.

Complications: hematoma formation, embolus (distal obstruction further down the artery), air embolus, infection, bleeding, loss of blood.

14.7.2. Central venous access

Indications: failure of peripheral IV access when access is emergently needed; cardiac arrest, critically ill, sepsis resuscitation protocols; goal-directed therapy (i.e. CVP and SvO_2 monitoring); need for pressors and/or multiple fluids/blood products; no peripheral access (IV drug abuse history, obesity, burns, long-term care).

Contraindications:

> **General:** distorted anatomy, extremes of weight, bleeding disorders, suspected proximal vessel injury, anticoagulation, thrombolytic treatments, combative patients, overlying infection at insertion site.

> **Subclavian site contraindications:** COPD (relative), chest wall deformities, contralateral pneumothorax.

> **Femoral site contraindications:** need for patient mobility.

Complications:

> **General:** infection, sepsis, dysrhythmias (stimulation of heart by the guidewire), arterial puncture, air embolus, large vein thrombus, catheter embolus (or wire), misplacement (i.e. subclavian ending up in internal jugular instead of superior vena cava [SVC]).

Subclavian/internal jugular route complications: Pneumothorax, hemothorax, chylothorax, neck hematoma, tracheal puncture or perforation, hemomediastinum.

Femoral route complications: Intra-abdominal placement, retroperitoneal hematoma, bowel perforation, psoas abscess.

14.7.3. Intraosseous (IO) insertion and infusion

Indications: failure of peripheral IV access when access is emergently needed; cardiac arrest, critically ill; generally used early in children and infants (difficult to start peripheral IV); access in adults as alternative to central venous line in emergent situation.

Contraindications: extremity fracture at IO site; evidence of cellulitis, infection, burn at desired insertion site.

Complications: incomplete or through-and-through penetration of bone; extravasation of medications/fluids, skin sloughing, compartment syndrome, epiphyseal injuries; infection; bleeding.

14.7.4. Peripheral venous cutdown

Use of a knife and other instruments to place an IV catheter so as to allow diagnostic testing of blood and also infuse IV fluids and blood products.

Indications: need for IV access but percutaneous/multiple IV attempts have not been successful.

Contraindications: none, unless other persons have already started a catheter.

Complications: pain, swelling, bleeding, infections.

14.8. Musculoskeletal procedures

14.8.1. Fracture/dislocation immobilization and reduction techniques

Indications: usually clear; pain with or without deformity following trauma should arouse suspicion for underlying bone or joint injury; swelling, discoloration, deformity, crepitus, or loss of neurovascular function.

Contraindications: no contraindications to splinting suspected fractures or dislocations; however, rapid transport may be more important than extremity splinting; averting loss of life takes precedence over averting loss of limb.

Complications: potential complications of splinting and reduction techniques include pressure necrosis, conversion of a closed injury into an open one, and loss of neurovascular function; compartment syndrome is possible although rare; reduction techniques have slight risk of worsening of neurovascular injuries and pain.

14.8.2. Compartment pressure measurement

Compartment syndrome is a condition of increased pressure within a limited space that results in compromised tissue perfusion and ultimate dysfunction of neural and muscular structures contained within that space. In patients with medical or traumatic etiology causing possible high pressure in muscle compartments, the pressure should be measured to determine if surgery is necessary or not. Regarding compartment pressure measurement/ monitoring:

Indications: early diagnosis is desirable and may be clinically obvious, and treatment (fasciotomy) may be done without measurement; however some are borderline, and some patients may benefit from measurement of compartment pressure, including unresponsive patients, uncooperative patients (intoxicated adults, young children), and patients with peripheral nerve deficits attributable to other causes.

Contraindications: none, except if the decision for going to the operating room for fasciotomy has already been determined then it may be unnecessary to do a painful test.

Complications: bleeding, swelling, infection, nerve injury, uncalibrated or inaccurate measurement devices/pressure monitors.

14.9. Obstetrics

14.9.1. Delivery of newborn

Indications: imminent delivery, active contractions with part of baby showing at perineum, and there is not adequate time to have the OB/GYN doctor come to the emergency room or other location of patient.

Contraindications: none.

Complications: usual delivery complications, retained placenta, prolapsed uterus, anemia, problems with newborn.

14.10. Thoracic

14.10.1. Emergency cardiac pacing (transcutaneous pacing [TCP]; transvenous pacing [TVP])

Use of electricity to induce cardiac contractions and improve the heart rate and hemo-dynamic status in patients with heart block, bradycardia, or other slow cardiac rhythm.

Indications: TCP is technically the fastest and easiest method of emergency pacing, and may be used for hemodynamically significant bradydysrhythmias that have not responded to atropine therapy. Chest pain, pulmonary edema, or evidence of decreased cerebral perfusion (altered mental status) are all indications.

Contraindications: in a conscious patient who is hemodynamically stable, TCP/TVP may not be necessary; TCP is somewhat painful; TVP is less painful.

Complications: pain from the electrical shocks, soft tissue injuries (burns, muscle spasm, other), failure to recognize the presence of underlying treatable ventricular fibrillation (V-fib; due to ECG screen artifact), induction of dysrhythmias.

14.10.2. Defibrillation

Application of electrical energy to restore a fibrillating ventricle to normal sinus rhythm.

Indications: V-fib or unstable ventricular tachycardia.

Contraindications: artificially induced appearance of V-fib or ventricular tachycardia (VT) (ECG lead wire shaking, seizure of patient, etc.).

Complications: soft tissue injuries (chest wall pain, burns) myocardial injury, and cardiac dysrhythmias.

14.10.3. Cardioversion

Application of direct electrical current across the chest or directly across the ventricle to normalize the conduction pattern of a rapidly beating heart.

Indications: cardioversion is indicated whenever there is a reentrant tachycardia causing chest pain, pulmonary edema, lightheadedness, or hypotension.

Contraindications: sinus tachycardia; and tachydysrhythmias that are known to be caused by digitalis toxicity.

Complications: soft tissue and chest wall pain, burns (superficial) from the electrical pads, myocardial injury ischemia (from prolonged tachycardia, stress), cardiac dysrhythmias, complications from procedural sedation.

14.10.4. Tube thoracostomy (chest tube placement)

Indications: pneumothorax (spontaneous, tension) with significant or worsening respiratory symptoms, or enlarging pneumothorax after conservative observation management, or if patient will require ventilator support; recurrence of pneumothorax after chest tube removal; hemothorax; empyema; chylothorax; pleural effusion (effecting oxygenation and/or ventilation).

Indications for surgical intervention after chest tube placement: massive hemothorax (>1000–1500 mL on initial drainage or ongoing bleeding of >300–500 mL in first hour or >200 mL/hr during first 3 or more hours); persistent hemothorax after 2 functioning chest tubes; large air leak preventing effective ventilation even after 2 chest tubes; inability to fully expand lung (relative).

Contraindications: no absolute contraindications in unstable, injured patient; relative contraindications in stable patient: coagulopathy (or severe thrombocytopenia); multiple pleural adhesions; emphysematous blebs; scarring; suspected loculation of pleural fluid (interventional radiology[IR]-guided drainage preferred).

Complications: infection, intra-abdominal organ injury, bleeding, tube malfunction, lung injury, re-expansion pulmonary edema, cardiac injury, subcutaneous or intra-abdominal placement, rib neurovascular bundle injury.

14.10.5. Needle thoracostomy for tension pneumothorax

Placement of a hollow needle or angiocatheter into the thoracic space in order to decompress the high intrathoracic pressure in patients with proven or suspected tension pneumothorax.

Indications: suspected tension pneumothorax.

Contraindications: none; this is a life-saving procedure that needs to be urgently performed if there are clinical signs or radiographic signs of tension pneumothorax.

Complications: infection, intra-abdominal organ injury, bleeding, lung injury, re-expansion pulmonary edema, cardiac injury, intra-abdominal placement, rib neurovascular bundle injury.

14.10.6. Emergency thoracotomy/resuscitative thoracotomy

"Cracking a chest" and "emergency department thoracotomy" are terms used for resuscitative thoracotomy. Anterolateral thoracotomy incision is most commonly used to open the thoracic cavity to allow diagnosis and repair of traumatic cardiac and pulmonary injuries in patients who develop full cardiopulmonary arrest with recently (within 3–5 minutes) confirmed signs of life (pulse, spontaneous movement); bimanual cardiac compression is the more effective method of cardiac massage.

Indications: acute penetrating chest trauma with recent loss of vital signs.

Contraindications: medical or blunt trauma mechanism is a relative contraindication due to very low survival rates; prolonged downtime or lack of documented signs of life in the prehospital setting will greatly decrease survival rate.

Complications: high risk for needle stick or cut to medical staff, infections, bleeding, pulmonary injury (during opening of thorax with knife).

14.11. Other techniques

14.11.1. Gastric lavage

Gastric lavage can be performed immediately on patients with a decreased level of consciousness once the airway is protected; ingested drugs that are removed by lavage are no longer available for absorption; major disadvantage is the time commitment of healthcare workers and risks of aspiration and esophageal injury.

Indications: overdose patients who present within 1 hour of ingestion of a toxin; a careful assessment of the risk-to-benefit ratio should be done.

Contraindications: unprotected airway, possible ingestion of strong alkalis, known esophageal strictures, ingestion of hydrocarbons (unless containing highly toxic substances such as pesticides, heavy metals, halogenated or aromatic compounds, or camphor); the regional poison control center can be of useful assistance and should be contacted.

Complications: upper airway injury (from tube), esophageal rupture, emesis, aspiration, pneumonia, hypoxia, electrolyte disturbance, esophageal spasm.

14.11.2. Gastrostomy tube replacement

Nursing home patients and others with chronic G-tube in upper abdomen are at risk for accidental or intentional removal, and will present to the emergency room for replacement; also some will "clog up" and become obstructed with food or medicines. A G-J tube and other more complicated feeding tubes are placed by IR or surgery, and these tube replacement patients should be admitted or arrangements should be made for outpatient surgery/IR to replace these.

Indications: feeding G-tube is pulled out or becomes obstructed/malfunctions. Seek information from the chart, patient, family, physician, nursing home when available about the placement and type of G-tube.

Contraindications: signs of infection; suspicion that the G-tube tract is disrupted; recently placed surgical G-tube procedure; bowel obstruction.

Complications: the major concern is that a new tube may be misplaced (i.e. into the peritoneal cavity); proper verification should be performed to document the correct location of a newly replaced G-tube.

14.11.3. Incision/drainage

Commonly done to drain an abscess or other fluid collection.
Indications: abscess, infection with fluid collection.
Contraindications: none.
Complications: wound infection, bleeding.

14.11.4. Wound closure techniques (skin glue; steristrips; staples; suture)

Indications: repair lacerations and close wounds that are open.
Contraindications: no absolute contraindications, but consider risk factors (below)
Complications: none expected.
Risk factors for wound infection:

Injury >8–12 hours and varies depending on following factors as well.
Location (risk in descending order): leg/thigh, arms, feet, chest, back, face, scalp.
Contamination with devitalized tissue, foreign matter, saliva, stool.
Crush/blunt mechanism.
Presence of subcutaneous sutures.
High-velocity injuries (bullets, shrapnel, high-pressure injections/factory).

Bibliography

Roberts JR, Hedges JR. *Clinical Procedures in Emergency Medicine*, 5th edn. Philadelphia: Saunders/Elsevier, 2010.

Chapter 15

Rapid review

Richard Frederick and Andrew Vincent

Cardiology emergencies

Tissue plasminogen activator (tPA) dose	10 mg Q30 minutes x2
Aortic dissection classes	Debakey-1: entire aorta Stanford-A and Debakey-2: proximal aorta Stanford-B and Debakey-3: distal aorta beginning at left subclavian
Electrical alternans associated with what condition?	Tamponade
Differential diagnosis of tachycardia with irregular narrow complex?	Multifocal atrial tachycardia, atrial fibrillation (A-fib), sinus tachycardia with premature atrial contractions
Differential diagnosis of tachycardia with wide complex? Treatment?	Ventricular tachycardia (VT), antidromic Wolff–Parkinson–White (WPW), supraventricular tachycardia (SVT) with aberrancy. Treatment: procainamide or amiodarone
Most common cause of mitral stenosis	Rheumatic fever
Most common cause of mitral regurgitation	Rheumatic fever
Most common cause of aortic stenosis	Calcific degeneration
Most common cause of death from aortic stenosis	Arrhythmia
Most common dysrhythmias in hypothermia	A-fib and sinus bradycardia
Treatment for β-blocker or calcium channel blocker overdose	Epinephrine, atropine, calcium chloride, glucagon, pacing
Pacer magnet does what?	Sets pacer to automatic baseline pacing rhythm (without sensing). It does not turn the pacer off.
Goal when decreasing blood pressure (BP) in hypertensive emergency?	Do not decrease mean arterial pressure (MAP) more than 20–25% within 2–6 hours
Most common viral cause of myocarditis	Coxsackie B
Most common ECG finding of myocarditis	Sinus tachycardia, low electrical activity, AV block, prolonged QT, MI pattern
Classic heart murmur of hypertrophic cardiomyopathy	Harsh systolic ejection murmur at left lower sternal border that increases with maneuvers that decrease preload

Pocket Guide to the American Board of Emergency Medicine In-Training Exam, ed. Bob Cambridge.
Published by Cambridge University Press. © Cambridge University Press 2013.

Maneuvers to increase and decrease the murmur of hypertrophic obstructive cardiomyopathy (HOCM)	Increase murmur: Valsalva, standing, β-agonist, amyl nitrate inhalation (maneuvers decrease preload) Decrease murmur: leg elevation, handgrips, squatting, α-agonists (maneuvers increase preload)
5 causes of high output congestive heart failure (CHF)	Thyrotoxicosis, anemia, AV fistula, beriberi (wet), Paget's disease
Medication causing pericarditis	Hydralazine, isoniazid, procainamide, anticoagulants
Class of drugs most effective for treatment of chronic CHF associated with dilated cardiomyopathies?	Angiotensin-converting enzyme (ACE) inhibitors
Treatment of hypertrophic cardiomyopathy	First-line: β-blockers Second-line: calcium channel blockers, amiodarone Diuretics with caution Do not use agents that increase contractility Do not use agents that decrease preload or vascular volume
Hs and Ts of pulseless electrical activity (PEA)	Trauma, Tamponade, Tension pneumothorax, Thrombosis, Toxins. Hypovolemia, Hypoxia, Hypoglycemia, Hydrogen ions (acidosis), Hypothermia, Hyper-/Hypokalemia,
ECG progression in acute MI	(1) Hyperacute T waves (2) Elevated ST (3) Inverted T (4) Q wave development
Hypertension (HTN) with subarachnoid bleed: agent of choice for BP control	Nicardipine: calcium channel blocker which decreases BP as well as decreases cerebral vasospasm
Medications for HTN with renal insufficiency	Nitroprusside, nifedipine, labetalol
Medications for HTN and MI/dissection	Nitrates, β-blockers
Medications for hypertensive encephalopathy	Nitroprusside, labetalol
Medications for HTN and CHF	Nitrates, furosemide, ACE inhibitor
Treatment for torsades de pointes	Magnesium (treatment of choice) Overdrive pacing Discontinue offending agent
ECG findings in digitalis toxicity	Premature ventricular contractions (PVCs) (most common, often bigeminal and multiform) Junctional tachycardia (common) SA and AV nodal block A-fib with a slow ventricular response SVT, especially premature atrial tachycardia with block Ventricular tachycardia or fibrillation Bidirectional VT (rare but highly suggestive of digitalis toxicity) Sinus bradycardia/sinus arrest
Arrhythmia highly specific for digitalis toxicity	Premature atrial tachycardia with 2:1 block (Do not cardiovert as you will get a ventricular malignant arrhythmia)
Medications to use in catecholamine-induced HTN crisis	IV labetalol, nitroprusside with β-blockers
Beck's triad	Hypotension, jugular venous distension (JVD), distant heart tones. Seen with tamponade

Contraindications to β-blockers in acute MI	Bradycardia <60 bpm, systolic blood pressure (SBP) <100 mmHg, CHF, chronic obstructive pulmonary disease (COPD)/asthma, signs of hypoperfusion, PR interval > 24 seconds and second/third-degree AV block, severe peripheral vascular disease
ECG findings in a posterior MI	(1) Large R wave with ST depression in V1, V2 (2) Mirror image anterior MI – exact opposite of septal MI (3) T waves in V1 and V2 are upright Note: usually associated with inferior MI
Causes of right ventricular (RV) failure	Left ventricular (LV) failure – most common Pulmonary artery hypertension (Cor pulmonale), R-sided valvular disease, cardiomyopathy, myocarditis, RV infarction, pulmonary embolism (PE), chronic pulmonary disease
Causes of LV failure	Coronary artery disease (CAD) (ischemia), idiopathic dilated cardiomyopathies, HTN, left-sided valvular disease, high-output states (anemia, AV fistula, thyrotoxicosis, beriberi, Paget's), congenital heart defect, coarctation aorta
Jones criteria for rheumatic heart disease (RHD): major (5), minor (5)	Major: (1) polyarthritis (2) carditis (3) chorea (4) erythema marginatum (5) SQ nodules Minor: (1) fever (2) arthralgias (3) elevated erythrocyte sedimentation rate (ESR), C-reactive protein (CRP) (4) leukocytosis (5) increased PR interval on ECG
Criteria needed for diagnosis of RHD	Evidence of group A β-hemolytic streptococcus (GABHS) (culture, anti-streptolysin antibody [ASO] titer, scarlet fever) AND (1) 2 major or (2) 1 major and 2 minor
Cardiac iso-enzymes: rise, peak, duration	Myoglobin: 1–2 hours, 4–7 hours, 24 hours CKMB: 3 hours, 12–24 hours, 2 days Troponin: 3 hours, 12–24 hours, 7 days

Respiratory emergencies

Most common causes of spontaneous pneumothorax	Idiopathic, COPD
Pneumothoraces that need chest tube	Traumatic, moderate to large in size, symptomatic regardless of size, increasing size after conservative management, recurrence after chest tube removal, need for ventilator support or general anesthesia, associated hemothorax, bilateral regardless of size, tension pneumothorax
Most common symptom of PE	Shortness of breath
Most common sign of PE	Tachycardia
Treatment for severe asthma	Epinephrine, bilevel positive airway pressure (BiPAP), albuterol and atrovent nebulizers, corticosteroids, IV magnesium, heliox
Ventilator settings for asthma	Low tidal volume, 6–8 mL/kg and prolonged expiratory phase
Massive hemoptysis definition	100–600 mL in 24 hours
Causes of hemoptysis	Infection, inflammation, PE, granulomatous disease, bronchiectasis, cancer, ectopic endometrial tissue (catamenial hemoptysis)

Virchow's triad	Hypercoagulability, stasis or turbulent flow, endothelial injury
Pulmonary Embolism Rule-Out Criteria (PERC) rule, indicating low-risk patient population	Lowest pretest probability for PE by the treating clinician's estimate (low risk by Wells' criteria), plus must be able to answer yes to all of the following (1) Age <50 (2) Pulse <100 bpm (3) Oxygen saturation >94% (4) No hemoptysis (5) No unilateral leg swelling (6) No recent major surgery or trauma (7) No prior PE or deep vein thrombosis (DVT) (8) No hormone use
Most common location for infection in AIDS	Pulmonary
Most common cause of opportunistic pulmonary infection in AIDS	*Pneumocystis jiroveci* pneumonia
Pleural fluid characteristics: exudates vs. transudates.	The effusion is likely exudative if at least one of the following exists: Ratio of pleural protein to serum protein >0.5 Ratio of pleural fluid LDH to serum LDH >0.6 Pleural fluid LDH level greater than two thirds of upper limit of normal for serum LDH
Causes of exudates	Infection, malignancy, pulmonary embolism, connective tissue disorders, pancreatitis, uremia, and pulmonary infarctions
Most common cause of exudative effusion	Parapneumonic
Causes of transudates	CHF, superior vena cava (SVC) obstruction, hypoalbuminemia, nephrotic syndrome, cirrhosis with ascites, peritoneal dialysis, myxedema, glomerulonephritis, PE
Most common cause of transudative effusion	CHF
Wells' criteria for PE : condition and points Low: less than 2 points Moderate: 2–6 points High: greater than 6 points	Clinically suspected DVT – 3 points Alternative diagnosis is less likely than PE – 3 points Tachycardia – 1.5 points More than 3 days of immobilization in last 4 weeks – 1.5 points History of DVT or PE – 1.5 points Hemoptysis – 1 point Malignancy or palliative treatment within past 6 months – 1 point
Cause of pneumonia when sputum is classically described as bloody or rusty	Pneumococcal, varicella
Cause of pneumonia when sputum is classically described as currant jelly	*Klebsiella*
Cause of pneumonia when sputum is classically described as foul smelling	Anaerobes
Cause of pneumonia when sputum is classically described as green colored	*Pseudomonas, Streptococcus pneumoniae, Haemophilus influenzae*
Systems involved in the presentation of Legionnaire's	Pulmonary (cough, dyspnea, pleuritic chest pain), gastrointestinal (GI) (watery diarrhea, nausea, vomiting, abdominal pain), and neurologic (altered mental status, gait disturbances, seizures)

Treatment for psittacosis	Doxycycline
Treatment for Q fever (*Coxiella burnetii*)	Doxycycline
Treatment for tularemia	Streptomycin
Chest X-ray (CXR) pattern for pneumonia caused by *S. pneumoniae*	Lobar
CXR pattern for pneumonia caused by *Klebsiella*	Bulging fissue in upper lobe
CXR pattern for pneumonia caused by *Staphylococcus aureus*	Cavitation
CXR pattern for pneumonia caused by atypical bacteria	Patchy infiltrates
Encapsulated bacteria which have a significantly higher mortality in what subset of patients	*S. pneumoniae, H. influenzae, Neisseria meningitides, Escherichia coli, Klebsiella, Pseudomonas* Population at risk: post splenectomy or functional aspenia (sickle cell disease), humoral immune dysfunction
Best location to assess for central cyanosis?	Perioral skin, oral mucosa, conjunctivae
What is a rapid and accurate way of detecting a pneumothorax?	Ultrasonography (expiratory CXR does not enhance detection)
Minimum amount of pleural fluid visible on CXR	200–500 mL
Primary tuberculosis (TB) infection occurs primarily in which lobes?	Can occur in any lobe and is often misdiagnosed as a bacterial pneumonia (look for hilar adenopathy as a clue). In reactivation (i.e. secondary TB), the upper lobes are preferentially infected
What percent of AIDS patients will develop pneumocystis pneumonia (PCP)?	80%
PCP is associated with what common complications in AIDS patients?	Death and pneumothorax
Having a pet bird puts you at risk for what kind of pneumonia?	Psittacosis
Working in a slaughterhouse puts you at risk for what kind of pneumonia?	Q fever
Working as a rabbit handler puts you at risk for what kind of pneumonia?	Tularemia
Coming in contact with rodent feces in the southwest USA puts you at risk for what kind of pneumonia?	Hantavirus
Treatment for *Chlamydia* pneumonia	Macrolide or fluoroquinolone

Gastroenterologic emergencies

Dysphagia	Difficulty swallowing (almost always organic cause)
Odynophagia	Pain with swallowing
Globus hystericus	Sensation that something is stuck in throat
Esophageal foreign body lodging sites	(1) Cricopharyngeus muscle (2) aortic arch (3) lower esophageal sphincter
A swallowed object >___cm wide and >___cm long should be removed even if in stomach	2 cm wide and >5 cm long
Disposition of button battery ingestion	(1) If in esophagus, do emergent endoscopy (2) If in stomach, OK for follow-up as outpatient (3) If battery not past pylorus within 48 hours, endoscopy needed (4) Once past pylorus may take 4–7 days to get to rectum

Full-thickness esophageal tear	Boorhave's (Mallory–Weiss is partial thickness with bleed)
Location of pleural effusion in (1) Mallory–Weiss tear (2) Boorhave's syndrome	(1) Right (2) left
Pharmacologic treatment for ruptured esophageal varices	Vasopressin, octreotide
Risk factors for peptic ulcer disease	*Helicobacter pylori*, NSAIDs/aspirin, ethanol, smoking, emotional stress, steroids
Fever, jaundice, right upper quadrant (RUQ) pain	Ascending cholangitis (Charcot's triad)
Charcot's triad	Fever, jaundice, RUQ abdominal pain. Add mental confusion and shock to get Reynaud's pentad. Seen in ascending cholangitis
Which types of hepatitis produce neither a chronic infection nor a carrier state?	Hepatitis A, E
Which form of hepatitis has no markers?	Hepatitis E
Drugs causing liver disease resembling viral hepatitis	Halothane, methyldopa, phenytoin, isoniazid
Definition of spontaneous bacterial peritonitis?	Varies, but about 500 granulocytes/mL or >250 polymorphonuclear neutrophils (PMNs)/mL in ascitic fluid
Hemorrhagic shock is a potential complication of which inflammatory GI disorder?	Pancreatitis
Most common cause of small bowel obstruction	Adhesions
Most common causes of large bowel obstruction	Tumor, diverticuli, volvulus
Most common causes of significant lower GI bleeding	Diverticulosis, angiodysplasia
The blood from which cause of GI bleeding is classically described as "brick red?"	Meckel's diverticulum
Rule of "2s" for Meckel's	Occurs 2% population, 2% symptomatic, 2 cm wide and long, 2 ft from ileocecal valve, occurs age 2
Characteristics of ulcerative colitis (UC)	Contiguous involvement of the submucosa/mucosa that always includes the rectum. Patient has frequent bloody diarrhea. Patient is at greater risk of colon cancer and toxic megacolon. Treatment is steroids and surgery.
Characteristics of Crohn's disease	Autoimmune cause of full-thickness skip lesions from the mouth to the anus. Patient presents with pain, weight loss and diarrhea. Crohn's carries an increased risk of fistula formation, perforation, and an increased risk of cancer although less than UC. Treatment includes steroids, flagyl, and sulfasalazine.
Antimotility agents are contraindicated in the treatment of infectious diarrhea (T/F)?	False
Invasive inflammatory diarrheas	*Shigella, Campylobacter, Salmonella, Yersinia*, enteroinvasive *E. coli, Vibrio vulnificans/parahaemolytica*
Enterotoxin-secreting diarrhea	*Aeromonas hydrophilia, Bacillus cereus,* ciguatera fish poisoning, *Clostridium perfingens,* enterotoxigenic *E. coli,* scromboid fish poisoning, *S. aureus, Vibrio cholerae*

Ciguatera fish poisoning	Occurs from consumption of grouper, snapper, kingfish, infected with dinoflagellate. Patient presents with neuromuscular, neurosensory deficits. Treatment is self-limited
Scromboid fish poisoning	Occurs from consumption of mahi-mahi or dark fleshed fish containing a heat stable histamine-like toxin. Patient presents with facial flushing, headache, abdominal cramps, nausea and vomiting, diarrhea, palpitations. Treatment is H1, H2 blockers
Which perirectal abscess can you drain in the emergency department?	Yes: perianal No: ischiorectal, intersphincteric, supralevator, perirectal

Neurologic emergencies

At what BP should hypertension be treated in acute stroke prior to tPA? Drug?	SBP remains >185 mmHg or diastolic blood pressure (DBP) >110 mmHg Treat elevated BP with labetalol as it preserves cerebral auto-regulation
Ischemic stroke is more common than hemorrhagic stroke. What subtype of ischemic stroke is most common?	Thrombotic. Of all ischemic strokes (80% overall), thrombotic are the majority, followed by embolic (20%) and systemic hypoperfusion (less than 1%). Hemorrhagic strokes are 20% overall and the majority of those are intraparenchymal.
What is the most common ECG abnormality associated with embolic stroke?	A-fib (seen in 60% of all embolic strokes)
Symptoms of cerebellar infarct	Dizziness, nausea/vomiting, nystagmus (vertical or bidirectional), ataxia, lateralizing dysmetria (trouble with finger/nose or heel/shin testing), dysdiadochokinesis (trouble with rapid alternating movements)
Symptoms of basilar artery occlusion	Severe bilateral motor and sensory deficits, quadriplegia, coma (locked-in syndrome)
Vertigo, dysphagia, facial pain/numbness, ipsilateral clumsiness, contralateral cool extremity distally, Horner's	Wallenberg syndrome. Posterior inferior cerebellar artery (PICA) infarct leads to infarct of lateral medulla
Current generally accepted window for use of thrombolytics in stroke is how many hours?	3 hours
Dose of tPA for acute stroke	0.9 mg/kg. Give 10% as bolus, then remaining 90% over 1 hour
Difference between Wernicke's and Broca's aphasias	Wernicke's: receptive (can't understand) Broca's: expressive (can't talk)
Incidence of stroke after transient ischemic attack (TIA) (1) 48 hours (2) 1 week (3) 1 month	(1) 5% (2) 8–9% (3) 10–12%
Most common bleeds secondary to closed head injury	Subarachnoid, subdural, epidural
Xanthochromia takes how many hours to develop	12 hours (metabolism of RBC)
Drug used to decrease incidence of rebleed in subarachnoid hemorrhage (SAH)	Nimodipine
Definition of status epilepticus	Seizure lasting >30 minutes or 2 or more episodes without full recovery in between

Treatment of status epilepticus	Diazepam 5–10 mg IV (0.2 mg/kg) Lorazepam 0.1 mg/kg Phenytoin 18 mg/kg Phenobarbital 15–20 mg/kg
Symptoms of complex partial seizures	Visceral sensations, memory disturbances, hallucinations, dream state, automatism, affective disorders
First-line treatment in neonate with seizures	Phenobarbital 20 mg/kg over 20 minutes then phenytoin if needed
Phenytoin toxicity: what symptoms generally develop at what levels?	Therapeutic: 10–20 mcg/dL Nystagmus: 20 mcg/dL Ataxia: 30 mcg/dL Lethargy/coma:> 40 mcg/dL
Most common cause of recurrent seizures	Noncompliance with medications
Most common cause of new-onset seizures	Metabolic derangements
What is Todd's paralysis?	Transient post-ictal paralysis. Thought to be due to exhausted neurons (lasts 1–2 hours). Symptoms can mimic a stroke.
Febrile seizure diagnosis	Lasts less than 15 minutes, seizure activity is non-focal, associated with high rising fever, only has 1 event, post-ictal
Age of patient with simple febrile seizure	6 months to 5 years
Dix–Hallpike maneuver	Patient sitting on stretcher, support head and rapidly lie patient flat first with head straight. Repeat the test with head rotated 45 degrees left then again with the head rotated 45 degrees right. Observe eyes at the end of each time laying the patient flat. If rotational nystagmus develops within 45 seconds then the test is positive for benign positional vertigo.
Triad of Meniere's disease	Vertigo, tinnitus, hearing loss
Horizontal nystagmus	Likely peripheral process
Vertical nystagmus	Central process
Guillain–Barré causes and characteristic presentation	Secondary to infections, toxins or autoimmune states. Look for ascending transverse myelitis (starts in legs)
Does Guillain–Barré exhibit a motor or a sensory deficit?	Both (polyneuropathy)
Tick paralysis characteristics	Ascending transverse myelitis with tick exposure (similar to Guillain–Barré)
Diagnosing myasthenia gravis	Edrophonium (temporarily prevents acetylcholine breakdown, patient's symptoms improve)
Myasthenic crisis vs. cholinergic crisis in myasthenia gravis	Myastenic crisis: acetylcholine deficiency. Severe weakness with respiratory compromise. Symptoms get better with edrophonium Cholinergic crisis: acetylcholine excess, muscarinic effects (SLUDGE [Salivation, Lacrimation, Urination, Diarrhea, GI upset, Emesis]; alternative mnemonic: "DUMBELS," Diarrhea, Urination, Miosis, Muscle weakness, Bradycardia, Bronchospasm, Emesis, Lacrimation, Salivation), worse with edrophonium

Achy weakness of pelvic girdle muscles, strength increases with repeat stimulation	Lambert–Eaton syndrome (associated with small cell lung cancer)
Botulism characteristics	Descending paralysis that starts with eye findings and bulbar palsy
Signs of Horner's syndrome	Unilateral ptosis, miosis, anhydrosis
Treatment of Bells' palsy	Controversial: steroid taper x10 days, acyclovir x10 days (within 48 hours of symptom onset), eye patch at night, artificial tears (dryness)
Four Ts of tetanus	Trismus, tetany, twitching, tightness of face (risus sardonicus)
Saturday night palsy is caused by injury to what nerve?	Radial nerve
Most common cranial nerve dysfunction in multiple sclerosis (MS)?	Optic neuritis
Cluster headache treatment	Triptans, oxygen by non-rebreather mask, ergotamines. Prednisone can be used as an adjunct
Cause of headache associated with polymyalgia rheumatica, excruciating at night. Patient also has decreased vision on same side as headache	Temporal arteritis
Acoustic neuroma triad	Vertigo, hearing loss, ataxia
Trigeminal neuralgia: "Tic douloureux"	Brief intermittent lancinating pain over distribution of V2 or V3 Triggers are usually eating, talking, face wash Treatment is carbamazepine
Pseudotumor cerebri characteristics	Young obese female with irregular menses and visual complaints with persistent headache. Papilledema can be seen on fundoscopic exam Treatment is spinal tap. Be sure to check opening pressures
Dorsal column disorders	Loss of position sense, vibration, and light touch. Classically seen in syphilis and vitamin B12 deficiency
Causes of altered mental status	"AEIOU TIPS" Alcohol, drugs Endocrine, Exocrine, Electrolytes Insulin (diabetes mellitus [DM]) Oxygen, Opiates Uremia (renal including high BP) Trauma, Temperature high or low Infection Psychiatric, Porphyria Stroke, Shock, SAH, Space-occupying lesion
Cushing reflex	HTN and bradycardia associated with increased intracranial pressure (ICP)
Pupillary finding in metabolic altered level of consciousness	Reactive but sluggish
Pupillary finding in structural altered level of consciousness	Non-reactive
Pupillary finding in herniation	Anisocoria

Pupillary finding in optic nerve injury	Marcus–Gunn pupil (afferent pupillary defect; tested with swinging flashlight test)
Pupillary finding in Horner's syndrome	Small pupil unilaterally but reactive
Pupillary finding in neurosyphilis	Argyll–Robertson (small bilaterally, reacts to near vision but not to light; prostitute's pupil – "accommodates but does not react")

Renal and urogenital emergencies

Blue dot sign	Torsion of testicular appendix
Most common side of varicocele	Left (because no valve in testicular vein on that side)
Initial treatment of priaprism	Subcutaneous terbutaline
Painless genital ulcer	Syphilis
Painful ulcer with tender inguinal lymphadenopathy	Chancroid
Appearance of rash of disseminated gonorrhea	Small papules turning into pustules on broad erythematous bases and necrotic centers. Face and mouth is usually spared
Patient presents with maculopapular brown plaques of palms and soles plus constitutional symptoms	Secondary syphilis
Are the venereal disease research laboratory test (VDRL) and rapid plasma regain (RPR) usually positive or negative during primary/chancre stage?	Negative

Endocrine, metabolic, and nutritional emergencies

Too rapid treatment of hyponatremia can cause?	Central pontine myelinolysis (if correct >12 mEq/24 hr)
Too rapid treatment of hypernatremia can cause?	Cerebral edema
Electrolyte abnormality causing perioral paresthesia	Hypocalcemia
ECG change with hypercalcemia	Short QTc
Causes of hypercalcemia	Mnemonic: "CHIMPANZEES" Calcium supplements Hyperparathyroidism (most common) Immobilization/Iatrogenic (i.e. from thiazide use) Milk alkali syndrome Paget's disease Addisons/Acromegaly Neoplasm Zollinger Ellison Excess vitamin D Excess vitamin A Sarcoidosis
Heat cramps are caused by deficiency of what electrolyte?	Sodium
Hypocalcemia is common with what overdose?	Ethylene glycol
Percent of (1) extracellular fluid (ECF) (2) intracellular fluid (ICF), and (3) total body water (TBW) in humans	(1) 20% (2) 40% (3) 60%
When using 0.9% normal saline IV how much remains intravascular and how much interstitial?	Intravascular: 25% Interstitial : 75%
Calculation of serum osmolarity	$Osm = 2Na^+ + (Glu/18) + (BUN/2.8) + (Ethanol/4.5)$
Definition of osmolar gap	Measured – actual osm = >10

Calculation of anion gap	$AG = Na^+ - (Cl^- + CO_2)$
Causes of anion gap metabolic acidosis	Mnemonic: "MUDPILERS" Methanol Uremia Diabetic ketoacidosis (DKA) Paraldehyde, propylene glycol Isoniazid, Iron Lactic acidosis Ethanol, Ethylene glycol Rhabdomyolysis Salicylates
Which substances can cause a large anion gap and a large osmolar gap?	Methanol Ethylene glycol
Differential diagnosis for increased osmolar gap	Mnemonic: "ME2DIGS" Methanol, Mannitol Ethylene glycol, Ethanol Diuretics Isopropyl alcohol Glycerol Sorbitol
Which substances cause high osmolar gap with NORMAL anion gap?	Ethanol, isopropyl, glycerol, sorbitol, mannitol, acetone
Calculation of Winter's formula	$pCO_2 = (1.5 \times HCO_3^-) + 8 \pm 2$ Evaluates respiratory compensation when metabolic acidosis is present. The formula gives an expected value for pCO_2 If calculated equals measured then compensation is adequate. If calculated is higher than measured then there is also a primary respiratory alkalosis. If calculated is lower than measures then there is also a primary respiratory acidosis
How to calculate corrected sodium during hyperglycemia	Measured sodium + (1.6 x (serum glucose – 100)/100)
A rise in pH of 0.1 would cause what change in potassium?	Potassium levels drop 0.5 mEq/L
Sodium correction rate in acute hyponatremia	1–2 mEq/L/hr
Sodium correction rate in chronic hyponatremia	0.5 mEq/L/hr
Treatment of hypovolemic hyponatremia	Normal saline
Treatment of hypervolemic hyponatremia	Water restriction, rarely use 3% normal saline
Characteristics of syndrome of inappropriate antidiuretic hormone secretion (SIADH)	Euvolemic hyponatremia, polyuria, elevated urine sodium with normal dietary intake, urine osmolarity >100 Osm/L Treatment is water restriction
Diabetes insipidus definition	Abnormal production (central) or response (nephrogenic) to antidiuretic hormone
ECG progression in hyperkalemia	Peaked T waves Loss of P waves QRS widening Sine wave development Ventricular fibrillation (V-fib)/asystole

Treatment of hyperkalemia	Mnemonic: "C A BIG K Drop" Calcium chloride or calcium gluconate for cardiac stabilization Albuterol nebulizer Bicarbonate (50 mEq of sodium bicarbonate) Insulin (10 units of regular insulin IV) Glucose (1 ampule of D50 IV) Kayexalate Dialysis
What effect does β-blocker overdose have on blood sugar?	Hypoglycemia
In a hypoglycemic patient, an elevated serum C-peptide level suggests the source of excess insulin is from where?	Endogenous
Differential diagnosis of refractory hypoglycemia	Sulfonylurea ingestion, adrenal insufficiency
Persistent hypoglycemia and hypotension despite treatment. Diagnosis?	Adrenal insufficiency
Initial treatment of adrenal insufficiency	Hydrocortisone 100 mg IV
Insulin drip rate in DKA	0.05–0.1 units/kg/hr
Desired drop in glucose per hour	Desired drop of 100 mg/dL/hr. More precipitous drop can cause cerebral edema
Relationship of anion gap to serum bicarbonate in DKA and lactic acidosis	In DKA the anion gap is roughly equal to serum bicarbonate. In lactic acidosis the anion gap will be greater than the serum bicarbonate
Classification of lactic acidosis	Type A: secondary to shock or anoxia (due to tissue hypoperfusion) Type B: secondary to disease states, drugs/toxins, or hereditary causes
Criteria for diagnosis of hyperosmolar coma	Glucose is >600 mg/dL, serum osmolarity >320 Osm/L, no ketones
Of the acidic ketones which is measurable?	Acetoacetate is measurable (β-hydroxybutyrate is not measurable)
Indications for bicarbonate administration in the setting of DKA	pH > 7.0 with the goal to correct to a pH of 7.1
Acute conditions that cause lactic acidosis	Hypoperfusion, exercise, hyperventilation, metformin, DKA, sepsis, hemorrhage
Chronic conditions that cause lactic acidosis	Severe CHF, liver disease, diabetes
Causes of non-anion gap metabolic acidosis	Mnemonic: "HARD-UP" Hyperalimentation, Hyperaldosteronism Acetazolamide use Renal tubular acidosis Diarrhea Ureteroenteric fistula Pancreaticoduodenal fistula
Treatment of thyroid storm.	ABCs. Give propranolol followed by propylthiouracil (PTU; can also use methimazole) followed by iodine. Propranolol minimizes sympathomimetic symptoms and decreases peripheral T4 to T3 conversion. PTU blocks further synthesis of thyroid hormone and also blocks peripheral conversion. Iodine blocks the release of preformed thyroid hormone but can be used by the body to form more

Most common cause of hyperthyroidism in the USA	Grave's disease
Findings in myxedema coma	Altered mental status, hypothermia, hypotension, bradycardia, hypoglycemia, hypoventilation
Treatment of myxedema coma	L-thyroxine (T4) 300–500 mg IV, hydrocortisone 100 mg IV, slow rewarming
Findings in primary adrenal insufficiency	Caused by nonfunctioning adrenals resulting in low cortisol, low aldosterone Patients have low sodium, low glucose, high potassium, hyperpigmentation, normal androgens Treatment is medication with mineralocorticoid and glucocorticoid activity
Findings in secondary adrenal insufficiency	Caused by lack of adrenocorticotropic hormone (ACTH) resulting in low cortisol, normal aldosterone Patients have low glucose, normal electrolytes, normal pigmentation, androgen deficiency Treatment is medication with glucocorticoid activity alone and androgen
Drug causes of hypoglycemia	Insulin, ethanol, sulfonylureas, β-blockers, salicylates
In addition to IV/PO glucose, what other medication should be given in the treatment of sulfonylurea-induced hypoglycemia?	Octreotide (to prevent rebound hypoglycemia)

Trauma

CT appearance of subdural hematoma	Concave (crescent shaped). Caused by tearing of bridging veins
CT appearance of epidural hematoma	Biconvex (lens shaped). Caused by tearing of arteries
Classic findings of uncal herniation	Ipsilateral third cranial nerve palsy, contralateral hemiparesis
Most common CT finding in moderate to severe traumatic brain injury	Subarachnoid hemorrhage
Cushing response to head injury	Hypertension, bradycardia, decreased respiratory rate
Calculation of CPP (cerebral perfusion pressure)	CPP = MAP – ICP (MAP: mean arterial pressure, ICP: intracranial pressure)
Clinical signs of basilar skull fracture	Hemotympanum, rhinorrhea/otorrhea, Battle's sign, raccoon eyes, cranial nerve palsies I, II, VII, IX
Indications for mannitol in head injury	Focal deficit, pupillary inequality, central nervous system (CNS) deterioration, Glasgow Coma Scale (GCS) < 6
Decorticate posturing	Cerebral dysfunction, arms flexed (in towards the core)
Decerebrate posturing	Brainstem dysfunction, arms extended and internally rotated
Triad indicating fracture of larynx	Hoarseness, subcutaneous emphysema, palpable crepitus
Minimum age for cricothyrotomy	12 years old
Jefferson's fracture	C1 blowout; caused by axial loading
Hangman's fracture	Bilateral pedicles of C2; caused by forcible extension with distraction

Facet dislocation	Flexion/rotation
Clay-shoveler's fracture	Spinous process; caused by direct blow or flexion
Types of odontoid fractures	Type I: tip dens (rare) Type II:transects dens at junction C2 (worst prognosis) Type III: involves the vertebral body of C2
Stable C-spine fractures	Clay shoveler, simple wedge
Unstable C-spine fractures	Mnemonic: "Jefferson Bit Off A Hangman's Thumb": Jefferson's fracture Bilateral facet dislocation Odontoid type II or III Any fracture-dislocation, Alanto-axial dislocation Hangman's fracture Teardrop fracture (flexion of spine with axial compression)
Most common C-spine level fractures in elderly	C1, C2, or C3
Most common C-spine fracture location in children	C1, C2
Chance fracture	Compression injury to anterior portion of vertebral body and transverse fracture through posterior elements of vertebra and body
Most common location and cause for Chance fracture	T12–L2; occurs with strong forward flexion, as seen in motor vehicle accident (MVA) when a lap belt restrains the patient but no shoulder belt
Pediatrics with paresthesia secondary to neck injury with negative X-ray. Treatment?	Spinal cord injury without radiographic abnormality (SCIWORA). Treatment is C-collar for 12 weeks. Uncommon diagnosis with the advances of MRI
SCIWORA facts	Most commonly >8 years old; Can be up to 2/3 of spinal cord injuries in children; Onset can be delayed up to 4 days
Signs of cervical cord injury	Flaccid areflexia, diaphragmatic breathing, ability to flex forearms but not extend, facial grimace to pain above clavicle, but not below, drop in BP with warming of extremities, priapism
Central cord syndrome	Weakness in upper extremities greater than lower extremities
Anterior cord syndrome	Complete loss of motor and pain with retention of deep pressure and vibratory sensation
Posterior cord syndrome	Loss of deep pressure and vibratory with retention of motor, pain, temperature sensations
Brown Sequard syndrome	Ipsilateral muscle paralysis, contralateral loss of pain and temperature
Dosing of methylprednisolone in spinal cord injury	30 mg/kg initially, 5.4 mg/kg/hr over 23 hours
Upper motor neurons (cord lesions)	Spasticity, hyper-reflexia. No regeneration
Lower motor neurons (root lesions)	Flaccidity, hyporeflexia. Possible regeneration
First and second rib fractures are associated with what kinds of injuries?	Traumatic rupture of the aorta, myocardial contusion, bronchial tear, vessel injury
Most commonly injured abdominal organ in blunt trauma	Spleen

Most commonly injured abdominal organ in penetrating trauma	Liver
Most common causes of fetal death secondary to trauma	Maternal death or placental abruption
Biggest life threat with pelvic fracture?	Exsanguinating pelvic injury
What is Kehr's sign?	Left shoulder pain secondary to splenic injury
Indications for thoracotomy in intrathoracic bleeding	Initial drainage from chest tube >1500 mL, continued output >200 mL/hr for 3 hours, persistent hypotension
Approximation of BP and pulses	Carotid only: SBP ~60 mmHg Femoral: SBP ~70 mmHg Radial: SBP at least 80 mmHg
Calculation of blood volume	Adults: 7% TBW or 70 mL/kg Pediatrics: 8–9% TBW or 80 mL/kg
Fluids for trauma resuscitation of pediatrics	20 mL/kg IV fluids x2 boluses, then 10 mg/kg packed red blood cells (PRBCs) if needed
Effect of rhabdomyolysis on electrolytes	Hypocalcemia, hyperkalemia.
Beck's triad	Hypotension, distended neck veins, muffled heart sounds
ECG sign of pericardial tamponade	Electrical alternans
Contraindications to urethral catheterization in trauma	Blood at urethral meatus, scrotal hematoma, high-riding prostate on digital rectal exam, perineal hematoma and pelvic fracture
"Ps" of compartment syndrome	Pain out of proportion to injury, paresthesia, paralysis, poikilothermia, pallor, pulselessness (late finding)
Compartment pressure requiring fasciotomy	30 mmHg
Negatively birefringent, spindle-shaped crystals	Gout (positive birefringent rhomboid crystals are associated with pseudogout)
Grades of nerve injury (least to greatest)	(1) Neuropraxia: blunt contusion (2) axonotemesis: severe contusion with distraction of nerve fibers, but intact myelin sheath (3) neurotemesis: complete transaction
Motor levels of the upper extremity	Shoulder abduction (C5) Elbow flexors (C6) Elbow extensors (C7) Wrist extensors (C6) Finger extensors (C7) Finger flexors (C8) Finger intrinsics (T1)
Reflexes of the upper extremity	Biceps (C5) Brachioradialis (C6) Triceps (C7)
Artery and nerves (2) injured in anterior shoulder dislocation	Axillary artery, axillary and/or musculocutaneous nerves
Most common type of anterior shoulder dislocation	Sub-coracoid
Hill–Sachs lesion	Compression fracture of lateral humeral head (associated with sub-coracoid dislocation)
Bankart lesion	Fracture of glenoid rim

Luxatio erecta	Inferior dislocation of shoulder (always associated with rotator cuff tear)
Most common type of posterior shoulder dislocation	Sub-acromial (associated with reverse Hill–Sachs lesion: compression fracture of anteromedial humeral head)
Muscles that make up the rotator cuff	Supraspinatus, subscapularis, infraspinatus, teres minor
Humeral shaft fracture that has a risk of injuring which nerve	Radial
Sail sign in pediatrics indicates? Adults?	Supracondylar fracture (pediatrics), radial head fracture (adult)
Nerve associated with medial epicondyle or olecranon fracture	Ulnar nerve
Colles' fracture	Transverse fracture of the radius with dorsal angulation and without fracture of the distal ulna
Opposite of Colles' fracture	Smith's fracture (volar angulation)
Barton fracture	Distal radius fracture with dislocation of radiocarpal joint
Monteggia fracture	Dislocation of radial head with fracture of proximal third of ulna (nightstick injury)
Galeazzi fracture	Fracture of radial shaft (between middle and distal third) and dislocation of distal radioulnar joint
Most commonly fractured carpal bone	Scaphoid
Ulnar base of thumb simple metacarpal fracture from fall on outstretched hand (FOOSH) (Most common thumb fracture)	Bennett fracture (call Orthopedics for surgery)
Same as above but comminuted fracture	Rolando fracture (call Orthopedics for surgery)
Skier/gamekeeper thumb	Involves injury to ulnar collateral ligament (connects thumb to metacarpophalangeal[MCP] joint), causing instability of that joint
Cardinal signs of partial tendon laceration	Pain with attempted use of tendon, slight decrease in tone with altered stance of digit at rest, weakness of tendon when actively flexed
Cardinal signs of flexor tendon tenosynovitis	Tenderness along and confined to flexor tendon sheath, flexion stance of finger at rest, pain on passive extension: marked at base of digit, symmetrical swelling of finger
Boutonnière deformity	Rupture of extensor tendon on flexor side of digit. Appearance: flexion of proximal interphalangeal (PIP) joint with hyperextension of distal interphalangeal (DIP) joint
Do you splint a Mallet finger in flexion or extension?	Extension
Bacterial pathogens in human bite infections	*S. aureus, Neisseria, Eikenella corrodens,* anaerobes
Contraindications for digit re-implantation	Amputations in unstable patients secondary to other life-threats; multiple-level amputations; self-inflicted amputations; single-digit amputations proximal to the flexor digitorum superficialis insertion; serious underlying disease, such as vascular disease, complicated DM, and CHF; extremes of age

Motor levels of the lower extremity	Hip flexors (L2, L3) Hip extensors (L4, L5) Knee extensors (L3, L4) Knee flexors (L5, S1) Dorsiflexion of foot (L4, L5) Plantarflexion of foot (S1, S2) Ankle eversion (L5)
Reflexes of the lower extremity	Patellar (L4) Tibialis posterior (L5) Achilles (S1)
In anterior and posterior hip dislocations what are the potentially associated nerve injuries, deep tendon reflex affected, muscle weakness, and sensory deficit?	Anterior: femoral nerve, decreased patellar deep tendon reflex, weak quads, decreased sensation to anteromedial thigh Posterior: sciatic nerve, weak muscles below knee, decreased ability to flex knee, decreased sensation of posterolateral leg and sole
Complications of posterior knee dislocation	Popliteal artery injury, peroneal and tibial nerves injury
Indicated study after posterior dislocation of the knee?	Angiography for popliteal artery injury
Nerve potentially injured in lateral tibial plateau fracture	Peroneal nerve
Knee ligament testing	Varus: adduction, lateral collateral ligament (LCL) Valgus: abduction, medial collateral ligament (MCL)
Maisonneuve fracture	Fracture of proximal fibula and distal tibia (associated with peroneal nerve injury: foot drop)
Measurement on X-ray for diagnosing subtle calcaneal fracture	Bohler's angle <20 degrees means fracture
Lisfranc injury	One or all of the metatarsal bones are displaced from the cuboid/cuneiform bones. Often occurs with fracture

Obstetrics and gynecology emergencies

Gray frothy, malodorous discharge, multiple punctuate hemorrhage on cervix ("strawberry cervix")	Trichomoniasis
Centers for Disease Control (CDC) recommendation for treatment of symptomatic patient with bacterial vaginosis or trichuriasis during pregnancy. Treatment?	Metronidazole 2 g PO x1
Most common hereditary disorder associated with menorrhagia	Von Willebrand's disease
Cardiovascular changes in pregnancy	Cardiac output increases 30–50% Blood volume increases 45% with plasma volume increasing more than RBC volume. HR increases 10–15 bpm BP decreases 5–10 mmHg systolic, 10–15 mmHg diastolic (during first trimester)
Pulmonary changes in pregnancy	Respiratory rate has no change or is slightly increased Total lung capacity decreases only slightly. Although diaphragm is elevated, hormonal effects loosen ligaments so anterior/posterior (AP) diameter increases and ribs become more mobile.
Gastrointestinal changes in pregnancy	Decreased tone and motility. Gastric emptying is slowed. Decreased tone of lower esophageal sphincter (causing reflux). Constipation and hemorrhoids are common.

Renal changes in pregnancy	Glomerular filtration rate (GFR) increases 50% BUN and creatinine decrease
Pregnant with sudden-onset hypotension, hypoxia, coagulopathy. Diagnosis?	Amniotic fluid emboli
Most common cause of post-partum hemorrhage after normal pregnancy	Uterine atony (<24 hours)
Late decelerations mean	Fetal hypoxia
APGAR scores	Scored at 1 and 5 minutes (if score is > 7 at 5 minutes, do more) Points 0, 1 or 2 for each item Appearance: cyanotic, acrocyanosis, pink Pulse: none, <100 bpm, >100 bpm Grimace: none, weak cry, strong cry Activity: none, some flexion, flexed limbs that resist extension Respirations: absent, irregular/gasping, strong cry
Indications for intubation and CPR in a newborn	(1) 2 minutes with HR <100 bpm and poor respirations = bag-valve-mask (BVM) (2) Not better 30 seconds = intubation (3) HR <60 bpm = CPR
Most common cause of maternal death overall	Trauma
Patient positioning for trauma resuscitation of pregnant patient	Position in left lateral decubitus position
Can see fetal heart by transvaginal ultrasound (TVUS)	6–8 weeks
Gestational sac seen by transvaginal ultrasound	5 weeks, 1200 mIU/mL beta human chorionic gonadotropin (β-HCG)
Gestational sac seen by transabdominal ultrasound	6 weeks, 5000 mIU/mL β-HCG
Preeclampsia before 24 weeks	Molar pregnancy
Uterine size greater than dates. Diagnosis?	Molar pregnancy
Premature rupture of membranes (PROM)	Definition: ROM >1 hour before labor starts Test : (+) nitrazine test or ferning Cautions: no bimanual
Events requiring Rhogam	Miscarriage, ectopic, trauma, placenta previa, abruptio placenta, vaginal bleeding
Rhogam dosing (by weeks gestation)	12 weeks gestation (300 mcg) <12 weeks gestation (50 mcg)
Mild preeclampsia definition	BP >140/90, >300 mg proteinuria
Severe preeclampsia definition	BP >160/100, proteinuria >5 g/day
Dose of magnesium for preeclampsia	4–6 g IV over 15 minutes, then drip at 1–2 g/hr
Signs of magnesium toxicity	Hyporeflexia, respiratory depression, bradydysrhythmias
Antidote for magnesium toxicity	Calcium gluconate
Most common cause of maternal death in preeclampsia	Intracranial hemorrhage (ICH)
Definition of eclampsia	Preeclampsia with seizures
Impending signs of eclampsia	Headache, visual changes, hyper-reflexia, and abdominal pain
Treatment of eclampsia	Magnesium sulfate 4–6 g IV. BP control with hydralazine or labetalol. Delivery

HELLP Syndrome	Hemolysis with abnormal smear or LDH >600 IU/L, Bilirubin >1.2 mg/dL, Elevated transaminases, Platelets <100 000/μL
X-ray risks in pregnancy	Fetal risks occur with 5–10 rads.
Risks of radiation exposure are highest to fetus at what weeks of gestation?	2–9 weeks
What are the drug classifications in pregnancy and what do they mean?	Class A: OK in humans Class B: OK in animals, no definite evidence for women Class C: not OK in animals, no definite evidence for women Class D: fetal risk, but benefit may outweigh risk Class X: definite fetal abnormalities – never use in pregnancy
Antihypertensives in pregnancy	Labetalol, hydralazine
Analgesia in pregnancy	Acetaminophen, codeine, hydrocodone, morphine. NSAIDs are OK during the second trimester only.
Anticoagulation in pregnancy	Heparin, Lovenox, and thrombolytics if indicated. Avoid warfarin as it crosses the placenta.
Preferred antibiotics in pregnancy	Penicillins, cephalosporins, azithromycin, nitrofurantoin
Contraindicated antibiotics in pregnancy	Tetracycline, sulfonamides, aminoglycosides
Treatment of urinary tract infection (UTI) in pregnancy	Treat even if asymptomatic. No single dose treatments. Treat for 3–7 days
Preferred antiemetics in pregnancy (Class B)	Ondansetron, metoclopramide, diphenhydramine
Pediatrics emergencies	
Tachycardia by age	Infant: >160 bpm; Preschooler: >140 bpm; 5–puberty: >120 bpm
Most common causes of abdominal mass in children	Neuroblastoma, Wilms' tumor, rhabdomyosarcoma
What films can be used to make the diagnosis of an airway foreign body?	If stable, lateral neck X-ray, CXR with inspiratory/expiratory views or bilateral decubitus views
What drug do you give for refractory seizure in a newborn who is not responsive to usual therapy?	Pyridoxine (B6), as pyridoxine deficiency can be an autosomal recessive trait
Endotracheal tube sizes	(age + 16)/4 or (age/4) + 4 for uncuffed (age/4) + 3 for cuffed
Most accurate method for determining endotracheal tube placement	Seeing tube go through the cords
Most sensitive/specific adjuvant for endotracheal tube placement?	End tidal carbon dioxide detector
Components of tetralogy of Fallot	Pulmonic stenosis, ventriculoseptal defect, overriding aorta, right ventricular hypertrophy
Causes of pediatric heart disease that become evident after an episode of syncope	Tetralogy of Fallot (patient is cyanotic), aortic stenosis (patient is not cyanotic)
Causes of cyanotic pediatric heart disease	Truncus arteriosus Transposition of the great vessels Tricuspid atresia Tetralogy of Fallot Total anomalous venous return

Hyperoxia test for cyanosis	Give 100% oxygen. If patient's P_aO_2 does not go above 100 mmHg then either patient has a right-to-left shunt or has methemoglobinemia
What is the emergent treatment of a ductal-dependent lesion to maintain patency of ductus arteriosus?	Prostaglandin E1 (0.05–0.1 mg/kg) Side effects: apnea, hypotension, hypoglycemia
Signs of CHF in infant	If right-sided, patient will have hepatomegaly If left-sided, patient will have tachypnea, dyspnea, poor feeding If both sides are affected, look for cardiomegaly, failure to thrive, tachycardia
Bounding pulses in an infant can suggest what cardiovascular structural abnormalities?	Patent ductus arteriosus, aortic insufficiency, arteriovenous malformation
Decreased pulses in an infant can suggest what cardiovascular structural abnormalities?	Coarctation or hypoplastic left ventricle
What pediatric heart disease presents as hypertension?	Coarctation
Diagnosis of a patient with presumed croup who then becomes toxic	Bacterial tracheitis
Common causative agent of bacterial tracheitis	*S. aureus*
Common causative agent of bronchiolitis in 2 month to 2 year olds	Respiratory syncytial virus (RSV)
Treatment for RSV	Humidified oxygen, trial of albuterol, inhaled epinephrine if severe. Otherwise treatment is supportive
Bronchiolitis is associated with apnea in what pediatric population?	Premature babies (less than 34 weeks)
Common agents causing pneumonia in newborns 0–2 weeks	Group B streptococcus, *E. coli*, *Klebsiella pneumoniae*, *Listeria*
Common agents causing pneumonia in patients aged 3–19 weeks	Viruses are most often the cause, of which RSV is the most common. *Chlamydia*, *S. pneumoniae* are also concerns.
Possible infectious agent in a patient that presents with staccato cough	*Chlamydia pneumoniae*
Common agents causing pneumonia in 4 months to 4 years	Viruses (of which RSV most common), *S. pneumoniae*, *H. influenzae*, *S. aureus*
Common agents causing pneumonia in 5 years to 15 years	*Mycoplasma*, viral, *S. pneumoniae*
What (2) common electrolyte disorders are commonly seen in cystic fibrosis?	Hyponatremia, hypochloremic hypokalemic metabolic alkalosis
Which sinuses are present at birth?	Ethmoid, maxillary (frontal and sphenoid develop by 6–7 years of life)
Diagnostic criteria for Kawasaki's	Fever greater than 5 days and 4 criteria from following list: Bilateral, painless conjunctival injection "Strawberry tongue" (pharyngeal injection and erythema) Rash on hands and feet with erythema Polymorphous truncal rash, desquamates Cervical lymphadenopathy
Kawasaki's treatment	IVIG (2 g/kg over 10 hours) and high-dose aspirin (100 mg/kg/day divided QID)

Most common cause of bacterial diarrhea	*Salmonella*
Definition of gastroschisis	Abdominal wall defect at birth with no peritoneal sac
Definition of omphalocele	Abdominal wall defect at birth with peritoneal sac
Meckel's diverticulum: rule of 2s	Occurs in 2% population, most patients present when they are younger than 2 years old, diverticulum is usually 2 cm long and 2 cm wide and located 2 ft from ileocecal valve
Ill-appearing infant presents with bilious vomiting, blood streaked stool, abdominal pain and distension. Diagnosis?	Midgut volvulus
Hirschprung's disease	Aganglionic lower colonic segment associated with chronic constipation since birth
Patient presents with cyclic abdominal pain, vomiting, "sausage-shaped" mass in RUQ, and "currant jelly" stool. Diagnosis?	Intussusception
Treatment of intussusception	Air enema is both diagnostic and curative, but surgeon should be available if it does not work
Most common cause of hip pain in childhood	Septic arthritis in 6–24 month old, transient synovitis otherwise
3- to 12-year-old White male with limp	Legg–Calvé–Perthes (avascular necrosis of femoral head)
10-year-old obese child with limp and hip pain. Diagnosis?	Slipped capital femoral epiphysis (SCFE)
Order of ossification in child's elbow	Mnemonic: "CRITOE" Capitellum (age 2) Radial head (age 4) Internal/medial epicondyle (age 6) Trochlea (age 8) Olecranon (age 10) External/lateral epicondyle (age 12)
Salter–Harris classifications	1: fracture through physis 2: fracture through metaphysis and physis 3: fracture through epiphysis and physis 4: fracture through epiphysis and metaphysis (crossing physis) 5: crush fracture of physis
Most common type of Salter–Harris fracture?	Salter 2 (75%)
Maxium dose of lidocaine without epinephrine	3–5 mg/kg
Maximum dose of lidocaine with epinephrine	7 mg/kg
Differentiating amide anesthetics from ester anesthetics	Amide anesthetics have 2 "i" in the name (e.g. lidocaine, bupivacaine, prilocaine). Ester anesthetics only have one "i" in the name (e.g. benzocaine, proparacaine)

Infectious emergencies

Common causes of erythema multiforme	Herpes simplex virus (HSV), drugs
Associated with rats in Southwest USA, causing painful axillary and inguinal lymph node swelling, fever, seizure	Bubonic plague, caused by the bacteria *Yersinia pestis*
Change in mental status, desquamation of skin, fever, hypotension	Toxic shock syndrome

Associated with ticks, caused by Gram-negative obligate intracellular bacterium. Presents like Rocky Mountain spotted fever (RMSF) with rash.	Ehrlichiosis
Minor wound, last tetanus >5 years ago but <10	Do nothing
Major wound, last tetanus >5 years ago but <10	Give Td (toxoid)
Major wound uncertain, previous immunity, or <3 total doses	Give Td + T IgG (repeat Td in 6 weeks and 6 months)
Is tetanus toxoid OK to give to pregnant women?	Yes
Rash of Lyme's	Erythema migrans
Tick of Lyme's	*Ixodes* (bacterium is *Borrelia burgdorferi*)
Outpatient antibiotic treatment for Lyme's	Doxycycline or amoxicillin
Pediatric patient with gastroenteritis who seizes. Cause?	*Shigella*
Abdominal pain that mimics appendicitis. Infectious cause?	*Yersinea* (causes ileocecitis)
Most common infectious bacteria in neonate	Group B streptococcus
Toxic pediatric patient with purulent discharge in the oropharynx, stridor. Diagnosis?	Bacterial tracheitis (life-threatening: endotracheal tube in operating room)
Fever, upper respiratory infection (URI), wheeze in neonate	Bronchiolitis/RSV (concern for apnea, death). Admit if >3 months old or hypoxic
Child who coughs enough to cause subconjunctival hemorrhage, leukocytosis (>30 000/µL) that is primarily a lymphocytosis	Pertussis
Purpose of erythromycin in the treatment of pertussis?	Prevents spread, but no change in symptoms for patients
Low-grade temperature, lacey rash, slapped cheek appearance, mother with arthralgias	Fifth disease/erythema infectiosum, caused by parvovirus B19
Most common cause of gastroenteritis	*Campylobacter*
Common cause of AIDS-related diarrhea	Cryptosporidiosis
Pneumonia in patient from Southwest USA	Hanta virus, Coccidiomycosis (fungal)
Pneumonia with GI symptoms	*Legionella*
Pneumonia in patient with CD4 >200/µL	*Pneumocystis jiroveci*
High fever x3 days, then sudden onset of rash after defervescence	Roseola (Human herpesvirus-6 [HHV-6])
Ocular and bulbar weakness with weakness descending from trunk to extremities	Botulism (floppy baby)
Mechanism of botulism toxin	Blocks release of acetylcholine
Honey-colored crusted lesions? Treatment?	Impetigo. Topical or PO antibiotics, treatment does NOT prevent glomerulonephritis
Toxic patient (old or young), with acute onset of hot, red, well-demarcated cellulitis with raised border	Erysipelas
Cause of erysipelas?	Streptococcal species (major cause: *S. pyogenes*)
Most common cause of septic arthritis	*S. aureus*
Malaria-like disease caused by tick bite	Babesiosis
Pasteurella multocida is associated with?	Cat bites (give Augmentin)

Toxicology

Dialyzable toxins	Salicylates, theophyline, uremia, methanol, barbituates, lithium, ethylene glycol
Aspirin overdose treatment	Multiple doses of activated charcoal (MDAC), alkalinize urine, hemodialysis if needed
Toxic dose iron?	20–60 mg/kg elemental iron
Pilocarpine, organophosphate, carbamates (polyurethane, insecticides) cause what toxidrome?	Cholinergic: "DUMBELS," <u>D</u>iarrhea, <u>U</u>rination, <u>M</u>iosis, <u>M</u>uscle weakness, <u>B</u>radycardia, <u>B</u>ronchospasm, <u>E</u>mesis, <u>L</u>acrimation, <u>S</u>alivation or SLUDGE (<u>S</u>alivation, <u>L</u>acrimation, <u>U</u>rination, <u>D</u>iarrhea, <u>G</u>I upset, <u>E</u>mesis)

Clinical feature associated with overdose

Fruity odor	Nitrites, isopropyl, alcohol
Bitter almond smell, brady-tachy-brady, change MS, cherry-red skin or cyanosis, same colored veins and arteries on retinal exam <u>OR</u> collapse at fire	Cyanide
Garlic smell	Organophosphates
Odor of rotten eggs	Hydrogen sulfide
Odor of mothballs	Camphor, naphthalene
Wintergreen smell	Methylsalicylate
Boiled lobster erythroderma rash	Boric acid
Jaundice	Acetaminophen, mushrooms
Flushing	Scromboid fish poisoning, anticholinergics, monoamine oxidase inhibitors (MAOIs), disulfiram reaction

End of clinical feature review

Extrapyramidal symptoms?	Tremor, trismus, torticollis, rigidity, dysphonia, dysphagia, opisthotonus
Extrapyramidal symptoms caused by what ingestion?	Chlorpromazine, thorazine, haldol, metoclopramide
Anticholinergic toxins	Atropine, antihistamines, scopolamine, tricyclic antidepressants
Prolonged QT differential diagnosis of toxicity?	Arsenic, class IA or class III antiarrhythmics, diphenhydramine, lithium, tricyclic antidepressant (TCA) overdose
TCA overdose features	Wide QRS, hypotension, tachycardia, pulmonary edema, confusion, seizure
TCA overdose treatment	Bicarbonate bolus, then drip
TCA overdose – do NOT use which anti-arrhythmic?	Class IA: procainamide (AV nodal blocker)
Differential diagnosis of pinpoint pupils	"CPR ON SLIME" <u>C</u>lonidine <u>P</u>henothiazines (chlorpromazine/thorazine, compazine/promazine) <u>R</u>est (sleep) <u>O</u>rganophosphates, <u>O</u>verdose <u>O</u>pioids <u>N</u>arcotics <u>S</u>eizure <u>L</u>iquors (ethanol, isopropranol) <u>I</u>nfarct (pontine: knock out sympathetics or SAH) <u>M</u>edications for sleep (sedative-hypnotics, barbiturates) <u>E</u>ye drops (pilocarpine)

Clonidine overdose – mimics what?	(Central-acting α2) mimics opioid overdose. Presents as change in mental status, miosis, hypotension, bradycardia, seizure
Clonidine is useful in the treatment of what withdrawal syndrome?	Opioid
Clonidine withdrawal treatment	α-blockers, re-start clonidine
GHB ingestion presents how?	Hallucinations. Patient becomes coma-like then rapidly awakens and cycle repeats
Multidose activated charcoal good for:	β-blockers, calcium channel blockers, TCAs
Antidotes for overdose	
Acetaminophen	N-acetylcysteine (NAC): 140 mg/kg bolus then 70 mg/kg Q4 x 17)
	Acetadote: 150 mg/kg in first hour, 50 mg/kg over next 4 hours, 100 mg/kg over next 16 hours
Anticholinergic overdose (not TCA)	Physostigmine
Arsenic, mercury, lead	BAL, dimercaprol or DMSA
Atropine	Physostigmine
Benzodiazepines	Flumazanil
Cyanide	Amyl nitrite, sodium nitrite, sodium thiosulfate
Ethylene glycol, methanol	Alcohol, fomepizole
Isoniazid	Pyridoxine (B$_6$)
Iron	Deferoxamine
Nitrites	Methylene blue
Organophosphates	Atropine, pralidoxime (2-PAM)
Oleander	Digibind
Phenothiazine	Benztropine, benadryl
End of antidotes	
Physostigmine: side effect	Seizures
Report of snowstorm vision	Methanol overdose
Positive birefringent calcium oxalate crystals in urine	Ethylene glycol
Ethylene glycol ingestion treatment	IV alcohol or fomepizole, hemodialysis
Isopropanol overdose features	Hemorrhagic gastritis, CNS depression, positive serum acetone
Ketonuria with normal glucose and osmolar gap	Isopropyl alcohol ingestion
Patient presents with delayed GI symptoms after eating mushroom, then develops jaundice and liver failure	Amatoxin
Severe hemorrhagic gastroenteritis after eating seeds. Treatment?	Concern for castor bean (ricin) ingestion. Treat with whole bowel irrigation
Signs of mercury inhalation	Acute (pulmonary edema), chronic (psychosis)
Disulfiram reaction occurs with alcohol + what medications?	Flagyl, chloramphenicol, chloral hydrate, griseofulvan, nitrofurantoin, sulfa drugs, sulfonylurea
What poisoning mimics tetanus?	Strychnine (rodenticide)
Methemoglobinemia improves or worsens in G6PD-deficient patient if given methylene blue?	Worsens

Environmental emergencies

Discrete exit wound from contact with an industrial electric source. Patient is in asystole and was thrown off of source. AC or DC exposure?	DC
Explosive exit wound from contact with a household electric source. Patient is in V-fib with tetany. AC or DC exposure?	AC
Parts of body that are good electric conductors	Tissues with electrolytes and low resistance such as muscles, blood vessels, nerves, and mucous membranes
Chemical treatment of hydrofluoric acid burns	Calcium gluconate
Parkland formula	4 mL/ kg per % total body surface area burned. Give half of amount over first 8 hours then second half over next 16 hours.
Key finding in heat stroke	Altered mental status
Hypothermia definition	Core temperature below 35 °C
Treatment for arrhythmias in hypothermic patient	Treat only life-threatening, others will resolve as rewarm
Do core rewarming for temp below what level?	<32 °C (88 °F)
What is the LD50 for whole body radiation?	4.5 Gy
The type of radiation ray that penetrates all tissue layers and causes acute radiation syndrome	Gamma rays
Lymphocyte count – poor prognosis for radiation exposed patient if___?	Absolute lymphocyte count at 48 hours is less than 1200/µL (or drops over 50% below baseline)
Best predictor of survival after radiation exposure	Absolute lymphocyte count at 48 hours
Vector for RMSF	Dermatocentor tick
Treatment of RMSF	Doxycycline in all ages
Treatment for high-altitude cerebral edema	Descent, dexamethasone, oxygen
Treatment for high-altitude pulmonary edema	Descent, oxygen, acetazolamide, nifedipine, hyperbaric oxygen
Anthrax treatment	Doxycycline + ciprofloxacin
Disease presenting with bulbar palsy, hydrophobia, salivation	Rabies
Treatment for rabies	Diploid vaccine plus rabies IG
Treatment for black widow spider bite	Usually supportive (narcotics and benzodiazepines); antivenin available
What kind of envenomation can cause abdominal wall rigidity?	Black widow spider
Local necrosis after spider bite	Brown recluse
What is loxoscelism?	Systemic flu-like syndrome from brown recluse spider bite
Snake bite causing coagulopathy	Pit viper (crotalinae; rattlesnake, copperhead, water moccasin)
Snake bite casing neurologic symptoms	Elapidae (coral snake)
Treatment of starfish, sting ray/lionfish sting	Hot water (limits toxin release)

Rheumatology/dermatology

Arthritis, urethritis, conjunctivitis, psoriatic lesions on palms and soles	Reiter's syndrome
Treatment for lupus erythematosus exacerbation	Steroids
Most common cardiac manifestation of systemic lupus erythematosus	Pericarditis
URI/upper airway granuloma + renal vasculitis	Wegener's granulomatosis
Findings of Henoch–Schönlein purpura	Abdominal pain, lower extremity edema and rash, arthritis, nephritis, hematuria
Rash associated with pitting and "oil spots" on nails	Psoriasis
Dermatologic maladies with Nikolsky sign	Toxic epidermal necrolysis, scalded skin syndrome, pemphigus vulgaris
Most common cause of toxic epidermal necrolysis	Drugs (sulfa)
Rashes that affect the palms and soles	Erythema multiforme, RMSF, secondary syphilis, toxic shock syndrome, Kawasaki's disease, hand/foot and mouth, measles
Herald patch, Christmas tree-like distribution skin rash	Pityriasis rosea

ENT

Type of sinusitis that can lead to periorbital cellulitis	Ethmoid
Signs of periorbital cellulitis	Erythema, swelling of eyelid, proptosis, limited extraocular muscles, fever
Most common presenting symptom of a brain abscess?	Headache
Sinusitis that can extend intracranially to the cavernous sinus	Ethmoid or sphenoid
Findings of cavernous sinus thrombosis	Proptosis, dilated episcleral veins, palsies of cranial nerves III–VI, altered mental status, fever
Cranial nerve most often affected by cavernous sinus thrombosis	Cranial nerve VI
Triad of Ménière's disease	Vertigo, tinnitus, hearing loss
Temporal arteritis is associated with what rheumatologic disease?	Polymyalgia rheumatica
Branches of the trigeminal nerve	V_1: Ophthalmic V_2: Maxillary V_3: Mandibular
Differential diagnosis of trigeminal neurolgia	Cerebellar pontine angle tumor, nasopharnygeal carcinoma, MS
Normal pre-dental space on lateral C-spine X-ray	5 mm in children, 3 mm in adults
Description of Lemierre's syndrome	Extension of peritonsilar abscess beyond peritonsilar space with septic thrombophlebitis
For otitis media (OM) with tympanic membrane (TM) perforation use corticosporin _____	Suspension (not solution)
Common bacterial causes of otitis externa	*Pseudomonas, S. aureus*
Vascular involvement for anterior epistaxis	Kiesselbach's plexus
Ellis classification for dental injuries	I: Enamel only II: Enamel, dentin III: Enamel, dentin, pulp

Treatment of avulsed tooth in an adult	<30 minutes: re-implant >30 minutes: Hank's solution for 30 minutes, then re-implant Refer to dentist
LeFort's classification for midface fractures	I: Nose to upper lip II: Eyes to upper lip III: Whole face (craniofacial dissociation)
LeFort fracture most associated with cerebrospinal fluid (CSF) leak	III
Components of "tripod" fracture	Zygomatic arch, zygomaticofrontal suture, infraorbital foramen
Mandibular deviation in (1) fracture and (2) dislocation?	(1) Mandible deviates to same side and (2) mandible deviates to opposite side
Narrowest part of airway (1) pediatric and (2) adult (foreign body obstruction)	(1) Cricoid cartilage and (2) vocal cords
Oral lesions of HIV	Candidiasis (can remove with tongue blade), hairy leukoplakia (cannot be removed with tongue blade), oral Kaposi's sarcoma (flat blistered lesions with irregular borders)
Bacterial etiologies for deep space infections of (1) Retropharyngeal (2) Peritonsilar (3) Peripharyngeal (4) Ludwig's (5) Masticator space abscess	 (1) *S. aureus*, GABHS (2) Mixed, GABHS dominant (3) Anaerobes and aerobes (4) *Bacteroides, Staphylococcus, Streptococcus* (5) *Streptococcus* and anaerobes

Ophthalmology

Characteristic fluorescein uptake pattern in herpes simplex	Dendritic pattern
CMV retinitis: (1) who is affected, (2) appearance, and (3) treatment?	(1) Immunocompromised (AIDS) (2) Funduscopy shows fluffy white retinal lesions, perivascular associated with hemorrhage (cheese and ketchup fundus) (3) Treatment IV ganciclovir or foscarnet and ophthalmology referral
Most common cause of blindness in HIV affected patients	CMV retinitis
Causes of neonatal conjunctivitis occurring in the first month of life	Days 3–5: *Neisseria gonorrheae* and/or HSV Days 7–30: *Chlamydia*, HSV, *Haemophilus*, *Streptococcus*, *Staphylococcus*.
Purulent conjunctivitis that can lead to perforated cornea in hours	*N. gonorrheae*
Treatment for adult gonorrhea conjunctivitis	Admit for IV ceftriaxone + topical erythromycin + oral azithromycin (for empiric *Chlamydia* coverage)
Hordeleum versus chalazion	Hordeleum: acute infection of eyelid (stye) Chalazion: acute or chronic granulomatous inflammation can progress from hordeleum; non-tender, usually mid position eyelid
Acute, painful swelling of the medial canthus	Dacrocystitis: acute infection of lacrimal sac secondary to obstruction

Causes of painful vision loss	Iritis, acute-angle glaucoma, optic neuritis, perforation, hyphema, lens dislocation, retrobulbar hemorrhage
What medications have produced sudden attacks of acute-angle glaucoma?	Topical cycloplegics, anticholinergics, β-agonists (including inhaled agents)
Why never give topical anesthetic to patient for home use?	Retards healing of cornea and can lead to ulceration
Painless loss of vision differential diagnosis	Central retinal vein or artery occlusion, solar retinopathy, retinal detachment, vitreous hemorrhage
Central retinal vein occlusion signs and symptoms	Painless, usually resolve in 3 months Fundus: "blood and thunder"
Central retinal artery occlusion signs and symptoms	Dilated pupil, acute painless vision loss, pale retina, cherry-red spot in macula (fovea)
Triad of retinal detachment	(1) Sudden increase in unilateral floaters (2) Photopsia (flashing lights) (3) Gray cloud or film over visual field
Spontaneous hyphemas are associated with what chronic medical condition?	Sickle cell disease
Major complications of hyphemas	Acute and chronic glaucoma, optic atrophy, rebleeding in 2–5 days
Definition of hypopyon	Pus in anterior chamber
Marcus–Gunn pupil	Dilated pupil not reactive to direct light, but reactive to consensual light. Indicator of optic nerve damage seen in central retinal artery occlusion
Anisocoria that is more pronounced in dim light	Horner's syndrome
Anisocoria that is more pronounced in bright light	Third nerve palsy
Cause of decreased visual acuity, decreased mobility, and proptosis after direct blunt eye socket trauma	Retrobulbar hematoma: blood behind globe due to trauma Treatment: lateral canthotomy, decompression by Ophthalmology
Signs of globe rupture	Teardrop-shaped pupil, Seidel's sign (fluorescein washed away by leaking humor), irregular globe shape

Hematology/oncology/immunology

Vitamin K-dependent coagulation factors	Factors II, VII, IX, X
Disease causing abnormal platelet aggregation.	Von Willebrand's disease
Differential diagnosis of elevated PT	Extrinsic pathway problem (factor VII deficiency), liver disease, warfarin use, vitamin K deficiency
Treatment of thrombotic thrombocytopenic purpura	Plasmaphoresis (with fresh frozen plasma [FFP]) or massive plasma exchange
Coagulation study changes associated with hemophilia	Prolonged PTT, normal PT, normal platelets and bleeding time
Factor deficiency associated with hemophilia A	Factor VIII
Factor deficiency associated with hemophilia B	Factor IX
Coagulation study changes associated with Von Willebrand's disease	Increase PTT, increase bleeding time, normal PT
Acute tumor lysis syndrome definition	Hyperuricemia, hyperkalemia, hyperphosphatemia, hypocalcemia 1–5 days after chemotherapy

Definition of neutropenia	Absolute neutrophil count <500/μL
Protamine dose	1 mg IV neutralizes 100 units of heparin
Recombinant factor 8 dose for massive hemorrhage in hemophiliac patient	50 U/kg
Purpura, thrombocytopenia in child after viral illness	Idiopathic thrombocytopenic purpura (self-limited)
Hemolytic uremic syndrome is associated with what bacterial precipitant in the USA?	*E. coli* O157:H7 (*Shigella* in Asia and Africa)
Most common extracranial solid tumor in children	Neuroblastoma
Most common malignancy in children	Leukemia
Preschool-aged child, painless abdominal mass, microscopic hematuria, HTN	Wilms' tumor (kidney)
Definition of aplastic crisis	Hemoglobin drop of 2 g/dL with a reticulocyte count <2%
Blood test to differentiate splenic sequestration and aplastic crisis	Reticulocyte count -Aplastic crisis associated with very low hemoglobin and low reticulocyte count from marrow failure -Splenic sequestration associated with low hemoglobin, but increased reticulocyte count
Define anaphylactoid reaction	Resembles anaphylaxis, but needs no prior exposure as it is not immune mediated
Name common offending agents of anaphylactoid reactions and treatment of the condition	Causes: radiographic contrast, aspirin, NSAIDs, codeine Treatment: same as anaphylaxis
Types of allergic/hypersensitivity reactions	Mnemonic: ACID Type I: Immediate (Anaphylaxis) Type II: Cytotoxic (blood transfusion) Type III: Immune complex-mediated (serum sickness) Type IV: Delayed cell-mediated (TB skin test)
Type I hypersensitivity reactions	Antigen exposure leads to sensitization. Upon re-exposure reaction occurs (mast cells release histamine. Reaction is IgE mediated) Examples: penicillin (most common), hay fever, foods
Type II hypersensitivity reactions (cytotoxic)	Antigen causes complement activation or direct injury to lymphocytes with release of mediators (IgG or IgM mediated) Examples: blood tranfusions, immune hemolytic anemias, idiopathic thrombocytopenic purpura (ITP)
Type III hypersensitivity reactions	Antigen–antibody (Ag–Ab) complex activated complements and platelets causing release of mediators and platelet aggregation (IgE) Example: serum sickness
Type IV hypersensitivity reactions	Delayed cell-mediated: Ag-specific T-cells go to site and release mediators (No Ab or complement, thus no anaphylaxis) Example: purified protein derivative TB skin test (PPD), contact dermatitis
Dose of epinephrine for mild and severe allergic reactions	Mild: 0.3– 0.5 cc of 1/1000 IM Severe: 1–5 cc of 1/10,000 IV over 10 minutes (consider dwindle)
Medications for treatment of anaphylaxis	Epinephrine, H1 and H2 blockers, steroids, albuterol, glucagon: useful for patient on β-blockers refractory to epinephrine

Biostatistics

For many statistics questions, you will need to construct a 2 x 2 table, then make calculations based on that table. Plug the numbers of patients in different groups into the following 2 x 2 table

		Has the disease	
		Yes	No
Test is Positive	Yes	A	B
	No	C	D

Description of groups	A: true positive B: false positive C: false negative D: true negative
Relative risk	$(A/(A + B))/(C/(C + D))$ Measures the risk of developing the disease when exposed to a factor versus not being exposed to a factor. The value is significant if greater than 1. If less than 1 the exposure may be protective against the risk This cannot be calculated from retrospective data
Sensitivity	$A/(A + C)$ Ability of the test to identify positive results. This is a good quality for a screening test but may have lots of false positives (i.e. D-dimer)
Specificity	$D/(D + B)$ Ability of a test to identify negative results. This is a good quality for a confirmatory test (i.e. Western blot for HIV)
Positive predictive value (PPV)	$A/(A + B)$ Proportion of positive test results that are true positives
Negative predictive value (NPV)	$D/(D + C)$ Proportion of negative test results that are true negatives
Likelihood ratios	If test result is positive, calculate ratio as: Sensitivity/(1 − Specificity) If test result is negative, calculate ratio as: (1 − Sensitivity)/Specificity Measures the ability of a test to determine whether the test result usefully changes the probability of a disease state existing. A ratio greater than 1 indicates the test is associated with the disease; a ratio of less than 1 indicates the test is associated with absence of the disease. Values around 1 are not helpful.
Definition of "mean"	Average of all values in a set
Definition of "median"	Middle value in a set when arranged by value
Definition of "mode"	Most frequently repeated value in a set
Type I error	When an investigator shows that there is a treatment effect when one does not exist
Type II error	When an investigator does not show a treatment effect when one does exist

Bibliography

American College of Surgeons Committee on Trauma. *Advanced Trauma Life Support for Doctors*, 8th edn. Chicago: American College of Surgeons, 2008.

Bahn, I. Nephromatic: Intelligent renal calculators [Internet]. 2012 [Cited: 2012 Jul 27]. Available from: http://www.nephromatic.com.

Marx JA, Hockberger RS, Walls RM, Adams J, Rosen P, eds. *Rosen's Emergency Medicine: Concepts and Clinical Practice*. Philadelphia: Mosby Elsevier, 2010.

Sinz E, Navarro K, Soderberg ES. *Advanced Cardiovascular Life Support: Provider Manual*. Dallas: American Heart Association, 2010.

Tintinalli JE, Stapczynski JS, Cline DM, *et al. Tintinalli's Emergency Medicine: A Comprehensive Study Guide*, 7th edn. New York: The McGraw-Hill Companies, Inc., 2011

Useful formulas

Calculated Osmolality

$$(Na \times 2) + \left(\frac{BUN}{2.8}\right) + \left(\frac{Glucose}{18}\right) + \left(\frac{Ethanol}{4.6}\right)$$

Anion Gap

$$(Na) - (Cl + HCO_3)$$

Sodium Correction for Hyperglycemia

$$(Measured\ sodium) + (0.016 \times (serum\ glucose - 100))$$

- A small study from 1999 suggested using a correction of 0.024 instead of 0.016. [1]

Calcium correction for hypoalbuminemia

$$(Serum\ Calcium) + (0.8 \times (Normal\ albumin - Patient's\ albumin))$$

Mean Arterial Pressure

$$\left(^1/_3 \times SBP\right) + \left(^2/_3 \times DBP\right)$$

1. Hillier TA, Abbott RD, Barrett EJ. Hyponatremia: Evaluating the correction factor for hyperglycemia. *Am J Med.* 1999 Apri; **106** (4): 399–403.

Index

A-a gradient 34
abdominal aortic aneurysm 30–1
abdominal emergencies 54–73, 149
abdominal trauma 120–1
abortion 135–6
abruptio placentae 137
acetaminophen toxicity 175–6
acetylcholinesterase inhibitor poisoning 174
achalasia 55
acute coronary syndromes (ACS) 18–23, 24–5
acute myocardial infarction (AMI) 18, 19, 20, 21, 22, 23
acute renal failure (ARF) 86–7
addictive behavior 153–4
Addison's disease 101
adrenal insufficiency 101
adrenal tumors 102
Aeromonas hydrophilia 65
AIDS 169–71
air embolism 185
airway(s)
    adjuncts/artificial 195–6
    infections 45–9
    irritants 50, 51
    obstruction 51, 197
    surgical 198
alcohol-related problems 153, 156
amebiasis 66, 69–70
amphetamine intoxication 176
amputation, traumatic 124
anal fissure 73
anal fistula 73
anal tumors 73
anesthesia 198–200
angina 23, 24
ankle injuries 125
anorexia nervosa 153
anoscopy 200–1
antiarrhythmic medications 13
anticholinergic toxidrome 174

anticoagulant overdose 176
antiepileptic drugs 83
antipsychotic toxicity 176
anxiety disorders 155–6
aortic disruption, traumatic 116–17
aortic dissection 31, 116–17
aortoenteric fistula 67–8
appendicitis 70
arterial blood gas (ABG) interpretation 33, 34
arterial catheter insertion 204
arterial injuries 131
arterial thromboembolism 32
arthrocentesis 201
ASA classification 199
asbestosis 50
ascariasis 70
asphyxiants 50
asthma 41–2, 43, 138
asystole 17
atrial fibrillation (A-fib) 8, 9
atrial flutter 10
atrioventricular (AV) block 2, 3, 4

Bacillus cereus 65
bacterial infections 64, 65, 66, 142, 165–6, 167–9
bacterial vaginosis 135
bag-valve-mask ventilation 196
balanitis/balanoposthitis 91
Bankart fracture 129
barotrauma 185
Bartholin's abscess 135
batteries, button, ingested 56, 149
Bell's palsy 74
benzodiazepine toxidrome 174
β-blocker toxicity 177
bilevel positive airways pressure (BiPAP) 196–7
bipolar disorder 154
bites 123, 183–4
black widow spider bite 183
bladder trauma 122

blood loss, estimating 106
blood products/transfusions 107–8, 200
Boerhaave's syndrome 56
botulism 167
bowel irrigation, whole 175
bowel obstruction 67, 71
bradyarrhythmias 1–2
breech presentation 139
bronchiolitis 45–6
bronchitis, acute 45
brown recluse spider bite 183
Brugada syndrome 13
bulimia nervosa 153
burns 189, 191

calcium channel blocker toxicity 177
calcium metabolism 94–5
Campylobacter (jejuni) infections 64, 166
candidiasis 55, 135
carbon dioxide monitoring 195
carbon monoxide poisoning 177
cardiac glycoside toxicity 177–8
cardiology emergencies 1–32, 212
cardiomyopathies 27
cardioversion 207
carotid artery dissection 75
central nervous system (CNS) infections/inflammations 77–8
central venous access 204–5
cerebral contusion 108
cerebral venous sinus thrombosis 75
cerebrovascular events 84–5
charcoal, activated 175
chest trauma 116–19
chest tube placement 207
chilblains 187–8
Chlamydia infections 132
cholangitis 62

cholecystitis 62
cholelithiasis/
    choledocholithiasis 62
chorioamnionitis 137
chronic obstructive pulmonary
    disease (COPD) 43–5
chronic renal failure 87
ciguatera fish poisoning 65, 167
cirrhosis 59
clavicle fracture 118
Clostridium difficile 69
Clostridium perfringens 65, 166
cocaine intoxication 175
cold injuries 187–9
cold water immersion
    syndrome 186
Colles' fracture 127
colorectal carcinoma 73
compartment syndrome 124,
    205–6
complete heart block 4
conduction pathway blocks 2–7
continuous positive airways
    pressure (CPAP) 196–7
conversion disorder 155
cord prolapse 139
corneal injuries 113–14
Crohn's disease 67
cryoprecipitate 108
Cryptosporidium infections 66
Cushing's syndrome 102
cyanide poisoning 178
cystitis 89–90
cystourethrogram 201–2

decompression syndrome 185
deep vein thrombosis (DVT)
    32
defibrillation 206–7
delirium 156
delirium tremens 153
delivery 138, 139, 205
dementia 156
dental injuries 112
depression 154
dermatology 235
desquamating rashes, pediatric
    143–4
diabetes mellitus 98
diabetic ketoacidosis (DKA) 98
dialysis complications 87
diaphragmatic injury 117
diarrhea
    antibiotic-associated 69
    Clostridium difficile 69
    infectious 64, 65, 66, 165–6

diffuse axonal injury (DAI)
    109–10
digoxin/digitalis toxicity 177–8
dilated cardiomyopathy 27
dislocations 128–30, 205
diverticulitis 71–2
diverticulosis 71
drowning, near 186
drug dependence 153
drug psychoses 156
drug-seeking behavior 155
dysbarism 185
dysfunctional uterine bleeding
    134
dystonic reaction 80

earlobe injury 114
early repolarization 15
eating disorders 153
eclampsia 82, 136
ectopic pregnancy 136
ehrlichiosis 168
elbow
    injuries 126, 129
    ossification centers 150
elder abuse 157
electrical alternans 16
electrical injuries 191–2
electrolyte disturbances 94–7
encephalitis 78
endocrine disorders 94–102,
    219–26
endometriosis 134
endometritis, post-partum 139
endotracheal intubation 197
endotracheal tubes, pediatric
    sizes 151
ENT emergencies 235–6
enterobiasis (pinworms) 66,
    146–7
envenomation 183–4
environmental emergencies
    183–93, 234
epididymitis 91–2
epidural hematoma 109, 110
epiphyseal fractures 127–8
epistaxis 204
erythema infectiosum 145
erythema multiforme (EM)
    spectrum 143–4
Escherichia coli
    enterohemorrhagic 64
    enterotoxigenic 65, 166
    O157:H7 166
esophageal disorders 55–7
esophageal perforation 117

esophagitis
    candida 55
    reflux 55
ethylene glycol poisoning 178
external genitalia, trauma 123
extremity injuries 124, 125–7
eye injuries 113–14

facial fractures 111–12
factitious disorders 155
factor VIII/IX 108
farmer's lung 50
febrile seizures 82
femur fractures 125–6
fetal distress 138
fetal malposition 139
fever
    neutropenic 161–2
    pediatric 141–2
fibroids, uterine 134
fifth disease 145
Fitz–Hugh–Curtis syndrome
    133
fluid disturbances 94–7
food-borne illnesses 65, 165–7
foot injuries 125
forearm fractures 126–7
foreign bodies
    airway 197
    ingested 56, 59, 149
    rectal 73
    vaginal 135
Fournier's gangrene 92
fractures 124–8, 205
fresh frozen plasma (FFP) 107
frostbite 188

Galeazzi's fracture 126
gallbladder tumors 62
gallstones 62
gas gangrene 167–8
gastric lavage 175, 208
gastritis 58
gastroenterologic emergencies
    54–73, 149, 214–16
gastroesophageal reflux disease
    (GERD) 55
gastrointestinal (GI) bleeds
    57–8
gastrostomy tube replacement
    208–9
genitourinary trauma 121–3
giardiasis 66, 70
Glasgow Coma Scale (GCS)
    105
glomerulonephritis 88

glucose metabolism 98–9
gonorrhea 132
greenstick fracture 128
grief reaction 154
growth, childhood 151
Guillain–Barré syndrome 80
gynecology 132–5, 219

hantavirus 172
head lice 147
head trauma 108–10
headache 75
heart
    contusion 117
    penetrating injury 119
heart failure 26–7
heat injuries 187
HELLP syndrome 136
hematology 237–8
hemoglobin oxygen saturation
    curve 35
hemolytic uremic syndrome
    (HUS) 88–9, 166
hemorrhage
    antepartum 137
    post-partum 139
hemorrhagic shock 106
hemothorax 118–19
Henoch–Schönlein purpura
    148
hepatitis 60, 61
hepatobiliary disorders 59–62
hepatorenal failure 60
hernias
    abdominal 54
    esophageal 57
herpes simplex virus (HSV)
    infections 133, 146
high-altitude illness 185–6
Hill–Sachs deformity 129
hip dislocation 129–30
hip fractures 125–6
Hirschsprung's disease 72–3
HIV infection 169–71
hookworms 66
human papillomavirus
    infections 133
humerus fractures 126
hydrocarbon
    inhalation/ingestion
    149–50
hydrocephalus, normal
    pressure 77
hydrogen sulfide toxicity 178
hypercalcemia 94–5
hyperemesis gravidarum 137

hyperglycemic hyperosmolar
    nonketotic coma (HHNC)
    98–9
hyperkalemia 95
hypermagnesemia 97
hypernatremia 96
hyperparathyroidism 100
hyperphosphatemia 97
hypertension, in pregnancy 136
hypertensive emergency 30
hyperthyroidism 99, 138
hypertrophic cardiomyopathy
    27
hyphema 113
hypocalcemia 94
hypochondriasis 155
hypoglycemia 99
hypoglycemic agent overdose
    178–9
hypokalemia 95
hypomagnesemia 96
hyponatremia 95–6
hypoparathyroidism 100
hypophosphatemia 97
hypothermia 188–9
hypothyroidism 100
hypoxia 34, 35, 36
hysteria 155

immunology 237–8
impetigo 145, 146
incision/drainage 209
infectious diseases 132–3, 137,
    142, 146, 159–72
infectious mononucleosis
    171–2
infective endocarditis 28
inflammatory bowel disease 67
inhalation injury 50–1, 191
injection, high pressure 123–4
intracranial hypertension,
    idiopathic 75
intracranial tumors 75, 85
intraosseous access 205
intussusception 68–9
iritis, traumatic 114
iron toxicity 179
irritants, airway 50, 51
isoniazid toxicity 179
Isospora infections 66

jaundice, neonatal 151
joint injuries 128–30
Jones fracture 125
junctional/ventricular escape
    rhythm 2

juvenile idiopathic/rheumatoid
    arthritis 148

Kawasaki disease 144
kerion 147
knee injuries 125, 130
Korsakoff psychosis 102, 153

labor 138
large bowel pathology 69–72
laryngeotracheal injury 116
lead toxicity 179
LeFort fractures 111
left anterior fascicular block 6
left bundle branch block
    (LBBB) 5
left posterior fascicular block 6,
    7
left ventricular hypertrophy 16,
    17
leiomyoma, uterine 134
lightning injuries 191–2
Lisfranc fracture/dislocation
    125
lithium toxicity 179–80
liver abscess 61
liver disease 59–62
liver injuries 120, 121
lumbar puncture 202
lung cancer 52

magnesium metabolism 96–7
malabsorption, intestinal 68
malaria 168
male genital tract 91–3
Mallory–Weiss syndrome 55–6
malrotation 68
mandible fractures 112
mania 154
marine organism bites/stings
    184
mastitis 139–40
mechanical ventilation 196,
    198
Meckel's diverticulum 68
meconium ileus 149
mediastinitis 37–8
meningitis 78, 79–84, 162–3,
    164
meningococcemia 162–3, 164
mesenteric ischemia 69
metabolic disorders 94–102,
    219–26
methanol toxicity 180
methemoglobinemia 181
Mobitz I heart block 3

Mobitz II heart block 3–4
monoamine oxidase inhibitors (MAOIs) 180
mononeuropathies 81
Monteggia fracture 127
mood disorders 154–5
multifocal atrial tachycardia (MAT) 11
multiple sclerosis 75
Munchausen syndrome/Munchausen by proxy 155
myasthenia gravis 80–1
myocardial infarction (MI) acute 18, 19, 20, 21, 22, 23 complications 25
myxedema coma 100

nasogastric (NG) tube 202
nasopharyngeal airway 195–6
neck trauma 115, 116
necrotizing enterocolitis 70, 151
neonatal jaundice 151
neonatal seizures 82
nephrotic syndrome 89
neuroleptic malignant syndrome 181
neurologic emergencies 74–85, 216–19
neuromuscular disorders 80–1
neurotic disorders 155–6
neutropenic fevers 161–2
non-accidental trauma 147–8
nuchal cord 139
nursemaid's elbow 129
nutritional disorders 102, 219–26

obsessive–compulsive disorder 155
obstetrics 135–40, 206, 219
obstructive uropathy 91
oncology 237–8
ophthalmology 236–7
opioid overdose 175
orbital fractures 112–13
orchitis 92
organophosphates 51
oropharyngeal airway 196
ossification centers, elbow 150
otologic trauma 114
ovarian pathology 133–4
oxygen supplementation 195

pacing, emergency cardiac 206
packed red blood cells (PRBC) 107
pancreatic injuries 120
pancreatic tumors 63
pancreatitis 62–3
panhypopituitarism 101
panic disorder 155
paracentesis 202
paralytic ileus 67
paraphimosis 93
parasitic infections 66, 69–70, 146–7
parathyroid disorders 100
Parkinson's disease 79–80
pediatric emergencies 127–8, 141–51, 228–31
pelvic fractures 127
pelvic inflammatory disease 133
peptic ulcer disease 58
pericardial tamponade 28, 119
pericardiocentesis 202–3
pericarditis 15, 27–8
peripheral neuropathies 81
peripheral venous cutdown 205
perirectal abscess 72
peritonitis, spontaneous bacterial 54
personality disorders 156–7
pharyngoesophageal injuries 116
phenytoin toxicity 180
pheochromocytoma 102
phimosis 93
phobia 156
phosphate metabolism 97
pilonidal cyst/abscess 72
pinworms 66, 146–7
pituitary dysfunction 101
pituitary tumors 101
pityriasis rosea 146
placenta previa 137
platelet concentrate 107–8
pleural effusion 38–9
pleurisy 38
pneumoconiosis 49
pneumomediastinum 37
pneumonia 46, 47–8
pneumothorax 36, 37, 119, 207
post-partum complications 139–40
post-traumatic stress disorder (PTSD) 156
potassium metabolism 95
preeclampsia 136

pregnancy 135–40
complications 135–7
high-risk 137–8
infections 137
labor and delivery 138–9, 205
premature labor 138
preterm premature rupture of membranes (PPROM) 138
priapism 93
procedures, emergency 194–209
proctitis 72
prolapse, genital 134
prostatitis 92
pseudotumor cerebri 75
psychobehavioral emergencies 153–7
psychoses 154, 156
psychosomatic disorder 155
pulmonary contusion 118
pulmonary embolism 39–40, 41
pulmonary tumors 52
pulse oximetry 194–5
pulseless electrical activity 17
pyelonephritis 90, 137
pyloric stenosis 58–9, 149

rabies 171
radiation injuries 71, 192, 193
rashes, pediatric 143–4, 146
rectal pathology 72–3
renal disease 86–93, 219–28
renal failure 86–8
renal trauma 122
renal tubular acidosis 89
respiratory emergencies 33–52, 212–22
restrictive cardiomyopathy 27
Rhesus (Rh) isoimmunization 137
rheumatic fever, acute 148
rheumatology 148, 235
rib fractures 118
right bundle branch block (RBBB) 5
right ventricular hypertrophy 17
Rocky Mountain spotted fever (RMSF) 169
roseola infantum 145, 172
rubella 172

salicylate poisoning 180
Salmonella infections 64, 165

Salter–Harris classification 127–8
scabies 147
scalp lacerations 110
scaphoid fracture 127
scarlet fever 144, 145
schizophrenia 155
scombroid fish poisoning 65, 167
scrotal gangrene 92
sedation 199–200
seizure disorders 82–3, 137
sepsis 159, 160
serotonin syndrome 181
sexual assault 157
sexually transmitted diseases 132–3
Shigella infections 64, 166
shock 106–8
shoulder dislocation 128–9
silicosis 49
sinus bradycardia 1
sinus tachycardia 7
skin trauma 123–4
slit lamp examination 203
small bowel pathology 64–9
snake bites 183, 184
sodium metabolism 95–6
spinal cord compression 83
spinal shock 106
splenic injuries 120
sprains 130
staphylococcal scalded skin syndrome 143, 144
Staphylococcus aureus
    food poisoning 65, 165
    toxic shock syndrome 164–5
statistics 239
status epilepticus 83
sternal fracture 118
stomach pathology 57–9
strains 130
streptococcal pharyngitis 145
streptococcal toxic shock syndrome 143, 164–5
stroke 84
subarachnoid hemorrhage 84, 108
subdural hematoma 75, 109, 110
submersion incidents 186
substance abuse 154
suicide risk 154
supraventricular tachycardia 8

synovial fluid analysis 148
syphilis 132, 168
systemic inflammatory response syndrome (SIRS) 159–60

tachyarrhythmias 7–13
temporal arteritis 75
tendon injuries 130–1
testicular torsion 93, 203–4
thoracocentesis 203
thoracotomy, emergency/resuscitative 208
thyroid disorders 99
thyroid storm 99, 138
thyroid tumors 100
thyroiditis, acute 100
tibial plateau fracture 125
tic douloureux 74–5
tinea capitis 147
tooth
    avulsion 112
    fractures 112
torsade de pointes 12
torus/buckle fracture 128
toxic epidermal necrolysis 143–4
toxic shock syndrome 143, 144, 164–5
toxicologic emergencies 149–50, 174–82, 232–3
toxoplasmosis 168, 169
tracheobronchial injury 117
tracheoesophageal fistula 57
transient cerebral ischemia 85
transverse myelitis 77–8
trauma 104–31, 214
    mortality 104
    primary survey (ABCDEs) 104–5
    secondary survey (head-to-toe exam) 105–6
    shock 106–8
trauma center designations 104
traumatic brain injury (TBI) 108, 109
traveler's diarrhea 65, 166
trench foot 187
trichomoniasis 132, 135
tricyclic antidepressant toxicity 181
trigeminal neuralgia 74–5

trophoblastic disease, gestational 134
tuberculin skin test 49
tuberculosis, pulmonary 48–9
tubo-ovarian abscess 133
tympanic membrane (TM) perforation 114

ulcerative colitis 67
ultrasonography, bedside 201
urethral trauma 122, 123
urethritis 92
urinary calculi 90–1
urinary catheterization 203
urinary tract infection (UTI) 90, 137
urogenital disorders 86–93, 219–28
uterine pathology 134, 138

vaginal pathology 135
valvular heart disease 29–30
varicella 145–6
varices, esophageal 57
vascular injuries 116, 131
ventricular fibrillation (V-fib) 18
ventricular tachycardia (VT) 12
ventriculoperitoneal shunt obstruction/infection 77
vertebral artery dissection 75
Vibrio infections 64, 65, 166
violence, interpersonal 157
viral infections 66, 145–6, 171–2
volvulus 71, 149
vulvar pathology 135
vulvovaginitis 135

warts, genital 133
Wenckebach phenomenon 3
Wernicke–Korsakoff syndrome 102, 153
whitlow, herpetic 146
Wolff–Parkinson–White (WPW) syndrome 14
wound closure 209
wrist fractures 126–7

Yersinia infections 64

zygomaticomaxillary complex fractures 111–12

Printed in the United States
by Baker & Taylor Publisher Services

Printed in the United States
by Baker & Taylor Publisher Services